Oxford Medical Publications

Quality of Life Assessment in Clinical Trials

Methods and Practice

Quality of Life Assessment in Clinical Trials

Methods and Practice

Edited by

Maurice J. Staquet

Brussels Free University, Faculty of Medicine, Brussels, Belgium

Ron D. Hays

Department of Medicine, University of California, Los Angeles, CA, USA

and

Peter M. Fayers

Unit for Clinical Research and Epidemiology, Norwegian University of Science and Technology, Trondheim, Norway

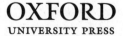

OXFORD
UNIVERSITY PRESS

OXFORD

UNIVERSITY PRESS

Great Clarendon Street, Oxford OX2 6DP

Oxford University Press is a department of the University of Oxford.
It furthers the University's objective of excellence in research, scholarship,
and education by publishing worldwide in

Oxford New York

Athens Auckland Bangkok Bogotá Buenos Aires Calcutta
Cape Town Chennai Dar es Salaam Delhi Florence Hong Kong Istanbul
Karachi Kuala Lumpur Madrid Melbourne Mexico City Mumbai
Nairobi Paris São Paulo Singapore Taipei Tokyo Toronto Warsaw

with associated companies in Berlin Ibadan

Oxford is a registered trade mark of Oxford University Press
in the UK and in certain other countries

Published in the United States
by Oxford University Press Inc., New York

© Oxford University Press, 1998

A catalogue record for this book is available from the British Library

Library of Congress Cataloging in Publication Data

R853.C55 Q34 1988 (Oxford medical publications)
1. Clinical trials—Social aspects. 2. Quality of life—Evaluation.
I. Staquet, Maurice J. II. Hays, Ron D. III. Series.
[DNLM: 1. Research. 2. Clinical Trials. 3. Quality of Life.
4. Outcome Assessment (Health Care) W 20.5 Q15 1998]
615.5'028'7—dc21 97-39560
Includes bibliographical references and index.
ISBN 0 19 262785 6

Printed in Great Britain by
Biddles Ltd,
Guildford and King's Lynn

Acknowledgements

The International Society for Quality of Life Research will receive all royalties from sales of this book. The contributors freely gave their time and received no renumeration. The editors are grateful to all of them.

Contents

Contributors

Jordi Alonso   Health Services Research Unit, Institut Municipal d'Investigació Médica, Calle Doctor Aiguader, 80, E-08003 Barcelona, Spain

Roger P. Anderson   The Bowman Gray School of Medicine, Medical Center Blvd, Winston-Salem, NC 27157-1063, USA

Richard A. Berzon   Department of Health Economics and Outcomes Research, Bayer Pharmaceuticals, 400 Morgan Lane, West Haven, CT 06516, USA

Bernard F. Cole   Department of Community and Family Medicine, Dartmouth Medical School, Dartmouth–Hitchcock Medical Center, Lebanon, NH 03756, USA

Desmond Curran   EORTC Data Center, Avenue E. Mounier, 83, Bte 11, 1200 Brussels, Belgium

Stephen Joel Coons   Center for Pharmaceutical Economics, College of Pharmacy, The University of Arizona, Tucson, AZ 85721-0207, USA

Diane L. Fairclough   AMC Cancer Research Center, Center for Research Methodology and Biostatistics, 1600 Pierce St, Denver, CO 80214, USA

Peter M. Fayers   Unit for Clinical Research and Epidemiology, Norwegian University of Science and Technology, N-7005 Trondheim, Norway *and* MRC Cancer Trials Office, 5 Shaftesbury Road, Cambridge CB2 2BW, UK

Richard D. Gelber   Department of Biostatistical Sciences, Dana-Farber Cancer Institute, 44 Binney Street, Boston, MA 02115, USA

Shari Gelber   Frontier Science and Technology Research Foundation, Inc., 303 Boylston Street, Brookline, MA 02146, USA *and* Center for Outcomes and Policy Research, Dana-Farber Cancer Institute, 44 Binney Street, Boston, MA 02115, USA

Aron Goldhirsch   Director, European Institute of Oncology, Department of Medical Oncology, Via Ripamonti, 435, I-20141 Milano, Italy *and* International Breast Cancer Study Group, Ospedale Civico, 6900, Lugano, Switzerland

Ron D. Hays   UCLA School of Medicine, Los Angeles, CA 90024-1736, USA *and* RAND Health Program, 1700 Main Street, Santa Monica, CA 90407-2138, USA

Sonja M. Hunt   Department of General Practice, University of Edinburgh, UK

Robert M. Kaplan Professor and Chief, Division of Health Care Sciences, 0622, Department of Family and Preventive Medicine, University of California, San Diego, La Jolla, CA 92093-0622, USA

Nancy Kline Leidy MEDTAP International, Inc., 7101 Wisconsin Avenue, Suite 600, Bethesda, MD 20815, USA

Elissa A. Laitin Frontier Science and Technology Research Foundation, Inc., 1244 Boylston Street, Suite 303, Chestnut Hill, MA 02167, USA *and* Department of Epidemiology, Harvard School of Public Health, 677 Huntington Avenue, Boston, MA 02115, USA

Eva Lydick Strategic Product Development, SmithKline Beecham Pharmaceuticals, UP4205, 1250 South Collegeville Road, Collegeville, PA 19426-0989, USA

David Machin National Medical Research Council Clinical Trials and Epidemiology Research Unit, 10 College Road, Singapore 169851 *and* MRC Cancer Trials Office, 5 Shaftesbury Road, Cambridge CB2 2BW, UK

Geert Molenberghs Limburgs Universitaire Centrum, Universitaire Campus, Building D, B-3590 Diepenbeek, Belgium

David Osoba BC Cancer Agency, 600 West 10th Avenue, Vancouver, BC, Canada V5Z 4E6

Dennis A. Revicki MEDTAP International, Inc., 7101 Wisconsin Avenue, Suite 600, Bethesda, MD 20815, USA

Carolyn E. Schwartz Frontier Science and Technology Research Foundation, Inc., 1244 Boylston Street, Suite 303, Chestnut Hill, MA 02167, USA *and* Department of Psychiatry, Beth Israel Deaconess Medical Center, Haward Medical School, Boston, MA, USA.

Frank A. Sonnenberg Division of General Internal Medicine, University of Medicine and Dentistry of New Jersey, Robert Wood Johnson Medical School, Clinical Academic Building, Rm 2312, 125 Paterson Street, New Brunswick, NJ 08903, USA

Maurice J. Staquet Brussels Free University, Faculty of Medicine, (DCS), CP 623, Route de Lennik, 808, B-1070 Brussels, Belgium

Barbara P. Yawn Olmsted Medical Center, 210 9th Street, SE, Rochester, MN 55903, USA

I

Introduction

1 Understanding and using health-related quality of life instruments within clinical research studies

Richard A. Berzon

Introduction

Health-related quality of life (HRQoL) is an increasingly used outcome measure in clinical trial research. With respect to evaluating new pharmacologic agents, this phenomenon reflects a shift away from an exclusive emphasis on safety and efficacy, and from research which in the past focused narrowly on laboratory and clinical indicators of morbidity and mortality. Within experimental designs today, it is more likely that the impacts of illness and treatment on functioning and well-being will be evaluated broadly.

In this chapter, HRQoL and related terms are discussed within the context of clinical trial research. HRQoL questionnaires (or instruments) characterize and measure what subjects experience as a result of their receiving medical care, and examination of these instruments is undertaken with the understanding that there is general agreement on how HRQoL is conceptualized (Moinpour 1994; Bullinger et al. 1996; Schipper et al. 1996). As a result of this consensus on HRQoL conceptualization and because they are regarded as useful and important supplements to traditional physiologic and biologic health status assessments, these instruments are today routinely included within experimental designs (Wilson and Cleary 1995; Cleary 1996).

An underlying postulate of this chapter is that in addition to relieving clinical symptoms and prolonging survival, a primary objective of any health care intervention is the enhancement of quality of life and well-being. Circumstances which contribute to this premise include the ageing of the population and the increasing prevalence of chronic diseases; the need to evaluate health care technologies with respect to individual and societal value; and the need to recognize the patient's own perception of changes in his or her health status. Indeed, for those individuals diagnosed with a chronic condition where cure is not attainable and therapy may be prolonged, quality of life is likely to be *the* essential outcome.

Health-related quality of life construct

The World Health Organization (WHO) defines health as 'not merely the absence of disease or infirmity, but a state of complete physical, mental, and social well-being' (WHO 1958). Just as this broad and inclusive definition of health transcends the medical model, so too does the term *quality of life* define all aspects of patients' well-being (including, for example, spiritual and economic health). For purposes of clinical trial research, however, *health-related quality of life* (HRQoL) is more specific and more appropriate; it refers to patients' appraisals of their current level of functioning and satisfaction with it compared to what they perceive to be ideal (Cella and Tulsky 1990). The concept, therefore, can be considered synonymous with subjective health status assessment, and points to those aspects of a person's experience which are affected only by health care interventions.

The purpose of an HRQoL instrument is not merely to measure the presence and severity of symptoms of disease, but also to show how the manifestations of an illness or treatment are experienced by an individual, whether that experience is descriptive or in terms of relative preferences for various health states. Within a clinical trial, therefore, HRQoL questionnaires can be used to evaluate health care treatments to assess an agent's clinical efficacy, its economic value, or both. The need for specific information by the decision maker(s) – whether that decision maker is a clinician, a policy maker, or someone else – often determines the type of instrument(s) required for the experimental design.

HRQoL can be assessed with health profile (descriptive) questionnaires that are either generic or specific. A health profile instrument denotes a health status questionnaire which measures, by means of a similar metric, different aspects of health-related quality of life and well-being defined across multiple health domains or areas (for example, physical function, emotional distress, social well-being, etc.) that the patient has identified as being important. Generally each domain is represented by a separate scale and the calculation of data from each scale produces a separate numerical value (or score) that, usually, is unweighted.

Both generic and specific health profile instruments have advantages and disadvantages and must be evaluated within the context of the needs of the particular study. Generic instruments allow comparisons to be made across conditions and interventions, but may not focus adequately on the area of interest for a specific intervention. Specific instruments are likely to be more responsive to change, but are not comprehensive, do not allow across-condition comparisons and may not be available for certain populations or interventions. These measures are designed to assess specific disease states, areas of function, or patient populations. Specific measures continue to be generated; guidelines for their development are readily available (Guyatt *et al.* 1991; Streiner and Norman 1989; Leplege *et al.* 1995; Juniper *et al.* 1996). In such cases, time and resources must be made available at an early stage in the protocol development process (that is, as soon as phase I clinical data are available and it appears likely that such instrument development is warranted) to assure that the work is completed in a timely fashion.

Operationally, a generic health profile instrument should permit a subject to assess his or her ability to perform every day activities across a broad range of domains; functional status in those key areas would therefore be assessed. Primary HRQoL domains include physical, social, and cognitive functioning; role activities; and emotional well-being (Stewart and Ware 1992; Shumaker and Naughton 1995). How a subject feels about the performance of each of those activities may be assessed separately by measuring satisfaction for each domain. Alternatively, overall well-being (life satisfaction) across all domains may be assessed by means of a global question. As is evident, the perspective of the patient is the essential component of the HRQoL construct.

Generic instruments need not be descriptive; alternatively, they can assess patient preferences (usually referred to as utilities) (Torrance 1987). While descriptive measures are based on a psychometric approach and are designed to provide separate scores for the key dimensions defined by HRQoL, the patient-preference approach is an attempt to weigh the dimensions of health and to provide a single unitary expression of health status as a global index or utility score (Kaplan and Bush 1982). Such utility scores are generally measured on a 0.0 to 1.0 scale in which 0.0 represents death and 1.0 is the quality of life associated with perfect health. Combining utility units with the cost of an intervention will result in a cost–utility analysis, with the utility expressed as quality-adjusted life-years (QALY).

To further contrast health profile and preference-weighted measures, one observes that descriptive questionnaires provide disaggregated measures of changes in patient functional status and satisfaction attributable to the intervention under study. *Individual* patient concerns and intervention effects are grouped into separate domains of patient function and satisfaction. On the other hand, patient preference questionnaires focus on *society* as a whole and the societal allocation of health care resources. Preference-weighted measures assign a single aggregated score for changes in health status based on patient relative preferences, and allow comparison of the impact of an intervention on HRQoL to the impact of other treatments for the same condition and/or to other treatments for different conditions.

Patient preference questionnaires share a disadvantage with health profile measures: they may not be responsive to small but important clinical changes experienced by the patient. In addition, patient-derived utilities can vary depending on how they are obtained – that is, measuring patient preferences via the different methodologies (standard gamble, time trade-off, or use of a rating scale) can lead to differences in scores. Discrepancies in score differences raise questions about the validity of any single measurement (Guyatt *et al.* 1991; Revicki and Kaplan 1995).

In the final analysis, important information for health care decision making is provided by both health profile and patient preference measures. Within a clinical trial, therefore, a case can often be made to collect HRQoL data in both aggregated and disaggregated forms (Drummond 1993). Findings from the use of these instruments address the need for broader, more sensitive patient-based outcomes, while the integration of treatment and disease effects which results from their use enables patients and other decision makers to consider the trade-offs that are unique to the specific illness under study (Wu and Rubin 1994).

HRQoL assessment within clinical trials

A clinical trial is an important medium through which treatment efficacy can be determined, and key variables within a trial's protocol inform and guide selection of an appropriate HRQoL instrument. Principal clinical trial variables include the study population, the intervention, and the clinical trial design (Gotay *et al*. 1992; Schron and Shumaker 1992).

The study population's demographics – its age, gender and educational level, for example – as well as its level of illness must be considered prior to selecting an instrument. As an example, a cohort of extremely ill persons will have greater difficulty than a cohort of moderately ill persons in completing a self-administered HRQoL measure. This situation will influence the integrity of the data, especially the degree to which data may be found to be missing. Under this circumstance, the manner by which a questionnaire is administered should be considered carefully (Wu *et al*. 1997). Modes of administration include self-administration, interviewer administration, telephone administration, and employing surrogate responders (Guyatt *et al*. 1996).

The treatment regimen should be understood within the context of other ongoing mitigating influences, such as time itself. For example, the immediate effects of the intervention of coronary artery bypass graft surgery on most HRQoL domains will be negative. However, six months postoperatively, patients will undoubtedly appreciate gains associated with reductions in chest pain, shortness of breath, and fatigue.

The clinical trial design should be considered with respect to issues of practicality. For example, if the trial is especially complex and the patients are especially ill, then the study's staff may be especially burdened. In such a case, the HRQoL measure that is selected should not contribute to that burden. However if HRQoL is the primary end-point, then patient and staff time should be directed to that end. As an example, when comparing two equally efficacious oncology agents, HRQoL may be considered to be the critical outcome variable; and patient and staff time and energies should reflect that design. Regardless of the nature of the end-point, the selected questionnaire should be brief and simple to complete.

The phase of the trial in which HRQoL is introduced is based on judgement. In small-scale phase II trials, HRQoL may seem unimportant. However, should dramatic differences in clinical outcomes become evident at an early stage in the treatment's evaluation, investigators may decide it is unethical to randomize patients in future trials (Pocock 1991). Piloting (that is, pretesting the measure on the specific population that is to be enrolled in the trial) HRQoL measures in phase II clinical trials is, therefore, a strategy that some investigators consider to gain initial insights into the intervention. Evaluation of these data from the pilot study can demonstrate both the feasibility of undertaking HRQoL assessment and the extent to which the study's design may require modification to accommodate it.

Evaluation of HRQoL instruments

Psychometrics, the science of assessing the measurement characteristic of scales, is used to evaluate HRQoL instruments. Psychometric properties for which an instrument should be evaluated include reliability, validity, and responsiveness (that is, sensitivity to clinically significant changes over time). Should an instrument not meet minimum recognized standards for measurement as defined by the literature (see, for example, numerous articles contained within Spilker 1996), data from its use are likely to be considered questionable because of a perceived bias. Any HRQoL questionnaire being considered for a particular clinical study should, if at all possible, be reviewed critically *prior* to its use in the study if results are to be taken as credible.

Reliability, validity, and responsiveness should be well understood prior to determining whether an instrument is psychometrically robust. Reliability refers to the extent to which an instrument is free of measurement error. The more reliable a measure is, the lower the element of random error. A measure found to be unreliable is not dependable. In practice, reliability refers to the extent to which the measure yields the same results in repeated applications in an unchanged population. This test–retest reliability is assessed by applying the measure to the same population at different points in time under the same conditions and looking at the statistical association between the two sets of results.

Another form of reliability, internal consistency, is relevant only to measures containing multiple items related to a single dimension. Internal consistency is assessed using Chronbach's coefficient alpha, a statistic which represents the degree to which items within a single scale are associated with one another. An alpha value of 0.70 or above is necessary to call a scale internally consistent; however, in general it is optimal to have alpha coefficients above 0.85 (Nunnally 1978). A Chronbach's alpha value provides an estimate of a domain's homogeneity.

Validity is defined by the extent to which an instrument measures what it is supposed to measure and does not measure what it is not supposed to measure. The concept refers to non-random or systematic measurement error. Of the several different types of validity, construct validity is especially relevant. Because in most cases no absolute criterion (that is, no *gold standard*) exists against which to validate an instrument, one becomes involved in collecting empirical evidence to support the inference that a particular measure has meaning. A measure of physical health may be tested against a measure of activities of daily living, with the prediction that the correlation should be positive. If this proves to be the case, it would be evidence of convergent validity. To the extent it can be demonstrated that the measure does not correlate with variables to which it should not be related, discriminant validity is made evident. For example, a measure of physical function should not be correlated highly with a measure of mental health. Another form of validity, content validity, refers to the adequacy with which a domain has been defined and sampled. While content validity is a more precise expression than face validity (which is defined by its reasonableness in representing a particular HRQoL domain), the two terms are often used interchangeably.

Responsiveness or sensitivity is the extent to which an instrument can detect true differences within the construct being measured. To evaluate treatment efficacy, it is essential, prior to its use within a clinical study, for an HRQoL instrument to have demonstrated an ability to detect small but meaningful changes over time. If such information is unavailable, then the study can be designed so that at its conclusion HRQoL changes can be compared with changes in clinical status, intervening health events, interventions of known or expected efficacy, or direct reports of change by patients or providers, among other items (Hays *et al.* 1995).

In the past, responsiveness has not received sufficient attention in the development of HRQoL questionnaires; but investigators are increasingly providing this information as part of an instrument's psychometric properties. In addition, the meaning of responsiveness statistics, how they relate to one another and to more established clinical measures of significance, has become a focus of much needed research (Jaeschke *et al.* 1989; Juniper *et al.* 1994; Lydick and Epstein 1996).

Cross-cultural HRQoL assessment

Clinical research today is international in scope and the demand for HRQoL instruments that can be utilized in the same trial cross nationally has dramatically increased. Prior to using an HRQoL questionnaire in a culture that is extrinsic from the country in which it was originally developed, however, consideration must be given to whether the measure conforms with the target culture or nationality. Variations in such factors as perceptions of health and sickness, the interpretation of symptoms, the meaning of 'quality of life', and expectations for care must be understood to assess HRQoL. Whether results from one culture can be applied to another will determine, for example, whether international HRQoL data can be pooled at the conclusion of the study (Hunt 1986; Bullinger and Hasford 1991).

Culturally adapting a HRQoL questionnaire indicates that the language and meaning within the instrument are consistent with that of the target country (Hunt and McKenna 1992). The approach that has been used most commonly to translate a measure from one culture to another involves a forward/backward translation process of an original source language document into the target language. In addition, focus groups are often used for critical evaluation of the translation (Bullinger *et al.* 1996).

There are specific methodologies to ensure cross-cultural comparability of HRQoL instruments; these include a sequential approach (examples include the Nottingham Health Profile, the SF-36, and the Sickness Impact Profile); a parallel approach (examples include the EORTC QLQ-C30 and the recently published herpes-specific HRQoL measure); and a simultaneous approach (examples include the WHOQOL and the recently published migraine-specific HRQoL measure) (Shumaker and Berzon 1995; Wild *et al*. 1995; Wagner *et al*. 1996). Guidelines for the adaptation of measures from one cultural context to another are found in the literature (Hui and Triandis 1985; Bullinger *et al*. 1993), and are reviewed elsewhere within this volume. The adapted questionnaire should be tested for cultural equivalence in patients within the target country prior to its use (Aaronson 1992; Hunt and McKenna 1992).

Collecting HRQoL data and assuring their integrity

The inclusion of HRQoL in clinical research yields three important results. First, it allows the investigator to characterize the impact of a given condition or disease in terms of clinically relevant humanistic attributes which are likely to be understood by the subject. Second, because HRQoL domains may be independent predictors of important clinical outcomes – such as treatment adherence, morbidity and condition severity, and mortality – these data may provide valuable insights into the natural history and progression of the condition or disease. And third, HRQoL measurement provides data on how a treatment influences an individual's daily functioning.

Subjective evaluation underlies HRQoL assessment and its measurement is delineated by an individual's perception of how he or she functions in specified domains, as influenced by his or her health status, health care, and health promoting activities. Additional aspects of HRQoL that stem from this understanding and should be incorporated into its assessment are the individual's perceived health and overall well-being. While the definition excludes from measurement contextual factors that influence HRQoL (for example, pain and other symptoms), these variables may play an important role in studies designed to understand better the impact of health care interventions on people's lives. Therefore, a broad range of variables should be considered in the context of their relevance to specific studies and populations. Pain, for example, while not a specific HRQoL domain *per se*, will influence perceptions of functional status and overall life quality; therefore it may be appropriate to measure it within specific study designs (Shumaker and Naughton 1995).

As with all data collected within a prospective clinical study, HRQoL data should be captured in a way that assures their quality and integrity and minimizes that which is missing. In particular, measures of HRQoL that are selected for a study should

(1) be consistent with the concept of HRQoL;

(2) collect data that can be assessed reliably and validly;

(3) collect data that are likely to exhibit sensitivity to change over time; and

(4) collect data that account for most of the variance in a subject's rating of his or her overall well-being.

Inadequate patient accrual and follow-up in trials that include HRQoL instruments introduce serious bias into the analysis of these data; such bias is likely to compromise the integrity of the study and may lead to uninterpretable results. If the collection of HRQoL data is deemed necessary to the conduct of a clinical study, these data should be obtained from all patients accrued into it.

Patient compliance with HRQoL questionnaires will be more likely if short, simple instruments are employed, if a relatively non-demanding data collection schedule is built into the protocol, and if specific individuals within the investigator's office or clinic are identified to coordinate and monitor HRQoL data collection. This strategy will ensure that the amount of data missing is kept to a minimum. In addition, the collection of these data should be planned around protocol-driven visits. For some study designs, the use of modes of questionnaire execution other than self-administration – such as interviewing subjects via telephone at home at a prearranged time – may be appropriate.

The individual designated to coordinate HRQoL data collection at the study site should be thoroughly familiar with the instrument prior to its being given to the subject. The coordinator may encounter, for example, a respondent with low literacy skills or poor eyesight which makes it difficult for the respondent to complete the questionnaire on his or her own. During that occurrence, HRQoL questions and their answer choices can be read to a respondent; and the coordinator's familiarity with the specific questions will assure deft accomplishment of the task. However, questions that appear in the instrument should not be interpreted or reworded because the meaning of a question can be altered unintentionally in this way, introducing a bias. If, upon review by the responsible individual, an item is found missing when the subject has completed the questionnaire, the subject should be asked if the item was intentionally unanswered. If so, the refusal should be noted on the questionnaire so that these data can be analysed separately from other HRQoL data.

The interpretation of HRQoL study results hinges on the translation of changes in these scores into clinically meaningful terms. Such translation may be undertaken using different approaches. One technique for both health profile and patient preference instruments is to compare the changes associated with the use of a new therapy with those changes associated with the use of therapies considered beneficial (using the same instrument). Recently, in a disease-specific health profile instrument, an attempt was made to identify the minimal important difference in a domain score which patients perceived as beneficial and which would likely mandate, in the absence of bothersome side-effects and excessive cost, a change in the patient's management (Jaeschke et al. 1989, 1991).

Methods to analyse and interpret HRQoL data are found in the literature (Schumacher et al. 1991; Zwinderman 1990; Hopwood et al. 1994) and are reviewed elsewhere within this volume (see pp. 227–298 for data analysis and see pp. 299–348 for data interpretation). Three related issues, however, are particularly noteworthy. The first is that missing data of both a random and non-random nature will probably result from the use of HRQoL instruments. The analysis of randomly missing data is generally well defined; but methods to analyse non-randomly missing data remain in development. The second issue related to analysis of HRQoL data is the multivariate nature of HRQoL studies and the dilemma created by it. That is, not only is HRQoL a multidimensional concept measured by multiple scales, but most studies are longitudinal. Separate analyses of each domain at multiple time points may make it difficult to communicate results in a meaningful fashion to clinicians and patients, while summary measures may reduce the multidimensionality of the problem without facilitating the complexity of interpretation. Weighting the items is likely to add to the intricacy of interpretation. The third quandary relevant to analysis of these data is how to integrate HRQoL and survival data such that the resulting information is clinically meaningful and easily interpretable (Fairclough and Gelber 1996).

Conclusion

Conceptual, methodological and practical considerations should precede HRQoL measurement within clinical research studies. Among the many considerations, those that seem especially pertinent include

- designing the study so that HRQoL data can be collected easily without interfering with the collection of other, equally important information;
- selecting an appropriate instrument (health profile, patient preference, or both) for the relevant audience (clinician, patient, managed care administrator, policy maker, or other);
- considering the unique aspects of the study population, particularly the burden of the illness under investigation;
- evaluating the instrument's psychometric strengths and weaknesses;
- assuring data integrity and minimal missing data through specific quality control procedures; and
- appraising how the HRQoL data will be analysed and interpreted prior to initiating patient accrual.

A variety of challenging issues are currently being studied. A few of those cited within this chapter include the integration of health profile measurement and patient preference weighting; the expeditious cross-cultural adaptation of HRQoL instruments for international trials; the analysis and meaningful interpretation of HRQoL data; and the development of guidelines to evaluate the psychometric properties of HRQoL questionnaires. The latter point is especially timely (if the audience for the data is a regulatory authority) because of the degree to which a measure must be identified as reliable, valid, and responsive – and therefore, unbiased and credible – prior to its use within a pivotal drug efficacy trial. Currently, the US Food and Drug Administration (FDA) has recommended that survival and quality of life data be accepted as key efficacy parameters for the approval of new anticancer agents. However, it is unclear which instruments will satisfy this requirement and whether the same instruments must be used across study designs.

Methods and tools to measure health-related quality of life are today readily available. Those who undertake such measurement within clinical research studies must continue to publish their findings in peer review journals and debate their work in public so that those unacquainted with the discipline can become familiar with it. The scientific rigor of HRQoL research, regardless of whether it is conducted within academia or within industry, will determine the extent to which the data are accepted by audiences to whom these outcomes are directed.

References

Aaronson, N.K. (1992). Assessing the quality of life of patients in cancer clinical trials. *Eur. J. Cancer*, **28**, 1307–10.

Bullinger, M. and Hasford, J. (1991). Evaluating quality of life measures for clinical trials in Germany. *Control Clin. Trials*, **12**, 91S–105S.

Bullinger, M., Anderson, R., Cella, D., and Aaronson, N. (1993). Developing and evaluating cross-cultural instruments from minimum requirements to optimal models. *Qual. Life Res.*, **2**, 451–9.

Bullinger, M., Power, M.J., Aaronson, N.K., *et al.* (1996). Creating and evaluating cross-cultural instruments. In *Quality of life and pharmacoeconomics in clinical trials*, (2nd edn), (ed. B. Spilker), pp. 659–68. Lippincott–Raven, Philadelphia.

Cella, D.F. and Tulsky, D.S. (1990). Measuring quality of life today: methodological aspects. *Oncology*, **5**, 29–38.

Cleary, P. (1996). Future directions of quality of life research. In *Quality of life and pharmacoeconomics in clinical trials*, (2nd edn), (ed. B. Spilker), pp. 73–8. Lippincott–Raven, Philadelphia.

Drummond, M. (1993). Quality of life measurement within economic evaluations. Paper presented at the ESRC/SHHD workshop on Quality of Life, Edinburgh, Scotland, April 27–28.

Fairclough, D.L. and Gelber, R.D. (1996). Quality of life: statistical issues and analysis. In *Quality of life and pharmacoeconomics in clinical trials*, (2nd edn), (ed. B. Spilker), pp. 427–35. Lippincott–Raven, Philadelphia.

Gotay, C.C., Korn, E.L., McCabe, M.S., *et al.* (1992). Building quality of life assessment into cancer treatment studies. *Oncology*, **6**, 25–37.

Guyatt, G., Feeny, D., and Patrick, D. (1991). Issues in quality of life measurement in clinical trials. *Control Clin. Trials*, **12**, 81S–90S.

Guyatt, G.H., Jaeschke, R., Feeny, D.H., and Patrick, D.L. (1996). Measurements in clinical trials: choosing the right approach. In *Quality of life and pharmacoeconomics in clinical trials*, (2nd edn), (ed. B. Spilker), pp. 41–8. Lippincott–Raven, Philadelphia.

Hays, R.D., Anderson, R., and Revicki, D.A. (1995). Psychometric evaluation and interpretation of health-related quality of life data. In *The international assessment of health-related quality of life: theory, translation, measurement and analysis*, (ed. S.A. Shumaker and R.A. Berzon), pp. 103–14. Rapid Communications, Oxford.

Hopwood, P., Stephens, R.J., and Machin, D. (1994). Approaches to the analysis of quality of life data: experiences gained from a Medical Research Council Lung Cancer Working Party palliative chemotherapy trial. *Qual. Life Res.*, **3**, 339–52.

Hui, C. and Triandis, H.C. (1985). Measurement in cross-cultural psychology: a review and comparison of strategies. *Cross Cultural Psychol.*, **16**, 131–52.

Hunt, S.M. (1986). Cross-cultural issues in the use of socio-medical indicators. *Health Policy*, **6**, 149–58.

Hunt, S.M. and McKenna, S. (1992). Cross-cultural comparability of quality of life measures. *Br. J. Med. Econ.*, **4**, 17–23.

Jaeschke, R., Singer, J., and Guyatt, G.H. (1989). Ascertaining the minimal clinically important difference. *Control Clin. Trials*, **10**, 407–15.

Jaeschke, R., Guyatt, G.H., Keller, J., *et al.* (1991). Interpreting changes in quality of life scores in N of 1 randomized trials. *Control Clin. Trials*, **12**, 226S–33S.

Juniper, E.F., Guyatt, G.H., Willan, A., and Griffith, L.E. (1994). Determining a minimal important change in a disease-specific quality of life questionnaire. *J. Clin. Epidem.*, **47**, 81–7.

Juniper, E.F., Guyatt, G.H., and Jaeschke, R. (1996). How to develop and validate a new health-related quality of life instrument. In *Quality of life and pharmacoeconomics in clinical trials*, (2nd edn), (ed. B. Spilker), pp. 49–56. Lippincott–Raven, Philadelphia.

Kaplan, R.M. and Bush, J.W. (1982). Health-related quality of life measurement for evaluation, research and policy analysis. *Health Psychol.*, **1**, 61–80.

Leplege, A. and Verdier, A. (1995). The adaptation of health status measures: methodological aspects of the translation procedure. In *The international assessment of health-related quality of life: theory, translation, measurement and analysis*, (ed. S.A. Shumaker and R.A. Berzon), pp. 93–101. Rapid Communications, Oxford.

Lydick, E.G. and Epstein, R.S. (1996). Clinical significance of quality of life data. In *Quality of life and pharmacoeconomics in clinical trials*, (2nd edn), (ed. B. Spilker), pp. 461–5. Lippincott–Raven, Philadelphia.

Moinpour, C.M. (1994). Measuring quality of life: an emerging science. *Seminars in Oncology*, **21**, 48S–63S.

Nunnally, J.C. (1978). *Psychometric theory*, (2nd edn), pp. 229–46. Basic Books, New York.

Pocock, S.J. (1991). A perspective on the role of quality of life assessment in clinical trials. *Control Clin. Trials*, **12**, 257S–65S.

Revicki, D.A. and Kaplan, R.M. (1995). Relationship between psychometric and utility-based approaches to the measurement of health-related quality of life. In *The international assessment of health-related quality of life: theory, translation, measurement and analysis*, (ed. S.A. Shumaker and R.A. Berzon), pp. 125–35. Rapid Communications, Oxford.

Schipper, H., Olweny, C.L.M., and Clinch, J.J. (1996). A mini-handbook for conducting small-scale clinical trials in developing countries. In *Quality of life and pharmacoeconomics in clinical trials*, (2nd edn), (ed. B. Spilker), pp. 669–80. Lippincott–Raven, Philadelphia.

Schron, E.B. and Shumaker, S.A. (1992). The integration of health-related quality of life in clinical research: experiences from cardiovascular clinical trials. *Prog. Cardiovasc. Nurs.*, **7**, 21–8.

Schumacher, M., Olschewski, M., and Schulen, G. (1991). Assessment of quality of life in clinical trials. *Stat. Medicine*, **10**, 1915–30.

Shumaker, S.A. and Berzon, R. (eds.) (1995). The international assessment of health-related quality of life: theory, translation, measurement and analysis. Rapid Communications, Oxford.

Shumaker, S.A. and Naughton, M.J. (1995). The international assessment of health-related quality of life. In *The international assessment of health-related quality of life: theory, translation, measurement and analysis*, (ed. S.A. Shumaker and R.A. Berzon), pp. 3–10. Rapid Communications, Oxford.

Spilker, B., (ed.) (1996). *Quality of life and pharmacoeconomics in clinical trials*, (2nd edn). Lippincott–Raven, Philadelphia.

Stewart, A.L., Greenfield, S., Hays, R.D., *et al.* (1989). Functional status and well-being of patients with chronic conditions. *J. Am. Med. Assoc.*, **262**, 907–13.

Streiner, D.L. and Norman, G.R. (1989). *Health measure scales: a practical guide to their use*. Oxford University Press, New York.

Torrance, G.W. (1987). Utility approach to measuring health-related quality of life. *J. Chronic Dis.*, **40**, 593–600.

Wagner, T.H., Patrick, D.L., Galer, B.S., and Berzon, R.A. (1996). A new instrument to assess the long-term quality of life effects from migraine. development and psychometric testing of the MSQOL. *Headache*, **36**, 484–92.

Wild, D., Patrick, D., Johnson, E., Berzon, R., *et al.* (1995). Measuring health-related quality of life in persons with genital herpes. *Qual. Life Res.*, **4**, 532–9.

Wilson, I.B. and Cleary, P.D. (1995). Linking clinical variables with health-related quality of life. *J. Am. Med. Assoc.*, **273**, 59–65.

World Health Organization (1958). The first ten years of the World Health Organization, WHO, Geneva.

Wu, A.W. and Rubin, H.R. (1994). Approaches to health status measurement in HIV disease: overview of the conference. *Psychol. and Health*, **9**, 1–18.

Wu, A.W., Jacobson, D., Berzon, R.A., *et al.* (1997). Effect of mode of administration on medical outcomes, study health ratings and Euroqol scores in AIDS. *Qual. Life Res.*, **6**, 3–10.

Zwinderman, A.H. (1990). The measurement of change of quality of life in clinical trials. *Stat. Medicine*, **9**, 931–42.

Further reading

Aaronson, N.K. (1989). Quality of life assessment in clinical trials: methodologic issues. *Control Clin. Trials*, **10**, 195S–208S.

Berzon, R.A., Donnelly, M.A., Simpson, Jr. R.L., Simeon, G.P., and Tilson, H.H. (1995). Quality of life bibliography and indexes: 1994 update. *Qual. Life Res.*, **4**, 547–68.

Berzon, R.A., Mauskopf, J.A., and Simeon, G.P. (1996). Choosing a health profile (descriptive) and/or a patient-preference (utility) measure for a clinical trial. In *Quality of life and pharmacoeconomics in clinical trials*, (2nd edn), (ed. B. Spilker), pp. 375–9. Lippincott–Raven, Philadelphia.

Deyo, R.A. and Centor, R.M. (1986). Assessing the responsiveness of functional scales to clinical change: an analogy to diagnostic test performance. *J. Chronic Dis.*, **39**, 897–906.

Deyo, R., Diehr, P., and Patrick, D. (1991). Reproducibility and responsiveness of health status measures: statistics and strategies for evaluation. *Control Clin. Trials*, **12**, 142S–158S.

Drummond, M. (1992). The role and importance of quality of life measurements in economic evaluations. *Br. J. Med. Econ.*, **4**, 9–16.

Fletcher, A. (1995). Quality of life measurements in the evaluation of treatment: proposed guidelines. *Br. J. Clin. Pharmacol.*, **39**, 217–22.

Gafni, A. (1989). The quality of QALYs (quality-adjusted-life-years): do QALYs measure what they at least intend to measure? *Health Policy*, **13**, 81–3.

Guyatt, G.H., Deyo, R.A., Charlson, M., Levine, M.N., and Mitchell, A. (1989). Responsiveness and validity in health status measurement: a clarification. *J. Clin. Epidem.*, **42**, 403–8.

Guyatt, G.H., Kieshner, B., and Jaeschke, R. (1992). Measuring health status: what are the necessary measurement properties? *J. Clin. Epidem.*, **45**, 1341–5.

Henderson-James, D. and Spilker, B. (1990). Quality of life: an industry perspective. In *Quality of life assessments in clinical trials*, (ed. B. Spilker), pp. 183–92. Raven Press, New York.

Jaeschke, R., Guyatt, and Cook, D. (1992). Quality of life instruments in the evaluation of new drugs. *PharmacoEconomics*, **1**, 84–94.

Katz, J.N., Larson, M.G., Phillips, C.B., Fossel, A.H., and Liang, M.H. (1992). Comparative measurement and sensitivity of short and longer health status measurement instruments. *Med. Care*, **30**, 917–25.

Loomes, G. and McKenzie, L. (1989). The use of QALYs in health care decision making. *Soc. Sci. Med.*, **28**, 299–308.

Mansfield, E. (1987). *Statistics for business and economics*. W.W. Norton and Co., New York.

Stewart, A.L. and Ware, J.E., (eds) (1992). *Measuring functioning and well-being*. Duke University Press, Durham, North Carolina.

Testa, M.A. and Lenderking, W.R. (1992). Interpreting pharmacoEconomic and quality-of-life clinical trial data for use in therapeutics. *Pharmacoeconomics*, **2**, 107–17.

Torrance, G.W. and Feeny, D. (1989). Utilities and quality-adjusted life years. *Intl J. Tech. Assess.*, **5**, 559–75.

Ware, J.E. (1984). The general health rating index. In *Assessment of quality of life in clinical trials of cardiovascular therapies*, (ed. N.K. Wenger, M.E. Mattson, C.D. Furberg, and J. Elinson). Le Jacq, New York.

Ware, J.E. (1987). Standards for validating health measures: definition and content. *J. Chronic Dis.*, **40**, 473–80.

Wilkin, D., Hallam, L., and Doggett, M. (1992). *Measures of need and outcome for primary health care*. Oxford University Press, New York.

II

Primary issues specific to quality of life trials

2 *Guidelines for measuring health-related quality of life in clinical trials*

David Osoba

Introduction

It is important to have a clear methodology for measuring health-related quality of life (HRQoL) in clinical trials. Although it is more common, at present, to measure HRQoL in randomized, controlled trials (phase III studies), there is an increasing need also to consider measuring HRQoL in earlier phase studies. How the nature of the study influences the methods of HRQoL assessment will be dealt with in the appropriate sections below.

The decision to assess (measure) HRQoL in the context of a clinical trial raises the need to answer several questions. Some of these questions are listed below.

- Is HRQoL the primary or a secondary end-point (outcome) in the study?
- Which method of measurement will be used – interview or questionnaire?
- To what extent will interviews be structured?
- If questionnaires are to be used, which instruments are best for the purpose?
- What is the sample size required to answer the study question?
- When will measurements be taken? Where will they be taken?
- How will compliance with questionnaire completion be documented?
- What are the feasibility issues to be considered?
- What are the actual steps in implementation?

Table 2.1 lists these and other questions that need to be considered. They have been grouped below into those questions that need to be answered during the writing of the trial protocol, and those that need to be answered during implementation and conduct of the trial.

The protocol

A description of all relevant aspects of the HRQoL measurement should be incorporated as an integral part of the main protocol for the study. The use of separate protocols or add-on studies to measure HRQoL implies that HRQoL measurement is not really an important part of the main study and can also

Table 2.1   Considerations for measuring HRQoL in clinical trials

1. Is HRQoL the major (primary) or minor (secondary) outcome (end-point) being studied?
2. Which method of HRQoL measurement – interview or questionnaire – will be used?
3. To what degree will interviews be structured?
4. If questionnaires are being used, which questionnaire(s) are best suited for the purpose of the study?
5. What are the eligibility requirements for the HRQoL position of the study, and are these different from the eligibility requirements for the study itself?
6. What is the required sample size and how is it to be determined?
7. When will measurements be taken?
8. Where will measurements be taken?
9. How will compliance be documented?
10. How will the measurement be implemented?
11. What should the trial protocol contain about HRQoL assessment?
12. How will the HRQoL assessments be monitored?
13. How will the results be analysed and reported?

lead to mislaying of material, forgetting to carry out HRQoL assessments, and so on.

Appropriate statements and instructions about the HRQoL assessments should be included under each of the usual protocol headings, such as introduction, objectives, eligibility criteria, etc. Detailed instructions for protocol writing have been published previously,[1] and will be reiterated here, along with a commentary providing the rationale for each instruction and other relevant comments. The importance of including clear instructions in the protocol cannot be overemphasized. Not only will clear instructions be necessary for the proper conduct of the trial, but also will help in the analysis of the data and the description of the study for publications arising from the trial.

Introduction and background

Why is measurement of HRQoL relevant in the trial? Is a hypothesis being tested or is the purpose to provide descriptive data for the generation of hypotheses? How will the results be used after the trial is completed? Will an interview or self-report questionnaire approach be used? Will an interview be open ended or structured? If the questionnaire method is used, which instrument(s) will be used and why was it (were they) chosen for this trial? Literature references must be given to support the choices and the reliability, validity, and responsiveness of the instruments that will be used.

Answers to all of the above can be provided in a reasonably short paragraph that establishes the background for measuring HRQoL in the trial. This will also establish that HRQoL is thought to be an important, integral component of the trial and not an add-on or an afterthought. A statement of whether hypotheses are being tested or merely generated will have a bearing on the subsequent analysis and reporting of the data.

Objectives

Is the measurement of HRQoL a major (primary) outcome (end-point) or a secondary end-point in the study? Within the HRQoL scores, will a particular domain be of more interest than another, such as emotional functioning, or will all domains be of equal interest?

Clearly stated objectives establish the importance of measuring HRQoL in the trial. HRQoL may be the primary, and only, end-point of interest in a trial involving palliative therapy. Thus far, there are few such trials reported in the literature,[2] but they will become much more frequent in the future. It is more usual, at present, to make the assessment of HRQoL a secondary end-point, often without a clear hypothesis-testing question. This approach has been very helpful in establishing the value of HRQoL assessments and providing hypothesis-generating data. In some trials, the HRQoL end-points of greatest interest may involve only certain domains, such as emotional functioning or physical functioning. If so, a hypothesis should be stated with regard to the domain of interest and the remainder of the HRQoL data can be descriptive. If only a single domain of HRQoL is to be measured, it should be stated why more comprehensive HRQoL data will not be collected: indeed, it should not be stated that the trial is measuring HRQoL, but that only emotional functioning or physical functioning, and so on, is being measured.

Eligibility criteria

Will patients be required to indicate their willingness to participate and answer questionnaires or to be interviewed at specified times? If a patient is not willing or unable to participate in HRQoL assessment, is the patient still eligible for the trial? Is a certain level of reading and comprehension required? Will oral translation of self-report questionnaires be allowed if a patient does not understand the language in which the questionnaire is written?

When HRQoL is an end-point in a trial (whether primary or secondary), there may be eligibility criteria required in addition to those that are normally included in protocols, such as the ability and willingness to answer HRQoL questionnaire(s). The degree to which these additional eligibility requirements should drive collection of HRQoL data is somewhat contentious. Clearly, if the assessment of HRQoL is required to answer the primary question in a trial, then the acceptance of patients who are unable or unwilling to answer HRQoL questions would be meaningless. However, in trials where the HRQoL question is a secondary one, should a patient who is eligible for the trial with respect to the primary end-point still be considered eligible if the patient refuses to answer HRQoL questions? The clinical trials group (CTG) of the National Cancer Institute of Canada (NCIC) has taken the view that HRQoL assessments are an integral and important aspect of its phase III trials, and patients who are unwilling, but otherwise able to answer questionnaires, are declared ineligible. In practice, this has turned out to be a rare occurrence. The situation is different if a patient is willing to answer questionnaires but unable to do so because of a physical handicap (poor vision, pain, etc.) or because he or she is unable to read and understand a questionnaire in the language in which it is available. Such patients are acceptable, if they are otherwise eligible, and HRQoL assessment is waived. Translation of the questionnaires by health care personnel, researchers, or family members is not allowed, since this may introduce uncontrolled bias and/or errors in the way the questionnaires are translated and answered. However, in certain situations, for example, where mental functioning may become impaired (as in brain cancer), the use of proxy respondents may be the only method by which HRQoL data can be collected and is preferable to not collecting any data at all. In these situations the investigators should use caution in interpreting the results, since they are not based on self-reported data.

Study design

Which assessment method will be used, interview or questionnaire? How structured will interviews be? If questionnaires are used, which instrument(s) will be used? When will the assessments be administered? Where will HRQoL administration take place, in the clinic or at home? If the latter, will it be conducted by telephone? Who will be responsible for administration of the interviews or questionnaires?

Interview methods using open-ended or semi-structured approaches are useful for initial development of items to be used subsequently in questionnaires, and to discover common themes, to list issues, and to describe patients' experiences. However, the interview method is labour intensive and the responses are difficult to quantify. Nevertheless, in phase I or II studies, when only small numbers of patients are involved, and particularly when exploratory detail is desirable, interviews (open or partly structured) may be preferable and/or of equal value to using questionnaires. Fully structured interview formats with quantitative response options are really the same as classical self-response questionnaires, with the only difference being that the questionnaire is administered by the 'interviewer' rather than being self-administered.

In large, phase III clinical trials, self-report questionnaires are the method of choice.[3,4] They are much less labour intensive than interviews and, hence, less expensive and more feasible. Also, the response options are structured to provide quantitative data as output.

Several psychometrically reliable and valid self-report questionnaires are now available, ranging from generic through condition-specific to disease-specific (see below for definitions) instruments. Therefore, it is no longer difficult to find psychometrically validated instruments for use in clinical trials. The task is to choose one that is suitable for answering the HRQoL questions posed in the trial. (A brief account of how to choose an appropriate instrument based upon the purpose of HRQoL assessment is given in the section titled 'choosing the instrument(s)' below.)

The *timing* of HRQoL administrations, that is, *when* HRQoL will be measured in relation to interventions and the course of the illness trajectory, is very important.[5] A baseline administration, *before* randomization and treatment initiation, should be mandatory in all trials in which HRQoL will be measured. The baseline administration is required not only to be able to make within-group comparisons for changes in HRQoL scores from before to after treatment, but also to check whether patients entered on the arms of a trial are balanced with respect to HRQoL characteristics. If baseline characteristics are balanced and if attrition of patients over time is equal in the groups being compared, then a simple comparison of mean scores between the various groups may be sufficient. However, if HRQoL characteristics are not balanced at baseline, then a comparison between groups will require a calculation and comparison of the changes in mean scores between the groups from baseline to the time points of interest and a careful interpretation of the results. It can be argued that change scores should be used even when baseline characteristics are reasonably balanced between groups, because the use of change scores takes into account small differences between individuals at baseline, which although not significant enough to produce a between-groups imbalance, should nevertheless be accounted for in a between-groups analysis at later times.

Baseline measurements are absolutely essential in phase II studies, since the comparisons will be between pretreatment, during treatment, and after treatment. The timing of measurements during the trial will be dependent on the questions being asked and the nature of the trial. If it is desirable to know how HRQoL changes during treatment then measurements will need to be taken at the appropriate times. These measurements may be intended to determine the effects of acute toxicity of therapy, or the effect of each cycle of a treatment, or the entire treatment course, on the progress of the disease. In the first situation, HRQoL measurements would be taken when acute toxicity would be expected to be greatest, for example, in the week after chemotherapy or at the end of a course of radiation therapy. In the latter situations, measurements should be taken when acute toxicity has subsided, such as on the last day of a three-week cycle of chemotherapy or a few weeks after the end of a course of radiation therapy. Ideally, to have a comprehensive view of HRQoL during and after treatment, several measurements should be taken so that all these situations are included. In addition, the timing of HRQoL assessments with respect to visits to the physician or for treatment should be specified. It is preferable to have the assessments completed at the same point in time relative to these events, that is before the physician's interview and examination, and before a scheduled treatment. If the assessments are completed just before these events, then the answers are not influenced by 'news' given by the physician or by the administration of a treatment or early side-effects of treatment (e.g. onset of nausea).

The protocol should state *where* assessments will take place, that is, in the doctor's office, in the clinic, or in the home. Completion in a physician's office or in the clinic is usually preferable to completion at home. The conditions under which the questionnaire is completed are more controllable in the former locations than in the latter. Personnel responsible for administering the questionnaire in a clinic can make certain that the respondent does not receive assistance from well-meaning family members or friends and the timing can be controlled to fit with the guidelines given above, whereas these factors can't be controlled at home. Nevertheless, there may be some circumstances when it is preferable to have questionnaires completed at home. For example, some centres have been successful in using telephone interviews routinely as a means of obtaining HRQoL data.[6] Telephone interviews can control for timing and self-completion, and also may be preferable when patients' office or clinic visits do not coincide with the timing of questionnaire administration. Another reason for completion of questionnaires at home is when the timing of questionnaire administration does not coincide with a visit to the office or clinic, and it is deemed too burdensome to have patients return to the clinic only for the purpose of answering questionnaires. Also, a questionnaire may need to be mailed to a patient if the questionnaire has not been given to a patient in the clinic due to administrative error. Despite these exceptions, the general rule is that as many as possible of the conditions surrounding questionnaire administration should be controlled and this is most easily done in the office, clinic, or hospital environment.

Instrument description

The protocol should contain a brief, but adequate description of the interview method or instrument and a full copy of the questionnaire(s) to be used. The anticipated time it will take patients to complete the assessment, as known from previous use of the interview or questionnaire, should be indicated. The questionnaire itself is best placed in an appendix (see below) to the main protocol so that it can easily be detached and copied, if desired.

Sample size

A clear statement of the sample size required to answer the HRQoL questions in the trial must be given. This subject is covered in detail in Chapter 3. All that will be stated here is that the protocol should contain a clear statement as to why the indicated sample size was chosen and how it was calculated. This is mandatory when HRQoL is the primary end-point in the study, but it is still important to make a statement about the adequacy of the sample size to answer the HRQoL questions even when HRQoL end-points are secondary.

Monitoring, stopping rules, evaluation, and analysis

Will the data be monitored during the course of the trial to determine whether enrolment of patients into the trial should be stopped or otherwise altered? If, so what are the rules for making such a decision? How will the responses in the questionnaires be scored and analysed? If more than one HRQoL outcome is being measured, what is the primary outcome (hypothesis) and how will it be analysed? How will other HRQoL outcomes be analysed?

Stopping rules are generally designed to ascertain whether unexpected, serious toxicity has occurred which would preclude the continuation of the trial. Also, they can be used to determine whether the efficacy end-point(s) in one arm of the trial is or are superior to that of any other to an extent that it is unethical to continue with the study. HRQoL data have not yet been used in this way but it can be envisaged their being used as such in the future, particularly in trials of palliative therapy.

A detailed description of analysis methods is presented elsewhere in this book (see Chapters 13, 14 and 15). Here it is enough to point out that phase III studies focus on HRQoL differences between the groups in the study (inter-group differences) whereas phase I and II studies focus on pretreatment and post-treatment differences within a group (intra-group differences). Of course, intra-group differences may also be assessed in phase III studies. The main temptation to avoid is going on a 'fishing expedition' by carrying out a large number of indiscriminate comparisons since, by chance, some may not satisfy the null hypothesis. Comparisons and probability estimates should be limited to the main hypothesis and any remaining analyses may be provided for descriptive purposes only. If statistical significance is to be provided for multiple comparisons, as may be necessary when a multidimensional instrument giving multiple scores is used at multiple time points, a statement about whether any correction will be made should be given. The statistical methods should be provided and, in the case of multiple measurements over time, whether the primary analysis output will be a comparison of scores at given times, a comparison of the change in scores from baseline scores, or some other output.

Consent form

The consent form for the trial should state that HRQoL is being measured and the purpose for which the data will be used. Whether or not there will be a potential benefit to the participant should be stated. The number of times that the subject will be required to complete HRQoL assessments and the length of time it will take for each assessment should be given. In addition, a statement as to whether the data are being collected for research purposes only or whether they will be used in the day-to-day care of the patient should be made. Other standard statements about confidentiality, who will see the data, and the right to refuse to participate or to drop out of the study at any time without jeopardizing future care should be included.

Cover sheet for monitoring compliance

A problem encountered with collecting HRQoL data is that missing data may affect the reliability of the results. In order to reduce missing data and, when this is unavoidable, to provide an explanation for it, a cover sheet for the questionnaire which is to be filled out by study personnel should be attached to the front of the HRQoL questionnaire. An example of part of the cover sheet used by the NCIC CTG is shown in Table 2.2. A completed cover sheet must accompany each questionnaire returned to the central data processing office, whether or not the HRQoL questionnaire has been completed.

Instructions for administration

Are detailed instructions provided so that personnel responsible for collecting the HRQoL data are fully aware of the procedures to be followed? How will the data be transmitted to the central office? Will direct electronic entry and transmission

Table 2.2   An example cover sheet*

Was questionnaire complete?

____Yes → Date questionnaire completed: ____ ____ ____
                                           yy   mm   dd
Were *all* questions answered? __Yes__No If no, reason_____
Was assistance required? __Yes__No If yes, reason_____
Where was questionnaire completed? ☐ home   ☐ clinic   ☐ another centre

____No → Please fill in today's date: ____ ____ ____
                                       yy   mm   dd
Specify reason(s) questionnaire not completed (tick those that apply):
____1. Patient kept appointment for examination, but could not complete questionnaire due to illness.
____2. Patient kept appointment for examination, but refused to complete questionnaire for reason other than illness. Specify reason_____
____3. Patient did not keep appointment. Specify reason_____
____4. Patient could not be contacted.
____5. Questionnaire not administered due to institution error.
____6. Other reason, specify:_____

* Adapted from cover sheet used in protocols of the National Cancer Institute of Canada clinical trials group.

be used? Detailed instructions on how to present the HRQoL instruments for completion should be provided for study personnel responsible for the collection of the data.[1] If desired, the method of questionnaire administration may be covered in an appendix to the main protocol. In addition, complete instructions should be given about how to return the HRQoL data to the central data processing office. Will the data be sent to the office as they are collected, or will they be kept in the participating centre office and sent in batches according to a predefined schedule? Will direct entry, using computers with touch-sensitive video monitors (screens), and electronic transmission be used? Instructions on preserving confidentiality, regardless of the data collection method used, should be given.

Appendix

As mentioned above, details about the characteristics of an instrument, the instrument itself with its cover sheet, and detailed instructions for the collection of the data can be included in one or more appendices to the main protocol.

Choosing the instrument(s)

Types of instruments

Several psychometrically validated, multidimensional questionnaires for measuring HRQoL are available. Some are intended for measurement of health status/quality of life in any illness or condition and are termed 'generic'. Others are more specific, intended for use in a set of similar conditions such as cancer, and can be termed 'condition-specific'. Questionnaires that are restricted to a particular cancer, for example breast cancer, are 'disease-specific', while those restricted even further for use in a particular treatment or clinical trial may be called 'treatment-specific' or 'trial-specific', or to use a phrase that will encompass both of these

Table 2.3 Examples of multidimensional instruments useful for clinical trials in patients with cancer

Generic	Medical outcomes study (MOS) short form (SF)[7,8]
	Sickness impact profile (SIP)[9,10]
Cancer-specific	Cancer rehabilitation evaluation system (CARES)[11]
(Condition-specific)	European Organization for Research and Treatment of Cancer (EORTC)
	core quality of life questionnaire (QLQ-C30)[12,13]
	Functional assessment of cancer therapy (FACT) scales[14]
	Functional living index–cancer (FLIC)[15,16]
	Linear analogue self-assessment (LASA) scales[17,18]
	Quality of life index (QLI)[19]
	Quality of life index (QL-Index)[20,21]
	Rotterdam symptom checklist (RSCL)[22,23]
Disease-specific	Prostate quality of life index (PROSQOLI)[2]
	Breast cancer chemotherapy questionnaire (BCCQ)[24]
	Various disease-specific modules
Situation-specific	Trial-specific modules and checklists[25,26]

situations, 'situation-specific'. Examples of some questionnaires belonging to the above categories are given in Table 2.3.

Desirable characteristics

There are several desirable characteristics of HRQoL measures (Table 2.4), the most important of which are reliability and validity. *Reliability* refers to the accuracy and consistency of the measure, that is, how accurately and consistently a test is measuring what it is supposed to measure. *Test–retest reliability and internal consistency* are classical measures of reliability; *split-test reliability* is a subtype of internal consistency. *Validity* is the extent to which a test measures what it is intended to measure. There are many types of validity; the most important are *content, construct*, and *criterion* validity. Further details are covered in Chapter 10.

A reliable test may not be a valid one, whereas a valid test is always reliable. For example, a set of questions pertaining to physical function may be reliable, that is, have internal consistency and excellent test–retest stability, but would be an invalid measure of cognitive function since these would not be appropriate for assessment of this domain. Most questionnaires in use today provide numerical data that are amenable to statistical analysis and to quantification. A textbook treatment of reliability and validity may be found elsewhere.[27]

Although *multidimensional* assessment is preferable to unidimensional assessment and is required to obtain a comprehensive assessment of quality of life, unidimensional or bidimensional assessment can be used, provided it is used as a measure of only the domain that is being measured and not touted as an assessment of overall HRQoL.

Within multidimensional instruments, a set of items dealing specifically with a global HRQoL domain is highly recommended. This is a useful way of obtaining the patient's assessment of overall quality of life without attempting to sum up, or aggregate, the scores from all the domains. The use of single, aggregate scores has pitfalls, for example, for the implicit assumption that each domain is equal to

Table 2.4 Desirable characteristics of quality-of-life measures

1. Should give *meaningful data*, that is, reflect the truth, and should
    (a) be based on patients' opinions, by
        (i) self-assessment (questionnaire or interview)
        (ii) construction and validation in appropriate samples of patients
    (b) use *understandable language*
    (c) have *reliability*, as demonstrated by
        (i) factor analysis
        (ii) internal consistency
        (iii) test–retest stability
        (iv) inter-rater reproducibility (when assessed by different raters)
    (d) have *validity*, which may be of several kinds, such as
        (i) content validity
        (ii) construct validity
        (iii) criterion validity
        (iv) concurrent validity
        (v) sensitivity and specificity
        (vi) being able to distinguish between effects of disease, toxicity of treatment, and co-morbid conditions
        (vii) predictive validity
    (e) provide *quantifiable data*, which
        (i) is amenable to statistical analysis
        (ii) allows comparison between data sets
    (f) have *clinical* significance as well as statistical significance
2. Should be *multidimensional*, including
    (a) physical/role function
    (b) emotional (mental)/psychological state
    (c) social (activity, support) interaction
    (d) symptoms (somatic discomfort)
    (e) global (summary) assessment
    (f) other dimensions, as necessary
3. Should consist of a 'core' of questions plus a specific module of questions for different situations, for example, a particular clinical trial
4. Should be *feasible*, that is,
    (a) short, so that it may be
        (i) administered repeatedly
        (ii) easy to score and analyse
    (b) acceptable to patients, by being
        (i) inoffensive
        (ii) unintrusive
    (c) usable in a busy, clinical setting

any other in the weight it provides to the aggregate score and in the dilution or masking of information which occurs when scores in some domains change in one direction while those in others change in the opposite direction within the same questionnaire completion. Thus, an aggregate score may not adequately reflect changes that may have occurred, that is, it may be insufficiently responsive, and does not provide sufficient detail to explain the effects of a disease or treatment on HRQoL. If a separate global domain score is available, a stepwise, multiple regression analysis may determine how much of the variance in the global response is attributable to any particular domain. In addition, correlations between other domains and the global domain may be examined. Since for most phase III clinical trials it is desirable to obtain information about overall quality of life as well as each domain, an instrument that provides sufficient detail about changes in several domains and symptoms is required. Thus, an instrument designed to give separate scores for domains and single items is preferable to one that provides only a single, aggregate score.

A '*core*' of questions refers to those that can be used for patients with many varieties of disease. However, if the core questionnaire is to remain relatively brief, it cannot contain all the questions that may be desirable in all situations for all patients. Therefore, it is recommended that a 'disease-specific' or, preferably, 'situation-specific' or even 'trial-specific' module or checklist of questions be constructed for each new situation.[26,28] Examples include a specific checklist for women with breast cancer receiving chemotherapy or a specific checklist for men with prostate cancer receiving hormones and analgesics. This 'modular approach' is now becoming the accepted standard in oncology clinical trials.

Finally, in many clinical trials situations, it is important that HRQoL questionnaires be easily administered to ill patients. Thus, they should be easily understood, and be reasonably short (less than 50 brief questions) so that they can be completed in a short time. In the author's experience patients who are feeling ill become tired after 15–20 minutes and lengthy questionnaires increase the risk of failure to complete an entire questionnaire or items near the end of a questionnaire.

Choosing questionnaires

Given that there are several reliable and valid questionnaires available today, how should a questionnaire or questionnaires be chosen for a particular trial? One approach is to base the choice on the perceived purpose of the trial. A taxonomy of purposes and an algorithm for selecting questionnaires have been detailed elsewhere.[4,29]

In brief, when the purpose of measuring quality of life is for *screening* a large sample to find cases of interest with particular HRQoL characteristics for subsequent study or intervention, or as a means of determining the incidence of particular characteristics, it may be desirable to use relatively brief instruments with characteristics that are likely to identify the persons of interest. However, when HRQoL will be assessed as part of a trial of a new therapy (compared to a standard therapy), it is desirable to use an instrument that can provide sufficient detail to provide HRQoL *status profiles* so that decisions can be made about the advantages of one therapy compared to another. When the purpose is to use HRQoL assessment as a *decision-making* tool in day-to-day clinical practice, even more detail as well as very high levels of internal consistency (Cronbach's alpha coefficient >0.90) are desirable. Furthermore, demonstrated responsiveness to change is clearly important. For *preference measurement*, a different set of tools is required. Preference is determined by utility assessment and psychometrically based instruments are probably not appropriate for this task (see Chapter 5).

A clear understanding of the purpose of the HRQoL assessment will assist greatly in choosing an appropriate measure to fit the need. Some additional criteria for assessing the suitability of questionnaires are, what is the question time frame? and what is the response structure? In general, time frames of a few days are preferable to those asking about the past few weeks or only 'today'. Those with a long time frame tend to be influenced by the patients' personality, while those with a very short time frame may provide information on very temporary phenomena.[30] The common response structures are categorical scales, varying from three to seven categories, or linear analogue scales. Both seem to work reasonably well and there is probably no clear advantage of one over the other.

The process of choosing an appropriate method and instrument is a complex process, and the novice should seek expert advice before attempting to delve, unassisted, into HRQoL assessment.

Implementation and monitoring

Overcoming barriers

Only a short time ago, it seemed reasonable to ask why HRQoL was not being measured more often. However, in the past few years, there has been a great deal of interest and activity in this area. Some of this activity has resulted from the successful breaking down of barriers to HRQoL assessment.

There are four types of barriers to the adoption of new technologies – attitudinal, conceptual, logical, and practical.[3,31] The attitudinal barrier to measuring HRQoL has diminished substantially. It was common for health care providers to raise such objections as 'Quality of life is subjective and, therefore, unquantifiable', or 'It can't be measured', 'I am too busy', and 'It's not my job'. These objections may still be heard but should be dispelled by the growing realization that HRQoL results provide valuable patient-centred outcomes in addition to the classical survival and toxicity outcomes, and by the demonstration that multidimensional HRQoL measures provide more information than can be obtained by assessing a single dimension such as performance status. Also, measuring HRQoL has provided new evidence in support of certain treatment strategies that may have seemed counter-intuitive initially, and has proved to be of prognostic value for survival.

The conceptual barrier to measuring quality of life versus quantity of life is no longer an issue. It is recognized that quality of life is as important as quantity of life and, although particularly cogent in those situations where treatment is primarily palliative in nature, is also important in most oncology clinical trials. Indeed, it may be generalized that the ultimate goal of all health care endeavours is the preservation or restoration of HRQoL.

There are still several methodological barriers that must be overcome. Some of these relate to the clinical meaningfulness of the results of HRQoL assessment, the need for a better understanding of the areas in which HRQoL assessment is applicable, and how to deal with the substantial amounts of missing data that are commonly reported in some studies.

Under practical barriers, one can list such issues as time, space, and personnel required and hence, the cost of collecting and analysing the information. These practical considerations (see below) have equal importance to the scientific considerations underlying HRQoL assessment and the choice of appropriate instruments.

Practical considerations

When the research question has been formulated, the method of measurement chosen and the population of interest identified, and the barriers to measurement removed, the next step is implementation. This involves primarily practical considerations and these are of such importance that inadequate attention to them can result in the failure of an otherwise well-planned project or programme.

Practical considerations will vary somewhat depending upon the context (setting) in which HRQoL will be measured. Will the measurement be carried out as part of a multi-institutional clinical trial, or in a single institution such as a hospital or clinic or in a private practice office? Many aspects of successful implementation will be the same, however, regardless of the setting. These include such considerations as

- ensuring support from appropriate personnel, administrators, and institutions before launching the project;
- writing appropriate protocols incorporating HRQoL measures;
- designating responsibility for tasks such as who writes the protocol, who collects the data, who analyses the data, and so on;
- ensuring an appropriate physical environment for data collection, storage, and analysis;
- establishing procedures for ensuring compliance with questionnaire completion;
- ensuring adequate funding for completion of all the tasks.

A major issue is to devise means to ensure completion of HRQoL assessments at the specified times throughout the trial. In the context of multi-institutional clinical trials, the clinical trials group of the NCIC has implemented a number of procedures designed to enhance questionnaire completion.[1,32] These include

- incorporation of HRQoL assessment as a specific trial objective;
- provision of a rationale for HRQoL data collection;
- establishment of the successful completion of the HRQoL assessment as an eligibility requirement;
- inclusion in the protocol of specific instructions about how to administer the instrument;
- modification of data collection forms to remind data managers to administer the instrument; and
- provision of specific reporting schedules.

All of the above are included in the protocol and case report forms. In addition, it is important to use pre-trial workshops for nurses and data managers to explain the rationale and procedures for HRQoL data collection. Regular feedback to participants via letter and newsletter on the HRQoL aspect of the clinical trials should be provided and, in some cases, computer-based reminders in advance of due dates for questionnaire completion can also be provided. The experience has been that these procedures have resulted in very high compliance rates (greater than 95 per cent) in several phase III trials in which HRQoL measurement was included.[25,32]

In a small hospital or clinic, most of the above will also apply, but less of the work can be shared with others, that is, the local investigators must set up the appropriate system within their own environment. Carrying out HRQoL measures in a private practice office should take into account the number of available patients and ensure that there are sufficient support personnel and adequate time to enable successful data collection and analysis.

Additional data collection

In addition to collection of the HRQoL questionnaire responses and other data required in the clinical trial, it is important to collect certain specific information that will be useful in the analysis and reporting of the trial. This information should include

- the number of patients eligible for HRQoL assessment and their relevant characteristics;
- how many eligible patients were accrued;
- the time over which accrual occurred;
- which patients were excluded from analysis and why (e.g. inadequate data, missing data, etc.);
- how many patients were adequately followed and assessed, and reasons for loss to follow-up;
- which patients died during the trial;
- which patients failed to complete the treatment protocol;
- what was the actual schedule of HRQoL assessments.

Monitoring the above will enable the analysis to take into account missing data and the reasons why it was missing. It will also ensure that compliance with questionnaire administration and completion can be evaluated. If there has been adequate data collection, results can be presented with respect to institutions that complied, number of patients that completed questionnaires out of the number that were eligible at defined time points, and the number of missing domains or items out of the number expected. This information, when reported,[33] (Chapter 18) will allow readers to obtain a complete picture of the HRQoL assessment procedure and assist in a well-informed interpretation of the results.

Conclusions

Measurement of HRQoL, whether within clinical trials or not, whether by interviews or questionnaires, is a task not to be taken lightly. All aspects of measurement should be integrated into the protocol for the study. A clear understanding of the reasons for measurement and the purpose to which the data will be put is necessary. Of equal importance is attention to practical aspects of feasibility and data collection, with particular emphasis being placed on mechanisms that will ensure a minimum of missing information. Finally, precise documentation of all aspects of data collection will ensure that the results can be reported completely and will decrease some of the current ambiguity surrounding interpretation of results.

Acknowledgements

I wish to thank all of the many people involved with the development of HRQoL assessment by the National Cancer Institute of Canada clinical trials group. In particular, Drs Joe Pater (Director) and Benny Zee (Senior Statistician) as well as the members of the quality of life committee and staff of the clinical trials group office have been most helpful. I also thank Jill Vardy for assistance in preparing the manuscript.

References

1. Osoba, D. The quality of life committee of the clinical trials group of the National Cancer Institute of Canada: organization and functions. *Quality of Life Research*, 1992; **1**: 211–18.
2. Tannock, I.F., Osoba, D., Stockler, M.R., *et al*. Chemotherapy with mitoxantrone plus prednisone or prednisone alone for symptomatic hormone-resistant prostate cancer: a Canadian randomized trial with palliative end points. *Journal of Clinical Oncology*, 1996; **14**: 1756–64.
3. Osoba, D. Measuring the effect of cancer on quality of life. In *Effect of cancer on quality of life*, (ed. D. Osoba). CRC Press, Boca Raton, 1991; 25–40.
4. Osoba, D., Aaronson, N.K., and Till, J.E. A practical guide for selecting quality-of-life measures in clinical trials and practice. In *Effect of cancer on quality of life*, (ed. D. Osoba). CRC Press, Boca Raton, 1991; 89–104.
5. Osoba, D. Rationale for the timing of health-related quality-of-life (HQL) assessments in oncological palliative therapy. *Cancer Treatment Reviews*, 1996; **22** (Suppl. A): 69–73.
6. Kornblith, A.B. and Holland, J.C. Model for quality-of-life research from Cancer and Leukemia Group B: the telephone interview, conceptual approach to measurement, and theoretical framework. *Monographs of the National Cancer Institute*, 1996; **20**: 55–62.
7. Stewart, A.L., Hays, R.D., and Ware, J.E. The MOS short form general health survey: reliability and validity in a patient population. *Medical Care*, 1988; **26**: 724–35.
8. Ware, J.E. and Sherbourne, C.D. The MOS 36-item short form health survey (SF-36): conceptual framework and item selection. *Medical Care*, 1992; **30**: 473–83.
9. Bergner, M., Bobbitt, R.A., Pollard, W.E., *et al*. The sickness impact profile: validation of a health status measure. *Medical Care*, 1976; **14**: 57–67.

10. Pollard, W.E., Bobbitt, R.A., Bergner, M., *et al*. The sickness impact profile: reliability of a health status measure. *Medical Care*, 1976; **14**: 146–55.

11. Coscarelli Schag, C.A., Ganz, P.A., and Heinrich, R.L. Cancer rehabilitation evaluation system – short form (CARES-SF). A cancer specific rehabilitation and quality-of-life instrument. *Cancer*, 1991; **68**: 1406–13.

12. Aaronson, N.K., Ahmedzai, S., Bullinger, M., *et al*. The EORTC core quality-of-life questionnaire: interim results of an international field study. In *Effects of Cancer on Quality of Life*, (ed. D. Osoba). CRC Press, Boca Raton, 1991: 185–203.

13. Aaronson, N.K., Ahmedzai, S., Bergman, B., *et al*. The European Organization for Research and Treatment of Cancer QLQ C-30: a quality-of-life instrument for use in international trials in oncology. *Journal of the National Cancer Institute*, 1993; **85**: 365–76.

14. Cella, D.F., Tulsky, D.S., Gray, G., *et al*. The functional assessment of cancer therapy scale: development and validation of the general measure. *Journal of Clinical Oncology*, 1993; **11**: 570–9.

15. Schipper, H., Clinch, J., McMurray, A., *et al*. Measuring the quality of life of cancer patients: the functional living index–cancer: development and validation. *Journal of Clinical Oncology*, 1984; **2**: 472–83.

16. Morrow, G.R., Lindke, J., and Black, P. Measurement of quality of life in patients: psychometric analysis of the functional living index–cancer (FLIC). *Quality of Life Research*, 1992; **1**: 287–96.

17. Selby, P.J., Chapman, J-A.W., Etazadi-Amoli, J., *et al*. The development of a method for assessing quality of life of cancer patients. *British Journal of Cancer*, 1984; **50**: 13–22.

18. Bliss, J.M., Selby, J.P., and Robertson, B. A method for assessing the quality of life of cancer patients: replication of the factor structure. *British Journal of Cancer*, 1992; **65**: 961–6.

19. Padilla, G.V., Presant, C., Grant, M.M., *et al*. Quality-of-life index for patients with cancer. *Research in Nursing and Health*, 1983; **6**: 117–26.

20. Spitzer, W.O., Dobson, A.J., Hall, J., *et al*. Measuring the quality of life of cancer patients: a concise QL-index for use by physicians. *Journal of Chronic Diseases*, 1981; **34**: 585–97.

21. Wood-Dauphinee, S. and Williams, J.I. The Spitzer quality-of-life index; its performance as a measure. In *Effect of cancer on quality of life*, (ed. D. Osoba). CRC Press, Boca Raton, 1991: 169–84.

22. de Haes, J.C.J.M. and Welvart, K. Quality of life after breast cancer surgery. *Journal of Surgical Oncology*, 1985; **28**: 123–5.

23. de Haes, J.C.J.M., Ratgever, J.W., van der Burg, M.E.L., *et al*. Evaluation of the quality of life of patients with advanced ovarian cancer treated with combination chemotherapy. In *The quality of life of cancer patients*, (ed. N.K. Aaronson and J. Beckmann). Raven Press, New York, 1987: 215–27.

24. Levine, M.N., Guyatt, G.H., Gent, M., *et al*. Quality of life in stage II breast cancer: an instrument for clinical trials. *Journal of Clinical Oncology*, 1988; **6**: 1798–1810.

25. Osoba, D., Dancey, J., Zee, B., *et al*. Health-related quality-of-life studies of the National Cancer Institute of Canada clinical trials group. *Monographs of the National Cancer Institute*, 1996; **20**: 107–11.

26. Osoba, D. Self-rating symptom checklists: a simple method for recording and evaluating symptom control in oncology. *Cancer Treatment Reviews*, 1993; **19**: 43–51.
27. Nunally, J.C. and Bernstein, I.H. *Psychometric theory*, 3rd edn. McGraw-Hill, New York, 1994.
28. Aaronson, N.K., Bullinger, M., and Ahmedzai, S. A modular approach to quality-of-life assessment in cancer clinical trials. In *Cancer clinical trials: a critical appraisal*, (ed. H. Scheurlen, R. Kay, and M. Baum), Recent Results in Cancer Research. Springer, Berlin, 1988; **111**: 231–49.
29. Osoba, D. Measuring the effect of cancer on health-related quality of life. *Pharmaco Economics*, 1995; **7**: 308–19.
30. Huisman, S.J., van Dam, F.S.A.M., Aaronson, N.K., *et al*. On measuring complaints of cancer patients: some remarks on the time span of the question. In *The quality of life of cancer patients*, (ed. N.K. Aaronson and J. Beckmann). Raven Press, New York, 1987; 101–9.
31. Deyo, R.A. and Patrick, D.L. Barriers to the use of health status measures in clinical investigation, patient care, and policy research. *Medical Care*, 1989; **27** (Suppl. 3), S254–68.
32. Sadura, A., Pater, J., Osoba, D., *et al*. Quality-of-life assessment: patient compliance with questionnaire completion. *Journal of the National Cancer Institute*, 1992; **84**: 1023–6.
33. Staquet, M., Berzon, R., Osoba, D., and Machin, D. Guidelines for reporting results of quality of life assessment in clinical trials. *Quality of Life Research*, 1996; **5**: 496–502.

3 Sample sizes for randomized trials measuring quality of life

David Machin and Peter M. Fayers

Introduction

In principle, there are no major differences in planning a clinical trial using quality of life (QoL) assessment as compared to that using, for example, a comparison of response rates between different treatments. Thus randomization remains as fundamentally important in this context as in others, as does the determination of an appropriate design and trial size.

An informed calculation of the sample size is an essential prerequisite for any trial, with guidelines from the Committee for Proprietary Medicinal Products (CPMP 1995) making it mandatory for all studies in the European Union; also, a number of medical journals, including those specializing in QoL, stipulate that a justification of the sample size estimate is required, in their statistical guidelines (British Medical Journal 1995; Staquet *et al.* 1996). It is unethical to over- or under-recruit patients. Over-recruitment is unethical as patients may be receiving a therapy that could be proved less effective with fewer patients; under-recruitment is unethical as clinically important effects may be hidden by there being insufficient numbers of patients. It is into this latter category that most trials with insufficient sample sizes fall, with authors, as Altman and Bland (1995) point out, perhaps incorrectly concluding that their 'lack of evidence' infers that there is 'evidence of absence' of any effect. However, it must be recognized that one is usually designing a study in the presence of considerable uncertainty surrounding the size of the anticipated effect – the greater this uncertainty the less precise will be our estimate of the appropriate study size.

The standard components of test size, α, and power, $1 - \beta$, need to be specified as does the anticipated benefit, that is, the size of the difference in QoL that may be expected between alternative treatments. However, in contrast to other end-points in clinical trials, such as survival time in patients with cancer, there is seldom sufficient prior experience to quantify such expectations with much precision. We return to this later. In addition, QoL is seldom summarized in terms of a single outcome variable; for example, the EORTC QLQ C-30 version 2.0 (Fayers *et al.* 1995) has 30 questions, some of which are combined to produce five functional, one global health status, and nine symptom scales (six of the latter are single items) – essentially 14 different outcomes. Not only are there these 14 different outcomes but they will typically be assessed on different occasions throughout the trial, thereby generating a longitudinal profile for each patient, typically starting immediately before randomization, occuring at relatively frequent intervals during active therapy, and perhaps extending less frequently thereafter until death.

As we have already indicated, unlike power and level of statistical significance, for which precedents dictate values, the anticipated effect size must be determined for each trial based on experience, published data, or pilot studies. However, it is first essential to identify and rank the QoL variables (scales or items) in order of importance for the specific trial under consideration. For example, the investigators may know, from previous observation of patients with the specific disease and receiving standard therapy for the condition, that patients experience considerable fatigue. If one objective of the new therapy is to alleviate symptoms, then fatigue would be regarded as the most important variable from those measuring aspects of QoL and would be used for sample size determination purposes.

Once the end-point variable has been established it is then necessary to identify how this is to be utilized to assess the outcome on a patient-by-patient basis. This may not be easy. As we have already indicated, this QoL variable is likely to be assessed several (perhaps many) times in each patient so that a summary is first required of each patient's profile. Thus Matthews *et al.* (1990) recommend that a series of observations, termed serial measurements, in our context QoL assessments, are themselves analyzed through a series of summary measures obtained from each patient. For example, this could be the change from the first QoL assessment to measurement at a key point – perhaps change from baseline assessment to that at the end of active therapy. Alternatively, the summary may be the time above a certain level; for example, the time for which the patient assesses QoL as being above the baseline assessment level – perhaps indicating the period of improvement following the start of therapy.

Once this summary is determined, then an average of this for both the control and test therapies needs to be determined. We assume that we are planning a randomized trial of two alternative therapies, a standard or control treatment (C) and a test treatment (T). Perhaps the control average can be obtained from previous experience of other or similar patients. It is then necessary to anticipate the benefit in the aspect of QoL just summarized, which may be expected by use of the test therapy in place of the standard. This too may be obtained from previous experience or perhaps may have to be elicited in some way using clinical opinion, as has been utilized by Parmar *et al.* (1995).

This benefit or effect size has been variously defined as the 'minimum value worth detecting' or a 'clinically important effect' or 'quantitatively significant' (Burnard *et al.* 1990, Juniper *et al.* 1994).

In patients with cancer, there is now a considerable body of data which enables one, for example, to describe the survival rates of particular groups receiving the current or standard therapy and sufficient experience of the size of survival advantages that may be plausible with a new therapy under test. Thus, if survival time is the main outcome measure, the anticipated effect size can usually be expressed in terms of the hazard ratio, and detailed tables such as those of

Machin *et al.* (1997) are available for determining sample size. However, in palliative trials involving patients with cancer, survival differences between alternative therapies may often be known to be small (Medical Research Council Lung Cancer Working Party 1993) and, in this context, therefore considered less important than QoL differences. In these situations aspects of QoL may be used as the main outcome measures. We will assume, for our purposes, that QoL is the main outcome measure but there is unlikely to be either the experience or agreement of what would constitute a meaningful benefit to the patient (Hopwood *et al.* 1994). This will often be the case as there is relatively limited experience of QoL assessment reporting the type of summary measures we advocate here.

Example

One method of assessing the psychological aspects of QoL which has been used widely in studies of cancer patients is the hospital anxiety and depression scale (HADS) (Zigmond and Snaith 1983). The HADS is a patient self-assessment questionnaire designed for use with physically ill patients, using a time frame of the past week. It comprises 14 items; each item is a four-point categorical scale. For example, the question 'I still enjoy the things I used to enjoy' has responses 'Definitely as much', 'Not quite so much', 'Only a little', and 'Hardly at all', which score 0, 1, 2, and 3 respectively. HADS divides into two seven-item subscales for scoring and analysis, covering the two domains of anxiety and depression. Each domain score is composed of the sum of responses to seven questions; a low score is indicative of absence of anxiety and/or depression. Hence, in a single questionnaire there is a finite number of discrete values that can be obtained. These scores are then summed to provide summary scores for the two domains, anxiety and depression.

A practical advantage of the HADS instrument is that an estimate of clinically important levels of distress can be made using recommended cut-off scores for each subscale. Thus a score of 11 or more is regarded as a potential clinical case, perhaps signalling more detailed clinical examination and possibly treatment; a score between 8 and 10 is regarded as borderline, and one of ≤ 7 regarded as normal. As a consequence, the major purpose of a randomized trial may be to ignore the actual score and only compare the proportions in these three categories in the different treatment groups.

For expository purposes, we assume that the HADS domain for depression is the most important of the two domains and that the summary measure of most relevance is the HADS assessment two months post-randomization. Thus the end-point of interest is one of the simplest possible.

In the formulae given below, we give the total number of subjects required for such a trial with equal numbers (randomized) per treatment group for a two-sided significance level α and power $1-\beta$. In these formulae, $z_{1-\alpha/2}$ and $z_{1-\beta}$ are the appropriate values from the standard Normal distribution for the $100(1-\alpha/2)$ and $100(1-\beta)$ percentiles, respectively. The calculations use a two-sided significance level of 5 per cent and a power of 80 per cent, thus $z_{1-\alpha/2}=1.96$ and $z_{1-\beta}=0.8416$.

Table 3.1 Frequency of responses on the HADS for depression for patients with small cell lung cancer two months post-randomization (data from MRC Lung Cancer Working Party 1996)

Category	Score	Number of patients with depression
Normal	0	4
	1	16
	2	12
	3	13
	4	12
	5	10
	6	19
	7	13
Borderline	8	11
	9	9
	10	4
Case	11	5
	12	11
	13	4
	14	2
	15	3
	16	4
	17	0
	18	0
	19	1
	20	0
	21	1
Total		154
Normal	0–7	99 (64.3%)
Boderline	8–10	24 (15.6%)
Case	11–21	31 (20.1%)
Mean		6.54
SD		4.39
Median		6

Julious *et al.* (1997) provide a detailed summary of such HADS anxiety and depression data generated from 154 patients with small cell lung cancer in a randomized trial conducted by the Medical Research Council Lung Cancer Working Party (1996). The data for the summed depression scores are given in Table 3.1. There are several possible approaches to calculating the sample size required for data such as those of Table 3.1. One is to assume the data have (at least approximately) a Normal distribution. The second is to categorize the data into binary form, for example, 'case' or 'not case'. A third is to categorize into more than two categories, for example, 'case', 'borderline', or 'normal' or to consider the full form of the data as an ordered categorical variable with, in our example, $\kappa = 22$ levels. Nevertheless, each approach requires specification of an anticipated effect size.

Sample size formulae

Comparing two means

In a two-group comparative study where the outcome measure has a Normal distribution form, a two sample *t*-test would be used in the final analysis

(Campbell and Machin 1993). In this case the (standardized) anticipated effect size is $\delta_{\text{Normal}} = (\mu_T - \mu_C)/\sigma$, where μ_T and μ_C are the anticipated means of the two treatments and σ the standard deviation (SD) of the QoL measurements and which is assumed the same for both treatment groups. On this basis, the number of patients to be recruited to the clinical trial is

$$N_{\text{Normal}} = \frac{4(z_{1-\alpha/2} + z_{1-\beta})^2}{\delta_{\text{Normal}}^2} + \frac{z_{1-\alpha/2}^2}{2}. \qquad (3.1)$$

The mean HADS depression score is 6.54 with SD 4.39 indicating, as does Table 3.1, a rather skewed distribution far from the Normal form, so that it may not be advisable to use this formula.

However, if the data are transformed using a logarithmic transformation then the transformed variable may have a distribution which approximates better to the Normal form. To avoid the difficulty of a zero HADS, each item on the scale can be coded 1 to 4 rather than of 0 to 3 – with corresponding changes in boundaries, so that $y = \log_e(x+7)$, where x is the HADS depression score on the original scale. In this case, the data of Table 3.1 lead to, $\bar{y} = 2.5546$ and $SD(y) = 0.3203$. The SD is now much smaller than the mean, suggesting the distribution has a more Normal form on this transformed scale, and eqn 3.1 could be utilized once the effect size, δ_{Normal} is specified. Unfortunately there is no simple interpretation of the inverse transformation back to the x scale, that is, $\exp(\bar{y}) - 7 = 5.8666$.

Since the object of therapy is to reduce problems of depression in the patients, that is, to increase the proportion classified as 'normal', then this corresponds to a desired reduction in HADS. We may postulate that the minimum clinically important difference to detect is a decrease in this equivalent to one unit on the HADS, that is, from 5.8666 to 4.8666. This is then expressed as an anticipated effect on the y scale as

$$\delta_{\text{Normal}} = (\mu_T - \mu_C)/\sigma = [\log_e(4.8666 + 7) - \log_e(5.8666 + 7)]/0.3203$$

$$= (2.4737 - 2.5546)/0.3203 = -0.25.$$

This would be regarded as a small effect, following the suggestions of Cohen (1988). Using eqn 3.1 with $\delta_{\text{Normal}} = -0.25$ gives $N_{\text{Normal}} = 504$ patients, or approximately 250 patients in each group.

The sample size obtained depends only on the absolute value of the anticipated difference between treatments and is independent of the direction of this difference. Thus the same sample size would be obtained if $\delta_{\text{Normal}} = +0.25$ corresponding to, for example, a new more toxic therapy being investigated in which an increase in HADS (corresponding to an increase in depression) was likely.

Comparing two proportions

The statistical test used to compare two groups when the outcome is a binary variable is the Pearson χ^2 test for a 2×2 contingency table (see Campbell and

Machin 1993). In this situation the anticipated effect size is $\delta_{\text{Binary}} = (\pi_T - \pi_C)$, where π_T and π_C are the proportions of 'normals' (however defined) with respect to depression in the two treatment groups. On this basis, the number of patients to be recruited to the clinical trial is

$$N_{\text{Binary}} = \frac{2(z_{1-\alpha/2} + z_{1-\beta})^2 [\pi_T(1-\pi_T) + \pi_C(1-\pi_C)]}{\delta^2_{\text{Binary}}}. \tag{3.2}$$

Alternatively, the same difference between treatments may be expressed through the odds ratio (OR) which is defined as

$$OR_{\text{Binary}} = \frac{\pi_T(1-\pi_C)}{\pi_C(1-\pi_T)}. \tag{3.3}$$

This formulation leads to an alternative to eqn 3.2 for the sample size. Thus

$$N_{\text{OR}} = \frac{4(z_{1-\alpha/2} + z_{1-\beta})^2/(\log OR_{\text{Binary}})^2}{\bar{\pi}(1-\bar{\pi})}, \tag{3.4}$$

where $\bar{\pi} = (\pi_C + \pi_T)/2$. Equations 3.2 and 3.4 are quite dissimilar in form but Julious and Campbell (1996) show that they give, for all practical purposes, very similar sample sizes, with divergent results only occurring for relatively large (or small) OR_{Binary}. Table 3.1 indicates that there are approximately 65 per cent of patients classified as 'normal' with respect to depression for treatment C. Suppose it is anticipated that this may improve to 75 per cent in the 'normal' category with treatment T. The anticipated treatment effect is thus $\delta_{\text{Binary}} = (\pi_T - \pi_C) = (75 - 65)$ per cent $= 10$ per cent. This equates to a total sample size of $N_{\text{Binary}} = 652$ from eqn 3.2.

Alternatively, this anticipated treatment effect can be expressed as $OR_{\text{Binary}} = (75/25)/(65/35) = 1.6154$. Using this in eqn 3.4 with $\bar{\pi} = (0.75 + 0.65)/2 = 0.7$ gives a total sample size of $N_{\text{OR}} = 650$ patients. As we have indicated previously, there is usually only a small and inconsequential difference between the calculations from the alternative formulae.

Ordered categorical data

The approach utilized above when dealing with a variable which does not have the Normal distribution form leads to difficulties in interpretation on the transformed scale and, in particular, the provision of an anticipated effect size. It would be easier if the original scale could be preserved for this purpose. In fact the data of Table 3.1 are from an ordered categorical variable and the statistical test used when the outcome is ordered categorical is the Mann–Whitney U test with allowance for ties (see Conover 1980). Thus it would be more natural to extend from the comparison of two proportions, which is a special case of an ordered categorical variable of $\kappa = 2$ levels, to $\kappa = 22$ levels for the HADS data. Formulating the effect size in terms of OR_{Binary} rather than δ_{Binary} enables this extension to be made.

The estimated sample size is given by Whitehead (1993) as

$$N_{\text{Categorical}} = \frac{12 \, (z_{1-\alpha/2} + z_{1-\beta})^2 / (\log_e \text{OR}_{\text{Categorical}})^2}{(1 - \sum_{i=0}^{\kappa-1} \bar{\pi}_i^3)}, \tag{3.5}$$

where the mean proportion expected in category i ($i = 0$ to $\kappa - 1$) is $\bar{\pi}_i = (\pi_{Ci} + \pi_{Ti})/2$, and π_{Ci} and π_{Ti} are the proportions expected in category i for the two treatment groups C and T respectively.

The categories are labelled as 0 to $\kappa - 1$, rather than 1 to κ, so that they correspond directly to the actual HADS category scores of Table 3.1. Here the $\text{OR}_{\text{Categorical}}$ is an extension of the definition of $\text{OR}_{\text{Binary}}$ given in eqn 3.3 and is now the odds of a subject being in category i or below in one treatment group compared to the other. It is calculated from the cumulative proportion of subjects for each category 0, 1, 2, ..., $(\kappa - 1)$ and is assumed to be constant through the scale.

The effect size in eqn 3.5, as summarized through $\text{OR}_{\text{Categorical}}$, implies an assumption of proportional odds which is, that for each pair of adjacent categories for which an OR can be calculated, that is, for the HADS resulting in OR_1, OR_2, ..., OR_{21}, all have the same true or underlying value $\text{OR}_{\text{Categorical}}$. Thus the odds of falling into a given category or below is the same irrespective of where the HADS scale is dichotomized. This appears to be a very restrictive assumption but, for planning purposes, what is of practical importance is that, although the ORs may vary along the scale, the underlying treatment effect is in the same direction throughout the scale. Thus all ORs are anticipated to be greater than 1 or all ORs are anticipated to be less than 1.

When using an ordered categorical scale the ORs are a measure of the chance of a subject being in each given category or less in one group compared to the other. For the HADS data there are 21 distinct ORs. However, the problem is simplified because the OR anticipated for the binary case, that is the proportions either side of the 'caseness' cut off, can be used in the ordered categorical situation (Campbell *et al.* 1995). Thus, if the trial size is to be determined with a Mann–Whitney U test in mind rather than the χ^2 test for a 2×2 table, then the anticipated treatment effect is still taken to be $\text{OR}_{\text{Binary}}$.

Julious *et al.* (1997) illustrate the evaluation of eqn 3.5. They first calculate Q_{Ci}, the cumulative proportions in category i for control treatment C, then the anticipated cumulative proportions for each category of test treatment T are given by $Q_{Ti} = \text{OR}_{\text{Categorical}} \, Q_{Ci} / [\text{OR}_{\text{Categorical}} Q_{Ci} + (1 - Q_{Ci})]$.

Similarly, the cumulative proportions can be calculated for the remaining categories and from these the anticipated proportions, $\bar{\pi}_{Ti}$, falling in each category can be determined. Finally, the combined mean of the corresponding proportions of treatments C and T for each category can be calculated.

We have assumed here that the alternative to the binary case ($\kappa = 2$) is the full categorical scale ($\kappa = 22$). In practice, however, it may be more appropriate to group some of the categories but not others to give κ categories, where $3 \le \kappa < 22$. For example, merging the HADS scores into the 'caseness' groups defined earlier would give $\kappa = 3$, while $\kappa = 5$ if the 'caseness' categories are extended in the manner described below. We will use these examples to illustrate the calculations.

Although there are 22 possible categories for the full HADS scales, it is reasonable to ask if the full distribution needs to be specified for planning purposes as, in many situations, it may not be possible to specify the whole distribution precisely whereas to anticipate the proportions in a somewhat fewer number of categories may be plausible. As indicated previously the HADS scale is often divided into three categories for clinical use: 'normal' (≤ 7), 'borderline' (8–10), and 'clinical case' (≥ 11). For illustration purposes only, we define two additional categories: 'very normal' (≤ 3) and 'severe case' (≥ 16). Thus HADS scores 0–3 are 'very normal', 4–7 'normal', 8–10 'borderline', 11–15 'case', and finally 16–22 'severe case'.

Table 3.2 gives, for the data of Table 3.1, the number of cases and cumulative proportions anticipated in each category for the depression dimension if we re-categorized the HADS depression scale into five categories (scores ≤ 3, 4–7, 8–10, 11–15, ≥ 16). If we assume $OR_{Categorical} = OR_{Binary} = 1.6154$, then, for example, the anticipated proportion for category two of test treatment T is

$$Q_{T2} = OR_{Categorical}Q_{C2}/[OR_{Categorical}Q_{C2} + (1 - Q_{C2})]$$

$$= 1.6154 \times 0.6429/[(1.6154 \times 0.6429) + 1 - 0.6429] = 0.8651$$

and the remaining values are summarized in Table 3.2. The final column of the table gives the corresponding values of $\bar{\pi}_i$. The denominator of eqn 3.5 is therefore $1 - [0.3462^3 + 0.3474^3 + 0.1384^3 + 0.1364^3 + 0.0318^3] = 1 - 0.0886 = 0.9114$ and finally $N_{Categorical} = 216$.

If we were to repeat the calculations but with the three categories for HADS (normal, borderline, case) the corresponding sample size is $N_{Categorical} = 298$. Finally, if the number of categories was reduced to 'normal' versus the remainder ('borderline' and 'cases') then $N_{Categorical} = 408$. This suggests that the more we can

Table 3.2 Number of patients with small cell lung cancer 2 months post randomisation categorised into 'caseness' groups following assessment using HADS for depression. Cumulative proportions observed on standard therapy C and anticipated with test therapy T (data from MRC Lung Cancer Working Party, 1996)

Category	Score	Number of C patients with 'depression'	Cumulative proportion Q_C	Cumulative proportion Q_T	$\bar{\pi}_i$
Very Normal	0–3	45	0.2922	0.4001	0.3462
Normal	4–7	54	0.6429	0.7441	0.3474
Borderline	8–10	24	0.7987	0.8651	0.1384
Case	11–15	25	0.9610	0.9755	0.1364
Severe case	16–22	6	1	1	0.0318
	Total	154			

assume about the form of the data and with the appropriate analysis then the smaller the study size can be.

Survival type data

Suppose the end-point of interest was the time from randomization until a patient achieves a particular value of their QoL. For example, suppose *all* patients had a score of 11 or more immediately before commencement of treatment, then one objective of treatment may be to improve QoL, as assessed by a HADS of 7 or less. In this artificial scenario, artificial since we know that only a proportion of these patients not depression prior to the start of treatment, we use the data of Table 3.1 for illustration and this indicates that with control therapy C, approximately 65 per cent are classified as 'normal' by two months. Our trial design anticipates that this will be improved to 75 per cent at two months using treatment T. However, in the actual study we will be determining the precise time at which the patient is classified as 'normal' so that the eventual analysis will involve Kaplan–Meier estimates of the corresponding cumulative survival curves, where 'survival' here is the time taken to become classified as 'normal', and comparisons will be made using the log rank test (Parmar and Machin 1995). In this situation the estimated size of the anticipated effect is determined by the hazard ratio (Δ), the anticipated value of which can be obtained from

$$\Delta = \frac{\log_e \pi_T}{\log_e \pi_C}. \tag{3.6}$$

The number of patients required to be recruited to the clinical trial is

$$N_{\text{Survival}} = \frac{2[(z_{1-\alpha/2} + z_{1-\beta})(1+\Delta)/(1-\Delta)]^2}{(2 - \pi_T - \pi_C)}. \tag{3.7}$$

For the current example, $\pi_C = 0.65$, $\pi_T = 0.75$, so that $\Delta = \log_e 0.75/\log_e 0.65 = 0.66$. Substituting these values in eqn 3.7 gives $N_{\text{Survival}} = 624$.

Choice of sample size method

It is important when designing any study to obtain a relevant sample size. In so doing it is important to make maximal use of the information available. Such information may come from that obtained in other related studies and may be quite detailed and precise or it may come from a reasonable extrapolation from other observations from unrelated studies, in which case it may be regarded as very imprecise. It is clear that the more we know, or more realistically assume, of the final outcome of our trial at the planning stage the better we can design the trial. In our example, we have detailed knowledge of HADS outcome at two months which is based on data from more than 150 patients. We may be fairly confident therefore, that provided the treatment C in a planned new trial remains unaltered and the patient mix remains the same, we can use this distribution for planning purposes. If the trial is to test the new therapy T, then possibly, apart from some very preliminary data, we may have little information on the effect of the treatment on QoL. In this case, we suggest that the investigator has to decide whether he or she wishes to detect (say) a 1, 2, or 3 point change in the average HADS score. This change then has to be expressed as an anticipated effect size before the sample size equations given here can be utilized. The smaller the anticipated benefit the larger the subsequent trial. If an investigator is uncomfortable about the assumptions then it is good practice to calculate sample size under a variety of scenarios so that the sensitivity to assumptions can be assessed.

It is important to emphasize that the sample sizes obtained by the different approaches described in this chapter may lead to markedly different estimates for what appears to be the same situation. It is crucial to remember that there is a different set of assumptions with each approach and these are best recognized through the analysis that is proposed at the end of the study – here the t-test, 2×2 χ^2, Mann–Whitney U, and log rank tests respectively. As we have indicated, careful consideration should be made when choosing the end-point – this should always be the most appropriate. For example, choice of the proportion 'normal' as the end-point would not be appropriate if one also wished to distinguish between the proportions 'borderline' and 'case'.

In general, when designing a clinical trial there will often be other variables (covariates), apart from allocated treatment itself, such as gender, age, stage of disease, or centre which may or may not affect the clinical outcome. Such variables may be utilized to create different strata for treatment allocation purposes and will also be used in the final analysis. If the QoL variable itself can be assumed to have a Normal distribution then the final analysis may adjust for these variables using a multiple (least squares) regression approach. If a binary type of measure of QoL has been utilized then the covariates can be assessed by means of logistic regression models (Collett 1991). Similarly, if a 'survival' time type of measure of QoL has been utilized then the covariates can be assessed by means of a Cox proportional hazards model, as described by Parmar and Machin (1995).

For illustrative reasons, we have used a transformation approach for non-Normal data by use of the logarithmic transformation and made the sample size calculations for that scale. Other common transformations for this purpose are the reciprocal or square root. However, use of transformations distorts the scales and makes interpretation of treatment effects difficult. In fact, only the logarithmic transformation (with, in order to remove zeros, each item on the HADS coded 1 to 4 instead of 0 to 3 – with corresponding changes in boundaries) gives results interpretable on the original scale (Keen 1995; Bland and Altman 1996). The logarithmic transformation expresses the effect as a ratio of geometric means but this ratio will vary in a way which depends on the geometric mean value of treatment C. For example, if the geometric mean for treatment C is 6, while treatment T induces a change in HADS of -1, this implies $\log_e(5/6) = -0.18$, whereas for a geometric mean of 14 for treatment C, a change of $+1$ implies

$\log_e(13/14) = -0.07$. The latter results in an effect size which is less than half ($-0.07/-0.18 = 0.39$) the former.

In any event, the rationale for the use of transformations was often to facilitate the use of least squares regression techniques to allow for covariates in the final analysis. However, this is no longer essential as, for example, the procedure PROC LOGISTIC in SAS (1991) now enables full regression modelling of ordered categorical data.

Another approach to avoiding the problem of a non-Normal distribution for a QoL variable was to dichotomize at a convenient point and design the study as though the objective was to compare two proportions. As we have just indicated, this is no longer necessary as new forms of analysis are now available and, as Julious et al. (1997) have pointed out, this may result in too many patients being recruited.

As we have indicated, it is not uncommon that when designing a trial where a QoL measure is the primary measure of interest, there is little prior knowledge of the full distribution of the scores. Thus, the very detailed information provided by Table 3.1 may not be available. However, this need not necessarily present a major problem for the full ordered categorical approach to sample size calculation to be utilized as Whitehead (1993) indicates that knowledge of the anticipated distribution within four or five broad categories is often sufficient. This information, which may be solicited from experience gained by the clinical team, can then be used to aid in the design of studies using HADS and other QoL instruments, perhaps adopting a Bayesian methodology combined with an internal pilot study, as has been suggested by Birkett and Day (1994), to attain the best estimate of the required sample size.

In general, statistics such as means and SDs are not suitable summary measures for non-Normal distributions, and neither are standardized differences a suitable basis for calculation of sample sizes. When giving normative data for QoL scores the frequency distributions should always be given and, in general, ordered categorical methods should be used for sample size calculations.

Although illustrated using HADS, the methods described in this chapter should enable investigators to plan a wide range of QoL studies more effectively and hence justify the sample size requirements for the ensuing protocol. Julious et al. (1995) describe sample sizes for studies with SF-36. Further work is needed to discover what changes in scores represent clinically important differences for health technology interventions.

Multiple end-points

Earlier in this chapter we indicated that it is very important to decide on a principal QoL end-point and suggested that it is of value, if there are additional end-points, to rank these in order of importance. We recognize that in most situations there may be a very long list of QoL variables but would urge that those that are to be included in a formal analysis should be confined to, at most, four or five. The remainder should be consigned to exploratory analyses or descriptive purposes only. However, if analysis of the four or five end-point variables are to be made, then some recognition of the multiple statistical testing that will occur should be taken into account in the planning process.

In practice, it is very unlikey that the anticipated effect sizes, we assume there are $k = 4$ (in rank order of importance) denoted $\Omega_{(1)}$, $\Omega_{(2)}$, $\Omega_{(3)}$, and $\Omega_{(4)}$, will be the same magnitude. Consequently, if these are used separately in four sample size calculations then four different estimates are likely to result. The final study size is likely to be a compromise between the sizes so obtained. Whatever the final size, it should be large enough to satisfy the requirements for the end-point corresponding to $\Omega_{(1)}$, as this is the primary end-point and hence the primary objective of the trial.

To guard against false statistical significance as a consequence of multiple testing it is a sensible precaution to examine the consequences of replacing the test size α in the various equations by a test size adjusted using the Bonferroni correction. The Bonferroni correction is

$$\alpha_{\text{Bonferroni}} = \alpha / k. \tag{3.8}$$

Thus α is replaced by $\alpha_{\text{Bonferroni}}$ in the sample size equations given above. So for $k = 4$, $\alpha = 0.05$ then $\alpha_{\text{Bonferroni}} = 0.05/4 = 0.0125$. Such a change will clearly lead to larger sample sizes.

Conclusion

In some of the sample size calculations described above we have used rather spurious numerical accuracy in some of the parameters utilized. This was to enable the reader to carry through the calculations. However, in practice, anticipated effect sizes are usually, by their very nature, rather imprecise as the objective of the trial itself is to determine the size of benefit, and so such precision is not justified.

When designing any study there is usually a whole range of possible options to discuss at the early design stage. We would therefore recommend that a range of anticipated benefits are considered, ranging from the optimistic to the more realistic and sample sizes calculated for several scenarios within the range. It is a matter of judgement, rather than an exact science, as to which of the options is chosen for the final study size.

The particular problems posed by QoL studies relate to the choice of the anticipated benefit in a diverse and growing field of enquiry in which there is relatively little understanding of what can be agreed to be a (modest) benefit yet one worth demonstrating. For example, would a therapeutic intervention designed to alleviate depression scores as measured by HADS of one unit be clinically worthwhile, if the sole purpose of the treatment was to relieve depression? This might be contrasted with a trial of a therapy designed to 'attack' the underlying disease but, at the same time, happens also to alleviate depression, in which case the reduction of one unit in HADS is a fortunate consequence.

It is also important, as we have stressed, that in QoL studies, where there are so many potential end-points, a clear focus is directed to identifying the major (at most five) ones. This is clearly important for sample size purposes but it is also necessary to state these clearly in the associated study protocol and to ensure that these are indeed the main focus of the subsequent report of the completed study.

Finally we would recommend, in the situation in which an ordered categorical variable such as HADS is the outcome measure for the QoL assessment, that the appropriate formula, eqn 3.5, is utilized directly, rather than seek a transformation of the scale to enable the formula for a Normal variable, (eqn 3.1) to be utilized. The major reason is that this will retain the 'benefit' on the original QoL scale and therefore will be more readily understood. Although the associated methods of analysis are less familiar the statistical software is now available for this purpose. It should be noted that if 'survival' type end-points are to be determined with any precision then careful choice of when the QoL assessments are to be made is essential. This is to ensure that a reasonably precise date can be given for the timing, in each patient, of the event determining the end-point. Such techniques are unlikely to be useful if the assessment intervals are lengthy.

Acknowledgement

We are grateful to the MRC Lung Cancer Working Party for the use of their data.

References

Altman, D.G. and Bland, J.M. (1995). Absence of evidence is not evidence of absence. *British Medical Journal*, **311**, 485.

Birkett, M.A. and Day, S.J. (1994). Internal pilot studies for estimating sample size. *Statistics in Medicine*, **13**, 2455–63.

Bland, J.M. and Altman, D.G. (1996). Logarithms. *British Medical Journal*, **312**, 700.

British Medical Journal (1995). Instructions to authors. *British Medical Journal*, **310**, 50–3.

Burnard, B., Kernan, W.N., and Feinstein, A.R. (1990). Indexes and boundaries for 'quantitative significance' in statistical decisions. *Journal of Clinical Epidemiology*, **43**, 1273–84.

Campbell, M.J. and Machin, D. (1993). *Medical statistics: a common sense approach*, (2nd edn). Wiley, Chichester.

Campbell, M.J., Julious, S., and Altman, D.G. (1995). Sample sizes for binary, ordered categorical and continuous outcomes in two group comparisons. *British Medical Journal*, **311**, 1145–8.

Cohen, J. (1988). *Statistical power analysis for the behavioral sciences*, (2nd edn). Lawrence Earlbaum, New Jersey.

Collett, D. (1991). *Modelling binary data*. Chapman & Hall, London.

Conover, W.J. (1980). *Practical nonparametric statistics*, (2nd edn). Wiley, New York.

CPMP Working Party on Efficacy of Medicinal Products (1995). Biostatistical methodology in clinical trials in applications for marketing authorizations for medicinal products. *Statistics in Medicine*, **14**, 1659–82.

Fayers, P., Aaronson, N., Bjordal, K., and Sullivan, M. (1995). *EORTC QLQ-C30: Scoring manual*. EORTC Study Group on Quality of Life, Brussels.

Hopwood, P., Stephens, R.J., and Machin, D. (1994). Approaches to the analysis of quality of life data: experiences gained from a Medical Research Council Lung Cancer Working Party palliative chemotherapy trial. *Quality of Life Research*, **3**, 339–51.

Julious, S.A. and Campbell, M.J. (1996). Sample size calculations for ordered categorical data. *Statistics in Medicine*, **15**, 1065–6.

Julious, S.A., George, S., and Campbell, M.J. (1995). Sample sizes for studies with SF-36. *Journal of Epidemiology and Community Health*, **49**, 642–4.

Julious, S.A., George, S., Stephens, R.J., and Machin, D. (1997). Sample sizes for randomised trials measuring quality of life in cancer patients. *Quality of Life Research*, **6**, 109–17.

Juniper, E.J., Guyatt, G.H., Willan, A., and Griffith, L.E. (1994). Determining a minimal important change in a disease specific quality of life questionnaire. *Journal of Clinical Epidemiology*, **47**, 81–7.

Keen, O.N. (1995). The log transformation is special. *Statistics in Medicine*, **14**, 811–19.

Machin, D., Campbell, M.J., Fayers, P.M., and Pinol, A.P.Y. (1997). *Sample size tables for clinical studies*. Blackwell Scientific, Oxford.

Matthews, J.N.S., Altman, D.G., Campbell, M.J., and Royston, J.P. (1990). Analysis of serial measurements in medical research. *British Medical Journal*, **300**, 230–5.

Medical Research Council Lung Cancer Working Party (1993). A randomised trial of three or six courses of etoposide cyclophosphamide methotrexate and vincristine or six courses of etoposide and ifosfamide in small cell lung cancer (SCLC) II: quality of life. *British Journal of Cancer*, **68**, 1157–66.

Medical Research Council Lung Cancer Working Party (1996). Randomised trial of four-drug vs less intensive two-drug chemotherapy in the palliative treatment of patients with small cell lung cancer (SCLC) and poor prognosis. *British Journal of Cancer*, **73**, 406–13.

Parmar, M.K.B. and Machin, D. (1995). *Survival analysis: a practical approach*. Wiley, Chichester.

Parmar, M.K.B., Spiegelhalter, D.J., Freedman, L.S., and the CHART Steering Committee (1995). The CHART trials: Bayesian design and monitoring in practice. *Statistics in Medicine*, **13**, 1297–312.

SAS(1991). SAS Institute Inc., Cary, NC, USA.

Staquet, M.J., Berzon, R., Osoba, D., and Machin, D. (1996). Guidelines for reporting results of quality of life assessments in clinical trials. *Quality of Life Research*, **5**, 496–502.

Whitehead, J. (1993). Sample size calculations for ordered categorical data. *Statistics in Medicine*, **12**, 2257–72.

Zigmond, A.S. and Snaith, R.P. (1983). The hospital anxiety and depression scale. *Acta Psychologica Scandinavica*, **67**, 361–70.

4 Cross-cultural issues in the use of quality of life measures in randomized controlled trials

Sonja M. Hunt

Introduction

The minimum requirements for a randomized controlled clinical trial, that is, randomization of subjects, standardization of procedures, and precision of measurement, are difficult to fulfil satisfactorily even when only a single centre is involved and when end-points are confined to the purely clinical. When a trial is expanded to encompass two or more centres, the achievement of the minimum requirements becomes more difficult the greater the number of countries and cultures involved. If the outcome measures also include quality of life, then meeting these requirements poses challenging and, in some instances, insurmountable barriers.

A complicating factor is that, although clinicians and other medical staff are, normally, familiar with the history, applicability, validity, and reliability of the clinical parameters to be used, they are much less likely to be cognisant of the technical and conceptual issues raised by the use of questionnaires. Typically, for example, the team running a trial will decide to use a particular questionnaire. This decision may be based on advice from others, availability, reputation, or, even, fashion, rather than serious consideration of the suitability of the questionnaire to the particular circumstances of the trial, such as patient characteristics, probable effects of the intervention, and ease of administration and response. Little thought may be given to the characteristics, development, and prior use of the questionnaire and its applicability in other cultures.

The inclusion of 'quality of life' measures in clinical trials escalated threefold during the four years from 1990 to 1994.[1] Today it seems almost mandatory to include some assessment outside the purely clinical. This escalation appears to have been fuelled mainly by commercial and political considerations. There are many similar pharmaceutical products aimed at the same disease which have similar clinical effects. A claim to improve 'quality of life', or at least not to adversely affect it, has advertising potential. In addition, health service providers have become increasingly concerned that therapies should bring some perceived benefit to patients and 'quality of life' outcomes may be used to justify priority setting. Currently, quality of life is a fashionable, if barely understood, term and many trials include questionnaires which purport to measure it, whether such measurement is justified by the intervention or not. As a *Lancet* editorial commented, the inclusion of quality of life measures in trial protocols may be based upon false premises,[1] the most obvious of which is that quality of life is of the same order as clinical end-points.

So-called quality of life measures almost always consist of self-completed questionnaires, simply because there has been a general agreement among researchers that patients are the best judges of this aspect of their condition. Accordingly, it is this means of measurement which will be addressed in this chapter. However, it is important to note that when a patient is given a questionnaire to complete, this does not guarantee that the responses necessarily reflect the concerns of the patient, since she or he may merely be responding politely to an agenda which has been set by health scientists, economists, or clinicians, who, in addition, may come from another culture. Matters of import-ance to the patient may not be represented at all.

The inclusion of patient-completed questionnaires in clinical trials that are conducted in more than one country, culture, or language raises two principal issues. First, whether or not quality of life can be defined and measured precisely enough to have scientific credibility in each country and, second, whether versions of the same measure in different languages can be regarded as equivalent for the purposes of the aggregation of data. In the case of clinical values, for example, blood pressure levels, white cell count, and so on, it is taken for granted that the measuring instruments in each country are equivalent. In relation to quality of life questionnaires this assumption cannot be made.

Some controversies in quality of life measurement

The problems which attend cross-cultural measurement, that is, those of definition and equivalence, are intertwined. The field of quality of life measurement is by no means as advanced as its popularity would suggest and the demand for questionnaires has far outrun philosophical enquiry and technical developments. This has led to the use of measures the connection of which to quality of life is equivocal at the very least. For example, all the following variables have been referred to as quality of life in recent clinical trials: psychiatric morbidity, number and severity of symptoms, cognitive ability, social contact, ability to work, physical capacity, and diarrhoeal frequency.[2-6]

One reason for this lack of precision is that until very recently there were no questionnaires in existence which were specifically designed to measure quality of life as such. Instead, the term 'health-related quality of life' appeared in the literature. This facilitated the use of existing measures of health status under a new name. The consequence was to reinforce the notion that quality of life is primarily about health and illness; a notion which has received considerable criticism from philosophers, sociologists, and health researchers.[7-9] In addition, the individual became isolated from the social and cultural context that can affect quality of life more than medical intervention.[10] These trends fed an assumption that 'quality of life' is a state of being which has the same sort of universality as physiology, that is, that it transcends culture.[11]

It is often taken for granted that quality of life is synonymous with human functioning, for instance, optimal physical ability, the satisfactory fulfilment of social roles, and the exhibition of 'normal' psychological states. However, the content of questionnaires is not only reflective of professional notions of 'normality', it may also be culturally biased in its implied conceptualization. Human beings are reflective, self-conscious agents who interpret the world and events in a manner which is partly a consequence of social and cultural background and partly idiosyncratic. It is not the presence of symptoms or limitations of function which affect quality of life so much as the meaning and significance of them for individual patients. Thus, it has been argued that patients with an identical health status may experience a range of existential states from despair to happiness.[12] Moreover, the relative weight given to different abilities and states of being differs from culture to culture. Socialization into a particular culture largely determines which features of existence are regarded as part of the human condition and which may be regarded as indicative of illness. Sorrow, anxiety, angst, melancholy may all, for example, be regarded as perfectly reasonable responses to unwelcome events and not necessarily evidence of the need for treatment or counselling or a life deficient in quality.

The cross-cultural applicability of questionnaires

The majority of questionnaires currently in use in clinical trials were developed mainly in English-speaking countries, primarily the USA and, to a lesser extent, the UK. The process of developing these questionnaires determined the kinds of people who contributed to the content, the samples used for field testing, and the ways in which validity and reliability were established. Any and all of these elements may limit the usefulness of the questionnaire for cross-cultural work.

When considering cross-cultural adaptation it is important to make a distinction between adapting a questionnaire for use in more than one language and culture, where there is no intent to compare outcomes cross-culturally, and taking a questionnaire and adapting it for use in several languages and cultures in order to compare or aggregate data across cultures. In this former case the original work is used merely as a methodological guide for the production of a culturally appropriate set of items. In the latter case there are quite different implications and serious ethical, conceptual, and technical problems are raised. This is because an absolute requirement for such an exercise is that both the items on the questionnaire and the responses to them are conceptually and functionally equivalent in every language and culture concerned. Moreover, it is necessary to be sure that the same phenomenon is being measured in each country. This implies that the underlying concept is present in and salient to the populations of all participating countries. For example, work in northern Scotland with chronic asthma sufferers showed that a high proportion of the sample did not understand the term 'quality of life' and there was little consensus on its meaning.[13] An attempt to adapt the Nottingham health profile for use in Arabic-speaking countries indicated that much of the content was unacceptable to local samples because it was perceived as irrelevant to daily life, not a salient topic, or even blasphemous.[14]

When the source of the questionnaire content derives from a single culture and, as is common, from highly selected groups within that culture, it is inevitable that at least some items will be culture-specific. Thus, items may be irrelevant or even offensive in another language, or the content may omit issues of importance to other cultures altogether. Psychological states and emotional experiences, especially, and the language in which they are expressed are profoundly shaped by cultural factors and are the most difficult to translate.[15] If it is accepted that quality of life is subjective, perceptual, and existential, then attempts to measure it will, inevitably, pose the most problems.

The influence of culture

The spread of modern technology and the 'globalization' of medical education have created a tendency to ignore cultural variations both within and between cultures. Yet perceptions of and reactions to physical, emotional, and social discomfort and distress, as well as the experience and expression of well-being, grow out of the particular cultural and social reality within which the members of any culture mature. Acculturation determines, to a large extent, such relevant attributes as, for example,

(1) customary behaviours and ways of spending time in relation to work, leisure, and social occasions; interactions with family, friends, and strangers, including the reactions of self and significant others to illness and to medical care;

(2) the relative value placed upon such behaviours and relationships; physical ability, health, independence, work, and so on;

(3) expectations of what it means to feel good, or to be healthy, or to be ill, and conventions about seeking health care. These expectations also form and interact with perceptions of pain, discomfort, and the relative seriousness of symptoms;

(4) the type of language which is used when recounting personal experiences and the conventions governing the communication of those feelings to other people. For example, it is well known that people from different backgrounds differ enormously in their propensity to complain of pain and the levels of intensity they report.[16,17]

These factors will also be influenced, at a minimum, by age, sex, religion, and socio-economic group.

It follows from these comments that the question of comparability of measures is inextricably bound up with the ways in which the content of questionnaires purports to reflect quality of life. The use of a single measure to gather data from, for example, a clinical intervention, with the intention of combining data sets across cultures, by its very nature reveals nothing about cultural differences since the assumption is that such do not exist in relation to the measure being used. Thus important information may be lost about differential effects of the intervention in different cultures.

Trends in the cross-cultural adaptation of measures

Cross-cultural measurement has shown clear developmental trends. Initially, due to the scarcity or absence of questionnaires in many countries, plus the expense in time and money involved in producing them, the adaptation of a questionnaire developed in the UK or USA was seen as the obvious way to obtain measures where none existed.

The choice of which questionnaire to translate has usually been based upon the reputation of the measure in the country in which it was developed (whether deserved or undeserved). Thus, the underlying assumption has been that if a particular questionnaire is widely used and appears useful in country A, it will be of equal use in country B. Much less consideration is given to the cultural relevance of the content and its source or the normative implications of the items. It could well be argued that the features of a questionnaire which give it appeal in its home culture are precisely those features which might make it inappropriate in another culture. This is an issue for measures of health status but it is even more so for so-called 'quality of life', an expression which may not even exist naturally in some languages and the notion of which may be puzzling or even alien in some cultures. Even where the term is widely used there may be little consensus within a culture as to the precise referent(s).[18]

Developments in the translation process

Cross-cultural measurement was first attempted in the fields of psychiatry, psychology, and cultural anthropology.[19,20] In the early days, translations were made by a single linguist and applied immediately afterwards. When the limitations of this became obvious, two or more translators were employed and several versions in the target language were produced. This was followed by discussion and negotiation until agreement on the best translation was reached. A further development was the introduction of back-translation, whereby several versions of an item in the original questionnaire were translated into the target language and then translated back into the original language to compare the closeness of fit. This range of methods is still in use.

When field testing of translations was introduced it was not unusual to find that respondents in cultures other than the one in which the questionnaire originated did not always understand the task in hand or identify with the form of language used. Sometimes the very questions themselves were regarded as irrelevant or too personal. This gradually led to more consideration being given to monolingual lay people in the translation process in preference to linguists or professional translators.[15,21,22]

The most complex types of translation process now involve extensive discussion between translation teams normally composed of bilingual people. Items may be translated into the target language and then back-translated into the original to judge the degree of equivalence. These translated items are presented to lay panels of people monolingual in the target language who are invited to comment freely on the meaning and acceptability of the translations. Normally, a single item can be translated in several ways, so there is a period of negotiating in order to find the 'best fit'. This process may include priority ratings.[23] Subsequently, there ensues a prolonged period of field testing with members of the general population, after which tests of reliability and validity in the target culture are carried out, together with the establishment of item weights where used and, eventually, the deriving of 'normal values'. In fact very few questionnaires have been subjected to this process and most of these are measures of some aspect of health status rather than quality of life, such as the Nottingham Health Profile,[15] the Sickness Impact Profile,[21] the SF-36,[24] the European Organisation for Research and Treatment of Cancer (EORTC).[22]

Unresolved issues in adaptation

Reports on randomized controlled trials in more than one country rarely contain details relating to the equivalency of the questionnaires used to assess quality of life, giving the impression that this is either a totally resolved matter, or an issue of no importance. Neither of these inferences is correct. It is a *sine qua non* of any controlled trial that participants are treated alike and subjected to **exactly** the same measurement procedures. Where data are to be aggregated across countries, this inevitably raises the issue of the adequacy of translation and adaptation of questionnaires. In fact, there are a number of outstanding issues in translation procedures and testing for reliability and validity which remain to be resolved.

Translation of questionnaire content has involved sole or primary use of bilingual people. However, in most countries, bilinguals are unrepresentative of the general population of a country in terms of education, socio-economic status, age, and health experience. Linguistic research has shown that bilinguals do not think in the same way for each of the languages they know and that the order in which languages have been learned is important in relation to the generation of translations from one language to the other.[25] There has been an over-reliance, in the translation of questionnaires, on people who learned English as a second, third, or even fourth language. Related to this limitation is the fact that most countries have more than one form of the official language, sometimes called 'high' or 'low', or standard and colloquial. The high or standard form is used for official communications, formal occasions, in professional exchanges, speeches, and so on, whilst the low or colloquial form is more common in every-day speech and, indeed, may form the only version for less well-educated members of the population (this is an important point since persons of lower educational attainment are over-represented in the ranks of the sick). Bilinguals almost always translate into the 'high' form of the target language, even where items on the original questionnaire are in a colloquial form. For example, an item from the Nottingham health profile, the content of which was drawn directly from lay expressions, is 'things are getting me down'. This had to be rendered as the equivalent of 'I find it hard to cope' in many of the European versions – an expression which does not have at all the same connotations.

In order to choose between alternative translations, the method of back-translation has been heavily utilized, but back-translation can be very misleading because there are often profound differences in the meaning of what appears to be the same word or concept. Thus, it is not sufficient to know that words are equivalent: it is necessary to understand to what extent equivalent words and phrases convey equivalent meanings.[26] The choice of one translation from the several likely to be produced by back-translation must be based upon clear criteria which are founded in the cultural concerns and concepts underlying the original version and their applicability in the target language. A good example of this point is in translations of the word 'friend' which can be found in an American questionnaire item: 'Does poor health prevent you from seeing friends?' The definition of a friend in different countries varies remarkably on a dimension of closeness. The German 'freund' is by no means equivalent to the American 'friend' and even more distant from the Spanish 'amigo' which can be used even of strangers. An American 'friend' is not the same as a French 'ami' and an English 'friend' is different again. Thus, the answer to the question would differ markedly depending upon cultural meaning.

A further issue is the geographical relevance of the translation. For example, on the borders of countries there may be more similarities between the form of language used in adjacent villages than there are between the official languages of the countries involved. For example, the type of French spoken on the borders of Spain, Italy, and Switzerland has more in common with the neighbouring villages of those countries than it does with the types of French spoken, for example, in Paris. In some areas language has political connotations. In Scotland, English is the official language but among Gaelic speakers English may be regarded as the language of oppression amd Gaelic is the preferred form for matters of intimacy and importance such as might apply to health issues. Asking questions relating to health in English thus puts such questions in a particular 'niche' in the respondent's mind and may lead to low compliance or indifference in responding. This issue is an important one in many parts of the world where the official language has been imposed, either by the majority group or by former (and current) colonizers.

In some countries even people of less than average education may grow up using four or five different languages depending upon the context, such as is the case in India, some African countries, and the Far East. Thus, the question of which language is most appropriate for gathering information about health is not a trivial one. The issue of which form would be most appropriate for questionnaires relating to so-called quality of life needs research that has so far been absent.

Similar issues arise in relation to the response systems typically used in questionnaires. These may range from a simple 'yes/no' system to scaled responses of the type 'always', 'very often', 'sometimes', 'rarely', or 'never'. Some measures use visual analogue scales where respondents are required to check a number or mark a line according to the degree or strength of the response, for example, pain.

Translations of questionnaires almost always attempt to preserve the original response system regardless of its applicability and acceptability in the target language. 'Yes', 'no', 'very often', 'sometimes', and even 'never' are not equivalent in many cultures.[27] Likewise, responding to instructions on visual analogue scales is subject to a great deal of intra- as well as inter-cultural variation. Where response categories form an apparent scale, as in the example given above, a problem exists in relation to the anchoring of the end-points and the distance between implied points on the scale. These may be different in different cultures. Moreover, in some countries there may be a tendency to agree, regardless of the question, because of conventions covering polite behaviour and deferential attitudes to the medical profession. Further, different cultures differ in their propensity to adopt a middle position on a response scale.

Cultural relevance of questionnaire content

In the past five years or so, several new approaches to cross-cultural measurement have been developed. One strategy in the developmental process of a new questionnaire has been to involve representatives from target countries prior to the finalization of the content of the questionnaire. Thus, although material is still gathered in one country only, items are screened for acceptability and translatability by representatives of other language groups before the definitive material is selected. This is followed by field testing simultaneously in each country with changes being made to items as necessary, after which testing for reliability and validity takes place. While this approach partially addresses the issue of the culture-bound content of questionnaires, it involves a huge administrative task which few are willing to undertake. Since the questionnaire must be identical in every country concerned, items which work well in one country have to be omitted if this is not the case in all target languages. For example, in the development of a questionnaire designed to assess quality of life in adults with growth hormone deficiency (GHD), source material was gathered from in-depth interviews with patients in England. This material was then subjected to screening by representatives from five other countries: Sweden, Spain, Italy, France, and Germany. This exercise led to 43 of the original 75 items being dropped, even though they had excellent face validity in England, simply because the expression did not exist in one of the other languages or the content was impossible to translate meaningfully, or the problem expressed was not salient in another culture.[28]

A further problem with this approach is that matters of importance in one or another country are left out because they are not salient in the country where the original material was gathered. Questionnaires which reflect culture-bound definitions will only, at best, ascertain the degree to which the same notions are absent or present in other societies and will miss the empirical significance of different cultural manifestations of health status or 'quality of life'. The work on GHD mentioned above showed that weight gain, which was a major preoccupation of people in England, was of little concern to people in Italy.

Similarly, the feelings of shame and guilt attached to a diagnosis of genital herpes in Spain were not apparent in Denmark.[29]

Recent work with asthma patients in Scotland has indicated very different priorities, in relation to health, from those customarily implied by questionnaire content.[13] Interviews conducted with AIDS patients in England elicited reactions to a range of standard questionnaires purporting to measure quality of life. Responses to the content varied from ridicule to indignation, so irrelevant was the content to the existential position of the patients. Rather, feelings of love and being loved; the ability to enjoy a joke; living free from discrimination; making spiritual, emotional, and practical adjustments to the fact of death; having enough money for one's needs; listening to music; having pleasant physical surroundings; and being assured of good medical care were mentioned as being of major import- ance.[30] Such concerns are not found on questionnaires currently used to measure quality of life. It is self evident that those issues of most importance to individuals will have the most influence on their quality of life and it is precisely these matters of concern that are shaped by culture.

There is still a lack of information on what problems of comparability of meaning occur when the same questions are addressed to people who differ in their every-day vocabulary, grammar, and social situation. Even within countries there are linguistic variations between social classes, ethnic groups, ages, sexes, regions, urban and rural segments, at a minimum. These problems have barely been addressed within countries and are even more exaggerated between countries.

Finally, during the translation and testing process it is customary to compare the original version to a single target language at a time. Thus, the new versions are not compared with each other. A situation can easily arise whereby, say, a Spanish translation of a questionnaire differs slightly from the original English in one direction while the Swedish version differs slightly in the opposite direction. On a continuum of meaning, the Spanish version is far removed from the Swedish even though neither are very far from the English. Ideally, every new version needs to be compared with every other version for equivalence of meaning before cross-cultural comparability can begin to be established. Obviously, the greater the number of languages involved the greater the task this poses.[26]

Sampling

The tasks of developing, testing, translating, and adapting measures have, most often, been carried out in university settings, in the context of health service, or by other organizations, such as pharmaceutical companies. Thus, the work is urban based, usually in big cities such as London, Paris, Washington, Stockholm, or Berlin. Translators come from a narrow circle and lay participants usually come from particular sub-cultures. Little attempt is made to involve people from rural areas or immigrant groups and yet most European countries have resident populations of ethnic minorities – from the Indian subcontinent and Africa in Britain; from Turkey and Greece in Germany; from North Africa in France. Field testing, reliability, and validity studies rarely extend to people from ethnic minorities or other language groups within the country. The relevance of this is that many such people, by reason of disadvantage or lower income, may be over-represented in the ranks of those requiring medical attention. Where they have not been included in the adaptation process, the relevance for them of the translated questionnaire may be minimal. There are no questionnaires currently available which have used, in their development, a sampling frame representative of the population at large. The reasons for this are the immensity of the task and the expense involved. Rather, it has been assumed that the final product will suit all or can be made to do so with minimal adjustment of the content and wording.

Testing the validity and reliability of a questionnaire in other language versions

Achieving a successful translation does not make a questionnaire culturally relevant and it would be quite wrong to make decisions about medical care on such a basis. It must be tested for validity and reliability in each language in which it is to be applied. As previously noted the validity of a measure cannot be divorced from the meaning of the underlying concept. If this is unclear then it is impossible to fulfil the first requirement for validity, that is, that the instrument measures what it is supposed to measure.

Three methods have most commonly been used for establishing validity in new versions of a questionnaire. These are

- examining the relationship between the scores on the new questionnaire and those on another, pre-existing, one in the target country which measures something similar;

- finding some external criterion of the phenomenon the questionnaire is attempting to measure, for example, use of health services and comparing scores with, say, number of medical consultations in a given year; and/or

- gathering a large amount of data from a random sample of the population and investigating group differences thought to be relevant to the content of the questionnaire, for example, differences by age, sex, the existence of a chronic illness.

The most scientifically sound of these procedures has been to use similar patient populations, study designs, and measures in different countries and to compare the psychometric properties of the responses; the assumption being that if these are equally good in all countries then the data are comparable.[31] However, drawbacks of these methods have received virtually no attention.

In the first instance, suitable questionnaires against which to test the validity of the new one may not exist. If they do it may well be that they too have been adapted from another language and are of doubtful or unknown validity. If there is a measure available it may not be a suitable comparator because of differences in underlying concept between the two measures. Testing the new questionnaire against an external criterion raises issues about differences between cultures in the criterion itself, for example, seeking medical attention. Taking a large population sample and analysing replies according to predetermined socio-demographic and disease categories raises a further set of problems. It tends to be assumed that if the pattern of responses is the expected one then the questionnaire is valid. A very similar pattern of responses to a questionnaire in two different cultures does not automatically imply that the meaning of those responses is the same. The pattern of responses may differ from country to country simply because of cultural differences. Thus, obtaining similar patterns of response in, for example, USA, Germany, France, and Italy on the same questionnaire may be evidence not of cross-cultural validity but rather of *lack* of validity and constraints on responses which relate to the content of the questionnaire and the irrelevance of the material or defects in the response system itself.

In addition, such exercises usually show quite large non-response rates and it is possible that the rate of refusals, uncompleted questionnaires, and the amount of missing data are a better guide to validity than any number of statistical tests.

The use of questionnaires in cross-cultural clinical trials

It is axiomatic that all subjects in a clinical trial must be treated in the same manner as far as possible. In multi-country trials, as has been indicated, there are two major pitfalls in relation to the use of questionnaires which may seriously compromise cultural comparability and, thus, the aggregation of data. The first of these is the conceptual and linguistic equivalence of the questionnaires in each language and the second is the cultural applicability of the content. As an example, a study of quality of life claims in clinical trials of antihypertensive therapy showed that several studies had used American questionnaires with UK samples without any prior testing for cultural acceptability or reliability and validity.[32] In two of the trials several European countries were involved and questionnaires had been translated into the relevant languages using only a bilingual translator and the method of back-translation,[33,34] both of which have been shown, as noted earlier, to be inadequate to produce culturally appropriate versions of questionnaires. Moreover, no field testing or tests of reliability or validity were carried out in the countries concerned prior to the trial. These studies reported aggregated data and drew conclusions which were, in fact, scientifically dubious.

Countries also differ in the 'questionnaire sophistication' of the population. In some countries questionnaires are so common in health services and medical care that patients take this part of the procedure for granted and, usually, understand well the reasons for the enquiry. In other countries questionnaires are very unusual and patients may not fully appreciate the task they are given.

Multi-country studies also entail problems of standardization of the administration of questionnaires since it may not be possible to recreate the same conditions in every country or centre. Standardization is also compromised by the degree of seriousness with which clinical staff regard questionnaires. Many randomized controlled trials take place over a large number of centres and several countries but few reports mention precautions taken to ensure that the administration of questionnaires is uniform throughout.

It is clear there can be substantial amounts of missing data in multi-country trials. Some of this will be a consequence of patients failing to understand the question fully and failing to answer and some will be a result of the inapplicability of some items. Although it is customary to report missing clinical values in some detail, missing data from questionnaires is rarely dealt with in depth, nor are the implications spelled out. For example, in one clinical trial 17 per cent of patients refused to answer one question and 35 per cent another.[35] Since these figures are likely to under-represent the number of people who were reluctant to respond, the implications for the relevance of the measures used are serious.

Conclusions

The foregoing comments highlight crucial issues that have received little attention. There are several reasons for this apparent indifference. First, the setting up and organization of clinical trials is primarily in the hands of people with training in clinical subjects or, sometimes, health economics and the trials are run and data collected, normally, by medical and related staff perhaps aided by a statistician. None of these people is likely to be deeply versed in ethnolinguistics, cognitive anthropology, or psychometrics, any more than the average social scientist is competent to practise cardiovascular surgery. Thus, the importance of the details of questionnaire construction, application, and interpretation is often underestimated.

Second, this lack of knowledge is combined with pressure from pharmaceutical companies and/or third-party payers to include 'quality of life' measures, whether this is either necessary or feasible.

Third, the availability of funding for such studies may induce those who have some awareness of the issues to 'turn a blind eye'.

In addition, there is a huge gap between the types of journals which publish the results of clinical trials and those publications which address the conceptual and methodological puzzles inherent in both quality of life and cross-cultural research. Thus, the former may be little informed by the latter. Moreover, papers submitted for publication to clinical journals are likely to be reviewed by clinicians who are also lacking the requisite information. Publication gives a spurious respectability to studies and certain 'traditions' about the way to conduct trials arise, turning what used to be merely scattered examples of ill-informed practice into near-universal bad habits which are difficult to break.

Perhaps the major issue in relation to the inclusion of quality of life measures into randomized controlled trials is that enthusiasm has outrun common sense. It may well be the case that there are universal phenomena in relation to health and disease which are not culture bound. This is more likely the closer such phenomena are to the biological and physiological characteristics of human beings. The further we move into subjective phenomena, the greater the extent of cultural variation. Moreover, the manifestations of cultural differences may be less apparent to those who mix with professionals from other countries who share a common background of education and status and who may be far from representative of the diversity of thought, custom, and mores in their home country.

Addressing the problems

There are several ways in which at least some of these problems can begin to be tackled.

1.   Where there is an intention, at some time, to conduct a cross-cultural clinical trial which might include self-completed questionnaires, the personnel involved in setting up and organization should be sent on training seminars which will cover the relevant information needed to make informed decisions about research design and content in the circumstances which pertain. Such seminars should include state-of-the-art comments on quality of life measurement and its attendant cross-cultural implications, together with alternative approaches to gathering patient data on relevant variables.

2.   The membership of ethics committees should include at least one person who is familiar with the major issues in quality of life and health measurement cross-culturally.

3.   The whole issue of whether quality of life measurement is truly relevant to the intention of the trial should be considered carefully. In what sense is 'quality of life' likely to be affected by the planned therapeutic regime, and will this apply in other countries? Indeed, several authors have questioned the feasibility and acceptability of trying to measure quality of life at all, in view of the conceptual, technical, and ethical problems it raises.[8,36-39] These problems are magnified in cross-cultural research. The notion of quality of life is, itself, a cultural construct, introduced originally by social scientists in the USA. It cannot be assumed to have universal relevance or meaning.

4.   As an alternative, where some kind of patient-based information is essential, it would be preferable to use questionnaires based upon more cross-culturally common phenomena such as disability, physical function, and symptoms, where it is also easier to achieve comparable translations across cultures. The crucial decision revolves around the choice of a measure which is appropriate to the medical condition and the probable consequences of the intervention and the patients involved. A new drug may relieve symptoms more quickly than its competitors. Can one extrapolate from this to argue that quality of life is thus improved? The evidence supports a verdict of 'not so'.[12,40,41] This is an existential, not a medical, question. It might be easier, more ethical, technically more feasible, and cross-culturally more appropriate simply to ask about symptom relief.

5.   Where questionnaires cannot be avoided, it is important that the development, source of the content, and response characteristics are carefully scrutinized. In addition, reports of previous use, under what circumstances, and in which countries, should be sought. Details of translation and adaptation procedures need to be studied and the cross-cultural acceptability judged, preferably by lay people from each country involved. Any standard questionnaire should be accompanied by a manual giving this information.

6.   There are options other than aggregating data across countries. For example, where translated questionnaires are available, it may be possible to conduct within-country analyses, even on small numbers of patients, and to compare data relating to changes over time within each country.

7.   In the longer term, it may be more important, for the eventual achievement of cross-cultural comparability, to develop scientifically sound measures *within each*

country, based upon a clear concept of what is to be measured and grounded in the experience of members of that country, rather than to begin with the assumption that a measure from a single country can be made applicable across cultures. In this situation the extent of change could also be measured separately in each country and the change data compared.

8.   An additional long-term solution could be to set up a project to gather a core set of items that are truly shared across cultures, together with a set of items specific to each culture or language group. Indeed, the World Health Organization is currently attempting this exercise on a worldwide basis.[42] However, the present content of the prototype questionnaire would not lend itself to a clinical trial situation and it would be necessary to develop an instrument aimed more directly at the needs and constraints of the trial situation.

9.   Another approach is represented by the 'individual quality of life assessment' approach, which allows each patient to express his or her own concerns, priorities, and values, albeit in a standard manner, and statistics applied to the results.[43] This might be feasible cross-culturally but cumbersome and costly to apply in the trial situation.

10.   Once decisions have been made about what and how to measure, it is vital that the personnel involved at data collection level in all countries are made aware of the importance of standard administration of measures and the various sensitivities of questionnaire-based research.

11.   Regardless of the choice of measure, the most crucial error that can be made in cross-cultural research is to conduct it according to the unstated norms and values of one particular culture, implying that the content is somehow culture free. To date, the content of so-called 'quality of life' and health status questionnaires has reflected a very narrow set of categories and assumptions from an even more limited sector within one or two countries. True cross-cultural comparability must begin from the position that culture does more than shape illness as an experience, it shapes the very way we conceive of illness and health-related states.[44]

If quality of life claims in cross-cultural research are eventually to have scientific credibility, then the care that is taken with the development and choice of measures and their administration must be at least as great as that taken over the clinical end-points themselves.

References

1. Editorial. *Lancet*, 1995; **346**: 1–2.
2. Bjork, S. Quality of life of adults with growth hormone deficiency: a controlled study. *Acta Pediatr. Scand.* (Suppl.), 1989; **356**: 55–9.
3. Dahlof, C. and Bjorkman, R. Diclofenac (50 & 100 mg) and placebo in the acute treatment of migraine. *Cephalgia*, 1993; **13**: 117–23.
4. Steiner, S.S., Friedhoff, A.J., Wilson, B.L., Wecker, J.R., and Santo, J.P. Antihypertensive therapy and quality of life: a comparison of atenolol, captopril and propranolol. *J. Hum. Hypert.*, 1990; **4**: 217–25.

5. Wassertheil-Smoller, S., Blaufox, D., Oberman, A., *et al.* Effect of anti-hypertensives on sexual function and quality of life: the TAIM study. *Ann. Int. Med.*, 1991; **8**: 613–62.
6. Walsh, R., Aranha, G., and Freeark, R. Mortality and quality of life after total abdominal colectomy. *Archives of Surgery*, 1990; **125**: 1564–6.
7. Leplège, A. La mesure de la qualité de vie des personnes séropositives au VIH. Questions épistémologiques et éthiques. *Ethique*, 1994; **12**: 27–36.
8. Drummond, N. Quality of life in asthma patients. PhD Thesis, 1996: University of Aberdeen, Scotland.
9. Hunt, S.M. Quality of life: an unsuitable case for measurement. Paper delivered at the Conference on Cancer, AIDS and Quality of Life, UNESCO, Paris, January 15–17, 1996.
10. Novak, P. 'Ways of living' and its contribution to quality of life research. In *Quality of life and health: concepts, methods and applications.*, (ed. Guggenmoos-Holzman, I., Bloomfield, K., Brenner, H. and Flick, U.), pp. 79–88. Berlin: Blackwell, 1995.
11. Hunt, S.M. Cross-cultural comparability of measures and other issues related to multi-country studies. *Brit. J. Med. Econ.*, 1993; **6C**: 27–34.
12. Pearlman, R. and Uhlmann, R. Quality of life in chronic diseases: perceptions of elderly patients. *Gerontol.*, 1988; **36**: 25–30.
13. Drummond, N. The concerns of asthma patients in Scotland. Paper delivered at the University of Aberdeen Health Services Research Unit, Aberdeen, Scotland; 1994.
14. Hunt, S.M., McEwen, J., and McKenna, S.P. *Measuring health status*. London: Croom Helm, 1986.
15. Hunt, S.M., Alonso, J., Bucquet, D., Niero, M., Wiklund, I., and Mckenna, S.P. Cross cultural adaptation of health measures. *Health Policy*, 1991; **19**: 33–44.
16. Brena, S., Sanders, S., and Motoyama, H. American and Japanese chronic back pain patients: cross-cultural similarities and differences. *Clin. J. Pain*, 1990; **6**: 118–24.
17. Strong, J., Ashton, R., and Chant, D. The measurement of attitudes towards and beliefs about pain. *Pain*, 1992; **48**: 227–36.
18. Hodge, J. The quality of life: a contrast between utilitarian and existential approaches. In *Quality of life: perspectives and policies*, (ed. Baldwin, S.), pp. 119–28. London: Routledge, 1990.
19. Triandis, H. Major theroetical and methodological issues in cross-cultural psychology. In *Readings in cross-cultural psychology*, (ed. Dawson, J. and Lonner, W.), pp. 26–38. Hong Kong: Hong Kong University Press, 1974.
20. Kleinman, A. Depression, somatization and the 'new cross-cultural psychiatry'. *Soc. Sci. Med.*, 1997; **11**: 3–10.
21. Hendrickson, W.D., Russell, J., Prihoda, T., Jacobson, J., Rogan, A., and Bishop, G.D. An approach to developing a valid Spanish language translation of a health status questionnaire. *Med. Care*, 1989; **27**: 959–66.
22. Aaronson, N., Ahmedzai, S., Bergman, B., *et al.* The European Organisation for Research and Treatment of Cancer (EORTC): a quality of life instrument for use in international clinical trials in oncology. *J. Nat. Cancer Inst.*, 1993; **85**: 365–76.
23. Aaronson, N., Ahmedzai, S., Bullinger, M., *et al.* The EORTC score quality of life questionnaire: interim results of an international field study. In *Effect of cancer on quality of life*, (ed. Osaba, D.), pp. 185–203. Boca Raton, Fl: CRC Press, 1991.

24. Ware, J. and Sherborne, C. The MOS 36-item short form health survey (SF36). International conceptual framework and item selection. *Med. Care*, 1992; **30**: 473–81.
25. Holme, J. *An introduction to sociolinguistics*. London: Longmans, 1992.
26. Hunt, S.M. Cross-cultural comparability of quality of life measures. In *Quality of life and health: concepts, methods and applications*, (ed. Guggenmoos-Holzman, I., Bloomfield, K., Brenner, H., and Flick, U.), pp. 15–26. Berlin: Blackwell, 1995.
27. Deutscher, I. Asking questions cross-culturally: some problems of linguistic comparability. In *Comparative research methods*, (ed. Warwick, D. and Osherson, S.), pp. 163–88. New Jersey: Prentice Hall, 1973.
28. Hunt, S.M. Developing a measure of quality of life for adults with growth hormone deficiency. *Drug Information J.*, 1994; **28**: 3–11.
29. Doward, L. Developing a measure of quality of life for use in genital herpes. Paper delivered at the Drug Information Association Meeting, Charleston, S. Carolina; April 14–16, 1993.
30. Hunt, S.M. Community care and quality of life of patients with HIV/AIDS. Report prepared for Trafford Health Authority, Manchester, England; 1994.
31. Bullinger, M. Ensuring international equivalence of quality of life measures. In *Quality of life assessment: international perspectives*, (ed. Orley, J. and Kuykken, W.), pp. 33–40. Berlin: Springer, 1994.
32. Hunt, S.M. The credibility of quality of life claims in clinical trials of anti-hypertensive therapy. Paper delivered at the Drug Information Association Conference, Charleston, S. Carolina; May 9–11, 1994.
33. Fletcher, A., Battersby, C., Adnitt, P., Underwood, N., Jurgensen, H.J., and Bulpitt, C.J. Quality of life on antihypertensive therapy: a double blind trial comparing quality of life on pinacidil and nifedipine in combination with a thiazide diuretic. *J. Cardiovasc. Pharmacol.*, 1992; **20**: 108–14.
34. Fletcher, A., Bulpitt, C.J., Chase, D.M., *et al.* Quality of life with three antihypertensive treatments: cilazapril, atenolol, nifedipine. *Hypertension*, 1993; **19**: 499–507.
35. Ameling, E.H., de Korte, D.F., and Man in't Veld, A.J. Impact of diagnosis and treatment of hypertension on quality of life: a double-blind randomized placebo-controlled cross-over study of betaxolol. *J. Cardiovasc. Pharmacol.*, 1991; **18**: 752–60.
36. Grimley Evans, J. Quality of life assessments and elderly people. In *Do we need measures other than QALYS?* (ed. Hopkins, A.), pp. 107–16. London: Royal College of Physicians, 1992.
37. Raspe, H. Quality of life measurement in rheumatology. In *Quality of life and health: concepts, methods and applications*, (ed. Guggenmoos-Holzman, I., Bloomfield, K., Brennes, H., and Flick, U.), pp. 97–106. Berlin: Blackwell, 1995.
38. Leplège, A. and Hunt, S.M. The problem of quality of life in medicine. *J. Am. Med. Assoc.*, 1997; **278**: 47–50.
39. Pearlman, R.A. and Jonsen, A. The use of quality of life considerations in medical-decision making. *Ann. Intern. Med.*, 1985; **97**: 420–5.
40. Bury, M. The sociology of chronic illness: a review of research and prospects. *Sociol. Health Illness*, 1991; **13**: 451–68.

41. Stimson, G. Obeying doctor's orders: a view from the other side. *Soc. Sci. Med.*, 1974; **8**: 97–104.
42. World Health Organization Working Group. The WHO quality of life assessment instrument. In *Quality of life assessment in health care settings*, (ed. Orley, J. and Kuyken, W.), Heidelberg: Springer, 1994.
43. McGee, H., O'Boyle, C., and Hickey, A. Assessing the quality of life of the individual: the SEIQoL with a healthy and a gastroenterology unit population. *Psychol. Med.*, 1991; **21**: 749–59.
44. Winch, P. *The idea of a social science and its relation to philosophy*. London: Routledge & Kegan Paul, 1958.

5 Profile versus utility based measures of outcome for clinical trials

Robert M. Kaplan

The measurement of quality of life outcomes in randomized clinical trials is becoming increasingly common. These measures are attractive because most illnesses and most treatments affect a variety of different health outcomes. In addition to its effects upon the life expectancy, disease intrudes upon the quality of life. Because of the important impacts upon health-related quality of life, a wide variety of measures has been proposed to quantify these effects.[1-5] These measures are similar in that each expresses the effects of medical care in terms that can be reported directly by a patient. However, the rationales for the methods differ considerably. Perhaps the most important distinction is between psychometric or 'profile' approaches and decision-theory based methods. The psychometric tradition typically creates a profile of patient outcomes. Some of the best known profiles measures in clinical trial research are the quality of life questionnaire C-30 (QLQ C-30) of the European Organization for Research and Treatment of Cancer (EORTC)[1] and the functional living index–cancer (FLIC).[2] The best known generic profile measures include the medical outcomes study 36-item short form (SF-36)[6] and the sickness impact profile (SIP).[7] Briefly, profile approaches characterize patients on a series of outcomes. Many profile approaches are empirically driven. They begin with a large number of items and the item pool is eventually reduced through factor analysis or other data reduction methods. Other profile approaches are conceptually based with items used to represent underlying concepts. Factor analysis is used to verify that the items are performing as would be expected if the constructs were measured adequately.

The concept of relative importance: dimensions of quality of life

Nearly all health-related quality of life measures have multiple dimensions such as physical functioning and pain. The exact dimensions vary from measure to measure. There is considerable debate in the field about which dimensions should be included.[8] For example, the most commonly included dimensions are physical functioning, role functioning, and mental health. The SF-36 includes eight health concepts.[6] These methods will be reviewed briefly.

Examples of profiles measures

Some of the more commonly used profiles measures are the sickness impact profile (SIP), the McMaster health index questionnaire, the SF-36, and the Nottingham health profile.

Sickness Impact Profile (SIP)

The sickness impact profile (SIP) is one of the best known and widely used quality of life measures and is a general measure applicable to any disease or disability group.[7] Furthermore, the SIP has been used successfully with a variety of different cultural subgroups.

The SIP includes 136 items, divided into 12 categories, that describe the effect of sickness on behavioural function. Each of the 12 categories is clustered into three groups: independent categories, physical, and psychosocial. Independent categories include sleep and rest, eating, work, home management, and recreation and pastimes. Physical categories include ambulation, mobility, and body care and movement. The psychosocial categories are social interaction, alertness behaviour, emotional behaviour, and communication. Table 5.1 shows the categories for the SIP.

Each SIP item has been evaluated by an independent group of judges on a 15-point scale of dysfunction. The judges' ratings determine the weighting of each item in the SIP scoring. The respondent does not consider the judges' weightings in deciding to endorse an item. The overall SIP percentage score is obtained by selecting the items endorsed by the respondent, summing their scale values, and dividing by the sum of all values for all items on the SIP. Then this proportion is multiplied by 100 to compute a total percentage impaired score. Similarly, scores are obtained for each category. Percentage scores for each category can be plotted on a graphic display that looks similar to a Minnesota Multiphasic Personality

Table 5.1   Sickness impact profile categories and selected items

Dimension
Independent categories
Physical
Psychosocial

Category

SR	Sleep and rest
E	Eating
W	Work
HM	Home management
RP	Recreation and pastimes
A	Ambulation
M	Mobility
BCM	Body care and movement
SI	Social interaction
AB	Alertness behaviour
EB	Emotional behaviour
C	Communication

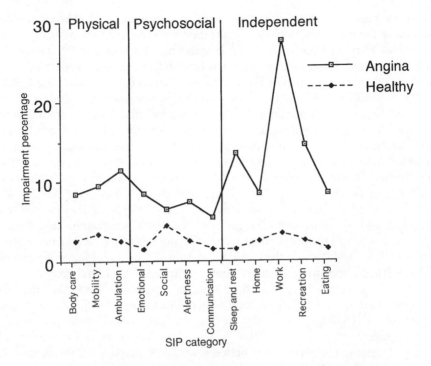

Fig. 5.1　SIP profile comparing patients with angina to healthy controls.

Inventory profile. A variety of studies attest to the reliability and validity of the SIP for various patient groups and clinical applications.[7] An example of an application of the SIP in cardiovascular disease is shown in Fig. 5.1. The figure compares 50 patients with angina against 50 healthy volunteers. Angina patients have more impairment in all categories. In comparison to healthy controls, those with angina are similar on social and alertness scales, but quite different for work and recreation.

The McMaster health index questionnaire

A similar approach has been developed by Chambers and colleagues[9] in Canada. The measure this group has developed is known as the McMaster health index questionnaire (MHIQ). In developing their questionnaire, a multidisciplinary group of specialists in internal medicine, family medicine, psychiatry, epidemiology, statistics, and social science reviewed existing health status questionnaires. Their goal was to develop an instrument that conforms to the World Health Organization's definition of health as 'not merely the absence of disease or infirmity'.[10] Similar to the SIP, the MHIQ has separate scales. For example, some of the physical health items were taken from the 'index of activities of daily living scale'.[11] The emotional function items were adapted or taken verbatim from a variety of sources, including the social readjustment rating scale.[12] This resulted in an original questionnaire of 172 items.

After validation testing, the pool of items was reduced to 59. The criteria for selection of the final items included association with observed functional changes before and after patients entered the hospital and correlation with ratings by family physicians. Later studies validated the MHIQ against a variety of other quality of life measures such as the Lee index of functional capacity, the Spitzer quality of life index, and the Bradburn psychological well-being scale.

The MHIQ is a self-administered questionnaire, and validity studies have demonstrated that these self-reports correlate significantly with ratings by external observers. In one study, it was demonstrated that the physical function portion of the index changes in response to therapies designed to affect physical function. The physical function portion of the MHIQ has adequate but not impressive reliability. In one study of patients in a physiotherapy clinic, the MHIQ was administered twice within a one-week period. The physiotherapists reported that functional status should not change over the short interval in this patient population. Using test–retest assessment, the interclass correlation coefficients were 0.53, 0.70, and 0.48 for the physical, emotional, and social function portions of the MHIQ, respectively. Another study evaluated the internal consistency of the MHIQ as assessed by Cronbach's alpha coefficients. For the physical, emotional, and social function indices, the coefficients were 0.76, 0.67, and 0.51, respectively. For group comparisons in large clinical trials coefficients in the 0.6 and 0.7 range may be acceptable, but they are less than optimal. Low reliability, causing attenuation in correlations between variables, may reduce the chances of detecting important relationships.

The medical outcome study 36-item short form (SF-36)

The SF-36 is the most commonly used health status measure in the world today. The SF-36 grew out of work by RAND and the medical outcomes study (MOS).[6] Originally, it was based on the measurement strategy from the RAND health insurance study. The MOS attempted to develop a very short, 20-item instrument known as the short form-20 or SF-20. However, the SF-20 did not have appropriate reliability for some dimensions. In particular, the SF-20 had floor effects and less than optimal reliability for its single item measures of pain and social functioning. The SF-36 includes eight health concepts: physical functioning, role–physical, bodily pain, general health perceptions, vitality, social functioning, role–emotional, and mental health. The SF-36 can either be administered by a trained interviewer or be self-administered. It has many advantages, for example, it is brief and there is substantial evidence for its reliability and validity. The SF-36 can be machine scored and has been evaluated in large population studies. The reliability and validity of the SF-36 are well documented.[13–14]

Despite the many advantages of the SF-36, there are also some disadvantages. For example, the SF-36 does not have age-specific questions and it is unclear whether it is equally appropriate at each level of the age continuum. The items for older retired individuals are the same as those for children, although the SF-36 is not usually recommended for studies of children.[14] Nevertheless, the SF-36 has become the most commonly used measure in contemporary medicine.

Nottingham health profile

One of the other major approaches is the Nottingham health profile (NHP), which has been particularly influential in the European community.[15] The NHP has two parts. Part one includes 38 items divided into six categories: sleep, physical mobility, energy, pain, emotional reactions, and social isolation. Items within each of these sections are rated in terms of relative importance. Items are rescaled in order to allow them to vary between 0 and 100 within each section. A paired preference method was used to derive the weights within categories, but not across categories.

Part two of the NHP includes seven statements related to the areas of life most affected by health: employment, household activities, social life, home life, sex life, hobbies and interests, and holidays. In the second portion of the NHP, the respondent indicates whether or not a health condition has affected his or her life in these areas. The NHP has been used in a substantial number of studies and there is considerable evidence for its reliability and validity.

There are many attractive features of the NHP. The scale is 'consumer' based and arises from definitions of health offered by individuals in the community. Furthermore, the NHP was designed to use language that is easily interpretable by people in the community and to conform to minimum reading requirements. Substantial testing has been performed on the NHP. The major difficulty with the NHP is that it does not provide relative importance weightings across dimensions. As a result, it is difficult to compare the dimensions directly with one another.[15]

Problems with the profile approach: relative importance of dimensions

The profile approach often uses factor analysis to establish construct validity. Most factor analyses of health status measures have been based on frequency data. The items, variables, or rates in such studies are aggregated into underlying 'dimensions'. Yet, these dimensions tell us very little about underlying aetiologies or causes. The analyses only demonstrate that many medical, health services, or symptom reports are correlated to some extent within different patient or population groups. The relationship between these factors and their importance to patient concerns is less clearly defined. Factor analysis cannot derive measures of relative importance from measures of relative frequency. The concepts of frequency and relative importance are conceptually and empirically independent. Factor analysis cannot go beyond the available data. A comprehensive quality of life measure must consider both the frequency of outcomes and their importance. Since factor analysis does not offer a means of combining the two components, the method may have only limited value in constructing health status measures. The problems with profile approaches are apparent for both clinical and policy applications.

Some of the problems in interpreting profiles are illustrated in Fig. 5.2. The figure shows three hypothetical profiles corresponding to three treatments for prostate cancer: surgery, radiation, and watchful waiting. Patients are measured

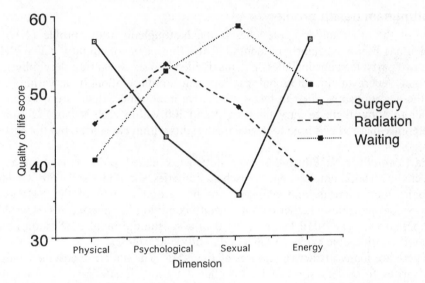

Fig. 5.2 Profiles of outcomes for three approaches to the management of prostate cancer.

along four dimensions: physical functioning, psychological functioning, sexual functioning, and energy. T scores (y axis) are standardized scores with a mean of 50 and a standard deviation of 10. Surgery may produce benefits for physical functioning but decrements for psychological and sexual functioning. Radiation may produce decrements for physical functioning and energy, but have less effect on psychological and sexual functioning. Waiting may result in few effects on physical functioning but may result in the highest scores among the treatments in psychological and sexual functioning. Ultimately, clinicians make some general interpretations of the profile by applying a weighting system. They might decide that they are more concerned about physical, rather than sexual functioning, or vice versa. Judgement about the relative importance of various dimensions is common and typically is done implicitly, arbitrarily, and in an idiosyncratic way. On the other hand, physicians may ignore a particular test result or a particular symptom because another one is more important to them, and the process by which relative importance is evaluated can be studied explicitly and be part of the overall model.

It is sometimes difficult to capture the total clinical picture using profiles measures because most treatments have side-effects as well as benefits. A successful surgery for prostate cancer, for example, might be associated with impotence and incontinence. The major challenge is in determining what it means when someone experiences a side-effect. Should the patient who feels sleepy discontinue his or her medication? How do we determine whether or not observable side-effects are important? Should a patient with insulin dependent diabetes mellitus (IDDM) discontinue therapy because he or she develops skin problems at the injection sites? Skin problems are a nuisance, but without treatment the patient would die.

Often the issue is not whether treatment causes side-effects, but how we should place these side-effects within the perspective of total health. Ultimately, we must decide whether treatment produces a net benefit or a net deficit in health status.

In addition to the problems in interpreting profiles for clinical decision making, it is difficult to use profiles for cost-effectiveness and cost–utility analysis. Comparison of different options for the use of common resources requires quantification of health outcomes using a common measurement unit. These multidimensional units must scale multiple attributes in terms of their relative importance. Despite many attempts, popular outcome measures such as the SIP, SF-36, MHIQ, and NHP have not been useful for cost-effectiveness analysis because they have multiple outcome dimensions. To a large extent, preference or utility is the most important feature of cost–utility analysis.

Measuring preference evokes many technical and methodological challenges.[16–19] Different methods of preference measurement can yield different results,[20] a finding that should not be surprising because the various approaches to preference assessment are based on different underlying conceptual models and the methods ask different questions. We will return to this issue later in the chapter and focus here on the common feature of decision-theory based methods, namely that they place wellness on a continuum between 0.0 and 1.0.

Decision-theory methods are refinements of generic survival analysis. In traditional survival analysis, those who are alive are statistically coded as 1.0 while those who are dead are statistically coded as 0.0. Mortality can result from any disease and survival analysis allows the comparison between different diseases. For example, we can state the life expectancy for those who will eventually die of heart disease and compare it to the life expectancy to those who eventually die of cancer. Thus, there is an advantage over disease-specific measures such as heart ejection fractions and tumour size. The difficulty is that everyone who remains alive is given the same score. A person confined to bed with an irreversible coma is alive and is counted the same as someone who is actively participating in athletics. Utility assessment, on the other hand, allows the quantification of levels of wellness on the continuum, anchored by death and optimum function.

Quality-adjusted life-years (QALYs) are required in order to perform cost-effectiveness analysis.[21,22] QALYs integrate mortality and morbidity to express health status in terms of equivalents of well years of life. If a woman dies of breast cancer at age 50 and one would have expected her to live to age 75, the disease was associated with 25 lost life-years. If 100 women died at age 50 (and each also had a life expectancy of 75 years), 2500 (100×25 years) life-years would be lost.

Death is not the only outcome of concern in cancer. Many adults suffering from the disease are left somewhat disabled over long periods. Although still alive, the quality of their lives has diminished. Quality-adjusted life-years take into consideration the quality-of-life consequences of these illnesses. For example, a disease that reduces quality of life by one-half will take away 0.5 QALYs over the course of one year. If it affects two people, it will take away one year (equal to 2×0.5) over a one year period. A pharmaceutical treatment that improves quality of life by 0.2 for each of five individuals will result in the equivalent of one QALY if the benefit is maintained over a one year period. This system has the advantage of considering both benefits and side-effects of programmes in terms of the common QALY units. Although QALYs are typically assessed for patients, they can also be measured for others, including care givers who are placed at risk because they experience stressful life events.

The concept of utility

The concept of quality-adjusted life-years (QALYs) has been in the literature for nearly 25 years. Perhaps the first application was suggested by Fanshel and Bush[23] and, at approximately the same time, Torrance introduced a conceptually similar model.[24] Since then, a variety of applications has appeared.[22]

Despite the differences in approach, some important assumptions are similar. All approaches set one year of life in perfect health at 1.0. Years of life with less than optimal health are scored as less than 1.0. The basic assumption is that two years scored as 0.5 add up to the equivalent of one year of complete wellness. Similarly, four years scored as 0.25 are equivalent to one completely well year of life. A treatment that boosts a patient's health from 0.5 to 0.75 produces the equivalent of 0.25 QALYs. If applied to four individuals, and the duration of the treatment effect is one year, the effect of the treatment would be equivalent to one completely well year of life. The disagreement is not over the QALY concept but rather over how the weights for cases between 0.0 and 1.0 are obtained.

Health utility assessment has its roots in the classic work of von Neumann and Morgenstern.[25] Their mathematical decision theory characterized how a rational individual should make decisions when faced with uncertain outcomes. Von Neumann and Morgenstern outlined axioms of choice that have become basic foundations of decision analysis in business, government, and health care. This work was expanded upon by Raiffa[26] and several others (see reviews 27–30). Torrance and Feeny[30] challenged the use of the term 'utility theory' by von Neumann and Morgenstern. To nineteenth century economists and philosophers, utility meant usefulness. Nineteenth century economists believed there was a fixed utility function that represented consumer satisfaction with goods or services that would be delivered with certainty. Early in the 20th century, Pareto demonstrated that ordinal utilities could represent consumer choice and argued against attempts to measure cardinal utilities.[31] Arrow further argued that there are inconsistencies in individual preferences under certainty and that meaningful cardinal preferences cannot be measured and may not even exist.[32] This came to be known as the 'impossibility theorem' and is often cited by economists to discredit preference ratings.[33-34]

There are several reasons why Arrow's impossibility theorem may not be applicable to the aggregation of utilities in the assessment of QALYs. First, utility expressions for QALYs are expressions of probabilistic outcomes, not goods received with certainty. Von Neumann and Morgenstern emphasized decisions under *uncertainty*, a theoretically distinct approach. The traditional criticisms of economists are directed toward decisions to obtain certain rather than uncertain outcomes.[30] Second, Arrow assumed that the metric underlying utility was not meaningful and not standardized across individuals. Substantial psychometric evidence now suggests that preferences can be measured using scales with meaningful interval or ratio properties. When cardinal (interval) utilities are used instead of rankings, many of the potential problems in the impossibility theorem are avoided.[35]

Different approaches to the calculations of QALYs are based on very different underlying assumptions. One approach considers the duration that someone is in a particular health state as conceptually independent from the utility for the state.[36] The other approach merges duration of stay and utility.[30] This distinction is central to the understanding of the difference in approaches and the required evidence for the validity of the utility assessment procedure.

In the approach advocated by Kaplan and Anderson,[37] utilities for health states are obtained at a single point in time. For example, suppose that the state of confinement to a wheelchair is assigned a weight of 0.5. The patients in this state are observed over the course of time to determine empirically their transitions to other states of wellness. If they remain in the state for one year, then they would lose the equivalent of 0.5 well years of life. The key to this approach is that the preferences only concern a single point in time and do not acknowledge duration. Transition is determined through observation and not by patient attitudes. The alternative approach emphasized by Torrance and Feeny[30] and others[34] obtains preference for both health state and for duration. These approaches also consider the more complex problems of uncertainty. Thus, they are consistent with the von Neumann and Morgenstern notion of decision under uncertainty in which probabilities and trade-offs are considered explicitly by the judge. In other words, the different approaches differ according to whether the subjective judgements explicitly include attitudes toward risk. Some authors distinguish between utility methods or methods that incorporate attitudes toward risk and preference methods that incorporate empirical rather than subjective probabilities of transitions between health states.[30] In the following sections, several preference and utility based outcome measurement systems will be reviewed.

Examples of utility based measures

In this section, brief summaries of two preference based measures will be presented: the 'quality of well-being scale' and the 'health utility index'.

Quality of well-being scale–general health policy model

The general health policy model grew out of substantive theories in economics, psychology, medicine, and public health. The model of health status includes components for mortality (death), morbidity (health-related quality of life), and time. The rationale for the model is that diseases and disabilities are important for two reasons. First, illness may cause the life expectancy to be shortened. Second, illness may make life less desirable at times prior to death (health-related quality of life).[38–41]

Central to the general health policy model is a general conceptualization of quality of life. The quality of well-being scale (QWB) is a method of measuring quality of life for calculations in the model. The QWB is a preference-weighted measure combining three scales of functioning with a measure of symptoms and problems to produce a point-in-time expression of well-being which runs from 0 (for death) to 1.0 (for asymptomatic full function).[42] The model separates aspects of health status and life quality into distinct components. These are life expectancy (mortality), functioning (morbidity), preference for observed functional states (utility), and duration of stay in health states (prognosis). The morbidity component is the core of the QWB measures. In addition to classification into observable levels of function, individuals are also classified by the symptom or problems. Symptoms, such as fatigue or a sore throat, might not be observable directly by others, while problems such as a missing limb might be noticeable by others. On any particular day, nearly 80 per cent of the general population is optimally functional. However, over an interval of seven days, only 12 per cent experience no symptoms. Symptoms or problems may be severe, such as serious joint pain, or minor, such as taking medication or following a prescribed diet for health reasons.

In order to obtain preference weights for observable health states, peer judges place the observable states of health and functioning on a preference continuum ranging from 0 for death to 1.0 for completely well.[43] A quality-adjusted life-year is defined as the equivalent of a completely well year of life, or a year of life free of any symptoms, problems, or health-related disabilities.[44] In addition to the QWB, the model requires mortality data from life tables.[45] The well-life expectancy is the current life expectancy adjusted for diminished quality of life associated with dysfunctional states and the durations of stay in each state. The model quantifies the health activity or treatment programme in terms of the quality-adjusted life-years that it produces or saves.

The general health policy model integrates components of the model to express outcomes in a common measurement unit. Using information on current functioning and duration, it is possible to express the health outcomes in terms of QALYs. The model for point-in-time quality of well-being is

$$
\begin{aligned}
\text{QWB} = 1 & - (\text{observed mobility} \times \text{mobility weight}) \\
& - (\text{observed physical activity} \times \text{physical activity weight}) \\
& - (\text{observed social activity} \times \text{social activity weight}) \\
& - (\text{observed symptom/problem} \times \text{symptom/problem weight})
\end{aligned}
$$

$$\text{QALY} = \text{QWB} \times \text{duration in years}.$$

The net cost/utility ratio is defined as

$$\frac{\text{net cost}}{\text{net QALYs}} = \frac{\text{cost of treatment} - \text{cost of alternative}}{\text{QALY}_\text{T} - \text{QALY}_\text{C}}$$

where $QALY_T$ and $QALY_C$ are the QALYs produced by the treatment and control groups respectively.

Health utility index

The health utility index (HUI) mark $I^{30,46}$ generates scores that can be used to adjust survival duration by reduced quality of life. The HUI mark I assesses four major concepts of health-related quality of life: physical function, which includes mobility and physical activity; role function, which includes self-care and role activity; social–emotional function, which includes well-being and social activity; and health problems. The concepts and levels of function within the concepts comprise a health status classification scheme. Individuals are categorized into one and only one level within each concept according to their functional status at the time the data are collected.

The HUI group has developed two additional versions of the HUI. These are known as the HUI mark II and the HUI mark III. The most recent version (mark III) contains eight attributes: vision, hearing, speech, ambulation, dexterity, emotion, cognition, and pain. Each of these attributes has five to six levels. A preference study involving 503 members of the general public is under development but has not yet been published. Preferences are measured using a 'time trade-offs' and 'standard gamble' instruments. Questionnaires are available in three formats: face-to-face interview, telephone interview, and self-administration. Overall, the HUI is a widely used and well-validated measure.[47,48]

The major differences between the QWB and HUI relate to the scoring systems. Both measures weight health states by human judgements. The QWB uses standardized preferences obtained from the general community while the HUI uses patient-generated preferences. Some studies show that the preferences obtained from patients and from the community are comparable. For resource allocation, it has been argued that community preferences are appropriate because it is community resources that will be consumed. Advocates for patient-level preference use suggest that the community cannot accurately represent the preferences for people who occupy specific health states. If the preferences of the community were discrepant from those of people who had experienced specific problems, this would be a major concern. However, the literature suggests that this may be a pseudo-issue. Although there are some differences between patient and community preference weights, the differences are typically small and often non-significant.[49]

Another difference between the HUI and QWB is that the QWB uses rating scales to obtain preference data while the HUI uses time trade-offs and standard gambles. These methods, particularly the standard gamble, are consistent with the von Neumann and Morgenstern axioms because they explicitly incorporate attitudes toward risk. Thus, they are more appropriately described as 'utilities' rather than preferences. There is a significant debate about which of these two methodologies is appropriate. Psychologists tend to prefer rating scales while economists argue in favour of standard gambles and time trade-offs. This issue will be addressed later.

A variety of other measures can also be used to estimate QALYs. For example, the EUROQoL is a commonly used health outcome measure. However, there are few published data on the sensitivity of the EUROQoL at this time.[50] One new measure is the 'health activity and limitation index' which is used to build years of healthy life for the US National Center for Health Statistics. This approach is attractive because it is linked to the US population via the National health interview survey.[51] However, the measure might not be able to pick up minor variations in wellness because it has too few questions. It has the advantage of simplicity, but the sensitivity remains to be demonstrated. We look forward to more research on each of these promising approaches.

In summary, the SF-36, SIP, MHIQ, NHP, QWB, EUROQoL, and HUI are each used in a significant number of studies. The SF-36 is clearly the most widely used measure in the field. The SF-36 has the advantage of linkage to a wide variety of databases. The SF-36 also provides a profile of outcomes. The major disadvantage of the SF-36 is that it does not provide data that are easily used in cost-utility or cost-effectiveness analysis. The deficiency is that it is not scored by preference. Fryback[52] has developed equations that can translate SF-36 scores into QWB and HUI scales. However, these translation equations leave much of the variance unaccounted for. The major criticism of the use of preference and utility measures is that they require subjective judgements. That issue will be explored in the next section.

Issues in preference measurement

Cost–utility analysis requires an assessment of utilities for health states. Several different techniques have been used to assess these utilities. Some analysts do not measure utilities directly. Instead, they evaluate health outcomes simply by assigning a reasonable utility (see ref. 53). However, most current approaches have respondents assign weights to different health states on a scale ranging from 0 (for dead) to 1.0 (for wellness). Although the importance of preference or utility measurement is well recognized, there is no consensus on how utilities should be measured. Below, we review three common approaches: rating scales, standard gamble, and time trade-off.

Rating scales

Rating scales provide simple techniques for assigning a numerical value to an object. There are several methods for obtaining rating scale information. One is the category scale. This is a simple partition method in which subjects are requested to assign each case a number selected from a set of numbered categories representing equal intervals. This method, exemplified by the familiar 10-point rating scale, is efficient, easy to use, and applicable in a large number of settings. Typically, the subjects read the description of a case and rates it on a 10-point scale ranging from 0 for dead to 10 for asymtomatic, optimum function. The end-points of the scale are typically well defined. Another common rating scale method is the visual analogue scale. The visual analogue method shows a subject a line, typically 100 cm in length, with the end-points well defined. The subject's task is to mark the line to indicate where their preference rests in relation to the two poles.

A large body of evidence indicates that rating scales provide meaningful metrics for the expression of these subjective preferences (see ref. 54). Although there have been some challenges to the use of rating scales, most biases can be overcome with the use of just a few simple precautions, such as clear definitions of the end-points and preliminary practise with cases that make the end-points salient.[54]

Standard gamble

Psychometric methods, such as category rating, assess wellness at a particular point in time and do not ask subjects to make trades or to consider aspects of uncertainty. Several methods more explicitly consider decision under uncertainty. The standard gamble offers a choice between two alternatives: choice A – living in a health state with certainty, or choice B – taking a gamble on a new treatment for which the outcome is uncertain. The respondent is told that a hypothetical treatment will lead to perfect health with a probability of p, or immediate death with a probability of $1 - p$. They can choose between remaining in a state that is intermediate between wellness and death or taking the gamble and trying the new treatment. The probability (p) is varied until the subject is indifferent between choices A and B. An example of the standard gamble is shown in Fig. 5.3.

The standard gamble has been attractive because it is based on the axioms of utility theory. The choice between a certain outcome and a gamble conforms to the tasks required for the theory proposed by von Neumann and Morgenstern. Although the interval properties of the data obtained using the gamble have been assumed, they have not been demonstrated empirically.[18] A variety of other problems with the gamble have also become apparent. For example, it has often been stated that the standard gamble has face validity because it approximates choices made by medical patients.[55] However, treatment of most chronic diseases

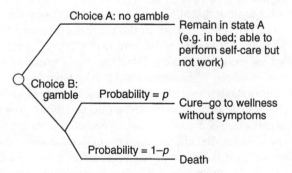

Fig. 5.3 Illustration of the standard gamble. (Adapted from Torrance and Feeny.[30])

does not approximate the gamble. Often there is no product that will make a patient completely well, nor is there one that is likely to kill her or him. In other words, the gambles used in the standard gamble tasks are dissimilar to the decisions that will be required of real patients. Further, the cognitive demands of the task are high.

Time trade-off

The concept of probability is difficult for most respondents and requires the use of visual aids or props to assist in the interview. Thus, an alternative to the standard gamble, which is also consistent with the von Neumann and Morgenstern axioms of choice, uses a trade-off in time. Here, the subject is offered a choice of living for a defined amount of time in perfect health or a variable amount of time in an alternative state that is less desirable. Presumably, all subjects would choose a year of wellness rather than a year with some health problem. However, by reducing the time of wellness and leaving the time in the sub-optimal health state fixed (such as one year), an indifference point can be determined. For example, a subject may rate being in a wheelchair for two years as equivalent to perfect wellness for one year. The time trade-off is theoretically appealing because it is conceptually equivalent to a QALY. However, several studies have questioned whether the tasks can be understood clearly by the average subject. For example, Stiggelbout and colleagues[56] found that many cancer patients are simply unwilling to trade at all.

Theoretical and methodological challenges

There are both theoretical and methodological challenges associated with the application of preference and utility based measures. Often, respondents and patients have a difficult time applying utility based methods. Recently, the task has been aided by new developments in computer software. One excellent example is the U-Titer program. U-Titer was developed as a hypercard stack for the Macintosh. Versions of the program are available to perform category scaling, standard gambles, and time trade-offs. The program was developed by Sumner and has been applied in a variety of studies assessing utilities for problems such as psoriasis[57] and chronic stable angina.[58] In addition to assessing the preferences, the program also records information on the process experienced by the user.[59]

The advantage of the standard gamble and time trade-off methods is that they are clearly linked to economic theory. However, there are also some important disadvantages. For example, Kahneman and Tversky have shown empirically that many of the assumptions that underlie economic measurements of choice are open to challenge.[60] Human information processors do poorly at integrating complex probability information when making decisions that involve risk.[61] Further, economic analysis assumes that choices correspond accurately to the way in which rational people put information together. Anderson[54] has presented evidence suggesting that methods commonly used for economic analysis do not represent the underlying mental processes used in human decision making.

Several papers in the literature have compared utilities for health states as captured by different methods.[34] In general, standard gamble and time trade-off methods give higher values than rating scales in most, but not all studies. In about half of the studies reported, time trade-off yields lower utilities than standard gamble. In one of the earlier studies, Patrick and colleagues[62] found that person trade-off methods gave the same results as rating scales. However, these findings were not confirmed in more recent studies.[33] Magnitude estimation has produced results which are highly variable across studies.[34] The variability of results across studies is hardly surprising. The methods differ substantially in the questions posed to respondents.

It is often assumed that rating scale methods ignore risk information. However, most methods for calculating QALYs using rating data do incorporate risk information. For example, the QWB includes a prognosis dimension. Prognosis is defined as the probability of transition between health states over the course of time. These transitions are empirical. Patients either get better, worse, or remain the same. The probabilities of these different events is determined through follow-up of large numbers of patients. The transitions are not a matter of value or preference. The subjective aspect is the perceived value of the end states. The model considers the value of the outcomes and multiplies by the actual number of events that occurred. Subjective judgements about the likelihood of outcomes are explicitly excluded from the model. In contrast, utility models take attitude toward risk directly into consideration and the weights explicitly reflect these attitudes toward risk. The true transitions between health states are not considered. Such analyses might be most appropriate for individual decision making.

Consider the example of an automobile dealer. The dealer has high demand for a variety of different models of the Ford line and he can sell all of the cars that are delivered. The preference for the product is reflected in the sales price. The actual income to the dealer is the price times the number of cars sold. Probability affects this income only in that it determines the number of each model that is eventually delivered.

Problems in reviewing the literature

In 1993, the US Department of Health and Human Services appointed a multidisciplinary group of methodologists to recommend standardized strategies for the evaluation of health care. The panel, which released its report in 1996,[63] suggested that standardized outcomes analyses be conducted to evaluate the cost-effectiveness of medical care. These analyses require preference-weighted measures of health-related quality of life. Although there has been considerable interest in measuring the cost-effectiveness of treatments, little is known about the validity of general outcomes measures and it is often difficult to choose between different approaches. Some authors have attempted to simplify the task by offering summary tables.

Despite the attractiveness of this approach, there are also some difficulties. In particular, creators of the tables typically examine the names of subscales, rather than the content of the measures. Consider the example of sensory function or loss. According to Table 5.2, sensory functioning is not included in the QWB. The creators of the table came to this conclusion because there is no subscale on the QWB named sensory function. However, the QWB includes symptoms for loss of vision, loss of hearing, impairment of vision (including wearing glasses or contact lenses), problems with taste and smell, and so on. Recently a new self-administered version of the QWB was developed. This is known as the QWB-SA. The development of new forms of the QWB has gone through several stages. First, a new list of symptoms and problems was developed. The interviewer-administered version of the QWB used a list of 26 symptoms or problems. The QWB-SA has 59 symptoms. This improved symptoms assessment not only better reflects health status, it more closely resembles a clinical review of symptoms, thus increasing the clinical utility of the QWB-SA. In fact the newer, self-administered QWB devotes a major portion of the questionnaire to items on sensation and sensory organs. The symptoms include any hearing loss, blindness in one eye, blindness in both eyes, any problems with vision (floaters, double or distorted vision), eye pain, sensitivity to light, ear aches, difficulty in balance, and a variety of others. Indeed, the QWB-SA includes much more content on sensory functioning than do measures that are identified as including content on sensory functioning.

Another example concerns mental health. Summaries, such as Table 5.2, almost always note that the QWB excludes mental health content. Despite widespread interest in the model among practitioners in many different specialties, the concept of a 'quality-adjusted life-year' has received very little attention in the mental health fields. This reflects the widespread belief that mental health and physical health outcomes are conceptually distinct. McHorney and Ware[14] emphasized that mental health and physical health are different constructs and that attempts to measure them using a common measurement strategy is like comparing apples with oranges.

Although many questionnaires include different dimensions, they still may be tapping the same constructs. For example, a measure without a mental health component does not necessarily neglect mental health. Mental health symptoms may be included and the impact of mental health, cognitive functioning, or mental retardation may be represented in questions about role functioning. Some measures have multiple dimensions for mental health symptoms while others include fewer items that ask about problems in general. It is not clear that multiple measures are more capable of detecting clinical differences. This remains an empirical question for systematic analysis. A common strategy is to report outcomes along multiple dimensions.

Several years ago Kaplan and Anderson argued that there are many similarities in mental health and physical health outcomes.[40] The preference and utility based measures that are assumed to ignore mental health include the basic dimensions of observable functioning, symptoms, and duration. Mental health problems, like physical health problems, can be represented by symptoms and by disrupted role functioning. Consider some examples. Suppose that a patient has the primary symptom of a cough. If the cough does not disrupt role function, the preference or utility weighted score might show a small deviation from 1.0. If the cough is more serious and keeps the person at home, the score will be lower. If the cough is very severe, it might limit the person to a hospital and may have serious disruptive effects upon role functioning. This would necessitate an even lower score. Coughs can be of different duration. A cough associated with an acute respiratory infection may have a serious impact on functioning which may last only a short time. This would be indicated by a minor deviation in QALYs. A chronic cough associated with obstructive lung disease would be associated with significant loss of quality-adjusted life-years because duration is a major component of the calculation.

Now consider the case of a person with depression. Depression may be a symptom reported by a patient, just as a cough is reported by other patients. Depression without disruption of role function would cause a minor variation of wellness. If the depression caused the person to stay at home the preference or utility weighted score would be lower. Severe depression might require the person to be in a hospital or special facility and would result in a lower score. Depressions, like coughs, are of different durations. Depression of long duration would cause the loss of more quality-adjusted life-years than would depression of short duration.

The QWB is an example of a measure assumed to exclude mental health. Some evidence supports the validity of the QWB in studies of mental health. One recent study evaluated the validity of the quality of well-being scale (QWB) as an outcome measure for older psychotic patients. Seventy-two psychotic patients and 28 matched controls from the San Diego Veterans Affairs Medical Center completed the QWB, the structured clinical interview for the DSM-III-R patient version (SCID-P), scales for the assessment of positive and negative symptoms (SAPS and SANS), and the global severity index (GSI) from the brief symptom inventory (BSI). The QWB correlated with the SANS -0.52 ($p < 0.001$); with the SAPS -0.57 ($p < 0.001$); and with the GSI -0.62 ($p < 0.001$). Patients and controls were significantly different on the QWB and we identified a linear relationship between QWB and severity of illness (as classified by the SANS and the SAPS). In addition, component scores of the QWB (i.e. mobility, physical activity, social activity, and worst symptom) were significantly lower among patients compared to controls, and declined systematically as psychiatric symptoms increased.[64]

Using the general health policy model, it is possible to estimate the benefit of any health care intervention in terms of the quality-adjusted life-years the treatment produces. Suppose, for example, that a treatment for anxiety elevates patients from a level of 0.65 to a level of 0.75. Suppose, further, that this treatment benefit lasted for one year. Each patient would gain 0.1 QALY ($0.75 - 0.65 = 0.10 \times 1$ year $= 0.1$ QALY) for each year the benefit was observed. The treatment benefit would be expressed in terms of general QALY units. The productivity of the providers could be compared with providers in other areas of health care. All providers in health care use resources. Dividing the cost of a treatment by the QALY productivity provides the cost–utility ratio. Measuring mental health productivity in QALY units would allow the assessment of investments in mental health services to be compared directly with those in other aspects of health care.

Summary

Measurement of quality of life outcomes is becoming increasingly important for clinical trials. A variety of different methods is now available to measure these outcomes. One important distinction is between profiles, which offer multiple scores, and preference or utility measures that attempt to reduce all outcomes to a single summary score. These different methods arise from different academic traditions. Profile measures are derived from psychometric theory and utility based measures are based on statistical decision theory.

Despite the advantage of profiles measures, they are difficult to use in studies of cost-effectiveness and cost–utility analysis. Thus, if the data may ultimately be used for economic analysis, a preference or utility based measure must be given central consideration. Many of the utility based methods can also produce a profile of outcomes. Within utility and preference based measures, there is debate about the most appropriate methods for utility assessment. Economists prefer methods linked to expected utility theory, such as the standard gamble or the time trade-off. Psychologists favour simple rating scale methods. Both camps argue that their approach is theoretically and empirically justified. More research is needed to clarify these issues.

Acknowledgements

Supported, in part, by Grant PO 1-AR-40423 from the National Institute of Arthritis, Musculoskeletal, and Skin Disorders of the National Institutes of Health and by a Scholars Grant from the American Cancer Society.

This chapter was completed while the author was a visiting professor at the Center for Evaluative Clinical Sciences, Dartmouth Medical School, Hanover, New Hampshire.

References

1. Aaronson, N.K., Ahmedzai, S., Bergman, B., Bullinger, M., Cull, A., Duez, N.J., et al. The European Organization for Research and Treatment of Cancer QLQ-C30: a quality-of-life instrument for use in international clinical trials in oncology. *Journal of the National Cancer Institute*, 1993; **85**: 365–76.
2. Shipper, H., Clinch, J., McMurray, A., and Levitt, M. Measuring the quality of life of cancer patients: the functional living index-cancer. *Journal of Clinical Oncology*, 1984; **2**: 472–83.
3. Greer, S. Improving quality of life: adjuvant psychological therapy for patients with cancer. *Support Care Cancer*, 1995; **3**: 248–51.

 4. Ganz, P.A., Schag, C.A.C., and Cheng, H.L. Assessing the quality of life – a study of newly diagnosed breast cancer patients. *Journal of Clinical Epidemiology*, 1990; **43**: 75–86.
 5. Bullinger, M., Anderson, R., Cella, D., and Aaronson, N. Developing and evaluating cross-cultural instruments from minimum requirements to optimal models. *Quality of Life Research*, 1993; **2**: 451–9.
 6. Kaplan, R.M. and Bush, J.W. Health-related quality of life measurement for evaluation research and policy analysis. *Health Psychology*, 1982; **1**: 61–80.
 7. Bergner, M., Babbitt, R.A., Carter, W.B., and Gilson, B.S. The sickness impact profile: development and final revision of a health status measure. *Medical Care*, 1981; **19**: 787–8.
 8. Kaplan, R.M. and Anderson, J.P. The quality of well-being scale: rationale for a single quality of life index. In *Quality of life: assessment and application*, S.R. Walker and R. Rosser (eds). London: MTP Press, 1988, pp. 51–77.
 9. Chambers, L.W. The McMaster health index questionnaire. In *Quality of life: assessment and application*, S.R. Walker and R. Rosser (eds). London: MTP Press, 1988.
10. World Health Organization. *Constitution of the World Health Organization*. Geneva: WHO Basic Documents, 1988.
11. Katz, S.T., Downs, H., Cash, H., and Grotz, R. Progress and development of an index of EDL. *Gerontologist*, 1970; **10**: 20–30.
12. Holmes, T.S. and Rahe, R.H. The social readjustment rating scale. *Journal of Psychosomatic Research*, 1967; **11**: 213–18.
13. Haley, S.M., McHorney, C.A., and Ware, J.E.J. Evaluation of the MOS SF-36 physical functioning scale (PF-10): I. Unidimensionality and reproducibility of the Rasch item scale. *Journal of Clinical Epidemiology*, 1994; **47**: 671–84.
14. McHorney, C.A. and Ware, J.E. Construction and validation of an alternate form general mental health scale for the medical outcomes study short-form 36-item health survey. *Medical Care*, 1995; **33**: 15–28.
15. McEwen, J. The Nottingham health profile. In *Quality of life assessment: key issues for the 1990s*, S.R. Walker and R.M. Rosser (eds). Dordrecht, The Netherlands: Kluwer, 1992.
16. Froberg, D.G. and Kane, R.L. Methodology for measuring health state preferences I: measurement strategies. *Journal of Clinical Epidemiology*, 1989; **42**: 345–52.
17. Froberg, D.G. and Kane, R.L. Methodology for measuring health state preferences II: scaling methods. *Journal of Clinical Epidemiology*, 1989; **42**: 459–71.
18. Froberg, D.G. and Kane, R.L. Methodology for measuring health state preferences III: population and context effects. *Journal of Clinical Epidemiology*, 1989; **42**: 585–92.
19. Froberg, D.G. and Kane, R.L. Methodology for measuring health state preferences IV: progress and a research agenda. *Journal of Clinical Epidemiology*, 1989; **42**: 675–85.
20. Revicki, D.A. and Kaplan, R.M. Relationship between psychometric and utility-based approaches to the measurement of health-related quality of life. *Quality of Life Research*, 1993; **2**: 477–87.
21. Russell, L.B., Gold, M.R., Siegel, J.E., Daniels, N., *et al*. The role of cost-effectiveness analysis in health and medicine. *Journal Of The American Medical Association*, 1996; **76**: 1172–7.

22. Weinstein, M.C., Siegel, J.E., Gold, M.R., Kamlet, M.S., *et al.* Recommendations of the panel on cost-effectiveness in health and medicine. *Journal Of The American Medical Association*, 1996; **276**: 1253–8.

23. Fanshel, S. and Bush, J.W. A health-status index and its applications to health-services outcomes. *Operations Research*, 1970; **18**: 1021–66.

24. Torrance, G.W. Social preferences for health states. An empirical evaluation of three measurement techniques. *Socio-Economic Planning Sciences*, 1976; **10**: 129–36.

25. von Neumann, J. and Morgenstern, O. *Theory of games and economic behavior*, Princeton, N.J.: Princeston University Press, 1944.

26. Raiffa, H. *Decision analysis: introductory lectures on choices under uncertainty*. Reading, MA: Addison-Wesley, 1968.

27. Bell, D.ωE. and Farquhar, P.H. Perspectives on utility theory. *Operations Research*, 1986; **34**: 179–83.

28. Howard, R.A. Decision analysis: practice and promise. *Management Science*, 1988; **34**: 679–95.

29. Cohen, B.J. Assigning values to intermediate health states for cost–utility analysis. Theory and practice. *Medical Decision Making*, 1996; **16**: 376–85.

30. Torrance, G.W. and Feeny, D. Utilities in quality-adjusted life years. *International Journal of Technology Assessment in Health Care*, 1989; **5**: 559–75.

31. Bator, F.M. The simple analytics of welfare maximization. *American Economic Review*, 1957; **47**: 22–59.

32. Arrow, K.J. *Social choice and individual values*. New York: Wiley, 1951.

33. Nord, E. Health status index models for use in resource allocation decisions. A critical review in the light of observed preferences for social choice. *International Journal of Technology Assessment in Health Care*, 1996; **12**: 31–44.

34. Nord, E. Methods for quality adjustment of life years. *Social Science and Medicine*, 1992; **34**: 559–69.

35. Keeney, R.L. A group preference axiomatization with cardinal utility. *Management Sciences*, 1976; **23**: 140–5.

36. Kaplan, R.M. The Ziggy theorem: toward an outcomes-focused health psychology. *Health Psychology*, 1994; **13**: 451–60.

37. Kaplan, R.M. and Anderson, J.P. The general health policy model: an integrated approach. In *Quality of life assessments in clinical trials*, B. Spilker (ed.). New York: Raven, 1990, pp. 131–49.

38. Kaplan, R.M. An outcomes-based model for directing decisions in women's health care. *Clinical Obstetrics and Gynecology*, 1994; **37**: 192–206.

39. Kaplan, R.M., Bush, J.W., and Berry, C.C. Health status: types of validity and the index of well-being. *Health services Research*, 1976; **11**: 478–507.

40. Kaplan, R.M. and Anderson, J.P. A general health policy model: update and applications. *Health Services Research*, 1988; **23**: 203–34.

41. Kaplan, R.M. and Anderson, J.P. The quality of well-being scale: rationale for a single quality of life index. In *Quality of life: assessment and application*, S.R. Walker and R. Rosser (eds). London: MTP Press, 1988, pp. 51–77.

42. Kaplan, R.M., Bush, J.W., and Berry, C.C. Health status index: category rating versus magnitude estimation for measuring levels of well-being. *Medical Care*, 1979; **17**: 501–25.

43. Kaplan, R.M. Human preference measurement for health decisions and the evaluation of long-term care. In *Values and long-term care*, R.L. Kane and R.A. Kane (eds). Lexington, MA: Lexington Books, 1982, pp. 157–88.

44. Kaplan, R.M. Quality of life assessment for cost/utility studies in cancer. *Cancer Treatment Reviews*, 1993; **19** (Suppl. A): 85–96.

45. Erickson, P., Kendall, E.A., Anderson, J.P., and Kaplan, R.M. Using composite health status measures to assess the nation's health. *Medical Care*, 1989; **27** (Suppl. 3): S66–76.

46. Torrance, G.W. Utility approach to measuring health-related quality of life. *Journal of Chronic Diseases*, 1987; **40**: 593–600.

47. Feeny, D., Furlong, W., Boyle, M., and Torrance, G.W. Multi-attribute health status classification systems: health utilities index. *Pharmaco Economics*, 1995; **7**: 490–502.

48. Torrance, G.W., Feeny, D.H., Furlong, W.J., Barr, R.D., Zhang, Y., and Wang, Q. Multiattribute utility function for a comprehensive health status classification system. Health utilities index mark 2. *Medical Care*, 1996; **34**: 702–22.

49. Kaplan, R.M. Value judgment in the Oregon Medicaid experiment. *Medical Care*, 1994; **32**: 975–88.

50. Brazier, J., Jones, N., and Kind, P. Testing the validity of the EuroQoL and comparing it with the SF-36 health survey questionnaire. *Quality of Life Research*, 1993; **2**: 169–80.

51. Erickson, P. Modeling health-related quality of life: the bridge between psychometric and utility-based measures. *Journal of the National Cancer Institute Monograph*, 1996; **20**: 17–22.

52. Fryback, D.G., Lawrence, W.F., Martin, P.A., Klein, R., *et al*. Predicting quality of well-being scores from the SF-36: results from the Beaver Dam health outcomes study. *Medical Decision Making*, 1997; **17**: 1–9.

53. Weinstein, M.C. and Stason, W.B. Foundations of cost-effectiveness analysis for health and medical practice. *New England Journal of Medicine*, 1977; **296**: 716–21.

54. Anderson, N.H. *Contributions to information integration theory*, Volumes 1–3, Hillsdale, NJ: Lawrence Erlbaum, 1991.

55. Mulley, A.J. Assessing patient's utilities: can the ends justify the means? *Medical Care*, 1989; **27**: S269–81.

56. Stiggelbout, A.M., Kiebert, G.M., Kievit, J., Leer, J.W., Habbema, J.D., and De Haes, J.C. The 'utility' of the time trade-off method in cancer patients: feasibility and proportional trade-off. *Journal of Clinical Epidemiology*, 1995; **48**: 1207–14.

57. Zug, K.A., Littenberg, B., Baughman, R.D., Kneeland, T., Nease, R.F., Sumner, W., *et al*. Assessing the preferences of patients with psoriasis. A quantitative, utility approach. *Archives of Dermatology*, 1995; **131**: 561–8.

58. Nease, R.F. Jr, Kneeland, T., O'Connor, G.T., Sumner, W., Lumpkins, C., Shaw, L., *et al*. Ischemic heart disease patient outcomes research team. Variation in patient utilities for outcomes of the management of chronic stable angina. Implications for clinical practice guidelines. *Journal of the American Medical Association*, 1995; **273**: 1185–90.

59. Sumner, W., Nease, R., and Litterberg, B. U-titer: a utility assessment tool. In *Proceedings of the Annual Symposium on Computer Applications in Medical Care*, 1991; pp. 701–5.

60. Kahneman, D. and Tversky, A. Choices, values, and frames. *American Psychologist*, 1983; **39**: 341–50.
61. Kahneman, D., Slovic, P., and Tversky, A. (eds) *Judgments under uncertainty: heuristics and bisases*. Cambridge, UK: Cambridge University Press, 1982.
62. Patrick, D.L., Bush, J.W., and Chen, M.M. Methods for measuring levels of well-being for a health status index. *Health Services Research*, 1973; 8228–45.
63. Gold, M.R., Siegel, J.E., Russel, L.B., and Weinstein, M.C. *Cost-effectiveness in health and medicine*. New York: Oxford University Press, 1996.
64. Patterson, T.L., Kaplan, R.M., Grant, I., Semple, S.J., *et al*. Quality of well-being in late-life psychosis. *Psychiatry Research*, 1996; **63**: 169–81.

III

Decision theory and preference assessment

6 *Introduction to decision theory and utilities*

Frank A. Sonnenberg

Introduction

Physicians are called upon to make dozens of decisions each day, including decisions to order diagnostic tests, to start or stop treatment, to change treatment, or to admit patients to the hospital. Most of these decisions are made easily, almost reflexively, because the diagnosis is obvious, and the chosen treatment is efficacious and without major risks. However, many other situations exist for which the correct decision is not obvious; for example, when there is more than the usual uncertainty about the diagnosis, when the possible tests or treatments are risky, when available treatments have uncertain benefit, or when there are significant trade-offs involved in all available choices. It is common in such cases for significant disagreement to take place among clinicians, even those called in as expert consultants, regarding the appropriate course of action. It is in such cases that decision analysis can provide additional insights. Also, increasingly, physicians are under pressure to practice medicine cost-effectively. This requires selecting clinical strategies that provide the greatest benefit from expended resources.

Decision analysis is a formal process for comparing available alternative strategies by delineating the relevant clinical events, determining the probability of each event, assigning a value (utility) to each outcome, and calculating an *expected utility*, which is the average utility expected if the decision were made repeatedly with a large number of identical patients. When decision analyses include costs, they can project the 'cost-effectiveness' of a clinical strategy; the additional benefit expected from an incremental expenditure of financial resources.

Detailed tutorials[1,2] and reviews[3,4] of decision analysis have been published. The purpose of this chapter is to describe

(1) the theoretical basis of decision analysis;

(2) trends in modelling and analysis techniques;

(3) what information can be obtained from a decision analysis;

(4) how subjective quality of life (utilities) can be measured and incorporated into an analysis; and

(5) how decision models are used in health economic analyses.

History of decision analysis

Decision analysis has its origins in the field of operations research and was initially applied to industrial problems. Ledley and Lusted, in a landmark paper, first proposed the use of decision analysis for medical applications in 1959[5] but it did not achieve prominence in the medical literature until the late 1970s. At that time, the Society for Medical Decision Making and its journal *Medical Decision Making* were founded to provide a scientific forum for advancement of decision-making techniques. In the mid-1980s, the Association of American Medical Colleges recommended adding decision analysis to the medical curriculum[6] and an editorial in the *New England Journal of Medicine* called for teaching it as a basic clinical skill.[7] It has also been applied successfully to individual patient cases as a consultative service,[8] but such use requires a readily available cadre of skilled analysts and has not been replicated elsewhere. However, decision analysis has been increasingly applied to health care policy and guideline development and studies employing it are frequently published in the medical literature.

Theoretical basis of decision analysis

Ron Howard, of Strategic Decisions Group of Menlo Park, California, defines decision analysis as a quantitative technique that 'specifies the alternatives, information and preferences of the decision maker and then finds the logically implied decision'.[9] In this definition, alternatives are the choices available to the decision maker, information consists of knowledge of the relevant events, and their probabilities and preferences are utilities, measures of the desirability of various outcomes to the decision maker. A decision is 'logically implied' when it is one which results in the greatest *expected utility*. The process of decision analysis uses a *decision model* that provides a computational basis for determining the expected utility of each available choice.

Expected utility is defined in terms of lotteries and utilities. A lottery (Fig. 6.1) is a chance event with two mutually exclusive and collectively exhaustive outcomes, each occurring with a specified probability. When each outcome is assigned a numeric value, the *expected value* of the lottery is the weighted average of the values of the two outcomes, found by multiplying each by its probability and

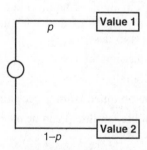

Fig. 6.1 A Simple lottery.

summing the products. One is said to 'own' the lottery when one is committed to experience one 'play' of the lottery with its attendant uncertainty and to live with the consequences. When the values assigned are *utilities*, the expected value is known as the *expected utility* and it is axiomatic that the expected utility is equal to the value of the lottery. However, expected utility is not necessarily equivalent to expected value because of the element of risk. A lottery with a given expected value is, in general, worth less than a certain outcome with the same value because most people will give up a certain amount of value in order to avoid risk. An important and prototypical example of this principle is the premium that people are willing to pay for insurance. They are trading money with a certain value in order to remove the risk of losing a larger amount of money. Risk is relevant to utility assessment as discussed below.

Decision analysis is a *normative* (prescriptive) technique. It specifies what choice, from among a list of alternatives, should be made. It is not a descriptive technique and does not specify how decisions usually *are* made by clinicians. Decision analysis is based on several *axioms of rational behaviour*. In their original form[10] these axioms are quite tedious and complex. However, each may be paraphrased in a simple and intuitive manner as follows.

1. Preferences for outcomes exist and can be ordered. The quantitative measure of the desirability of an outcome is known as its utility.

2. Given a choice between two simple lotteries (only two outcomes for each), a rational decision maker will always prefer the lottery with the greater chance of the prize.

3. The preference for an intermediate outcome may be quantified by determining the probability (of achieving the best possible outcome in a simple lottery between best and worst outcomes) at which the decision maker is indifferent between ownership of the lottery and ownership of the intermediate outcome.

4. Preferences are transitive: a logical decision maker who prefers A to B and B to C, will prefer A to C.

5. The 'substitution principle': if a decision maker is indifferent between two outcomes, his or her solution to a decision problem cannot be affected by substitution of one of these outcomes for another.

6. A decision maker's preferences among the consequences of a decision should not be affected by knowledge as to whether he or she merely may or certainly will have to make the decision.

Note that these are axioms, not empirical facts. Utilities are defined in such a way that these axioms hold true. Given these axioms, the best decision is one yielding the highest expected utility when alternatives are compared using a decision model.

Steps in the decision analytic process

The steps in a decision analysis are illustrated in Fig. 6.2. The steps of constructing, evaluating, and interpreting the model are done iteratively as the

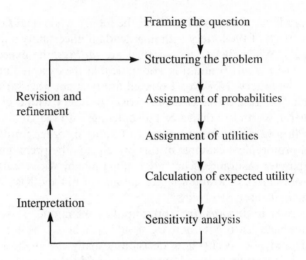

Fig. 6.2 The decision analysis cycle.

evaluation and sensitivity analysis reveal insights or shortcomings in the model which lead to progressive refinement. The individual steps are as follows.

Framing the question

The question for analysis must be a specific choice among available options. A vague question such as 'What should one do?' is not specific enough to permit analysis. The question must delineate the alternative strategies (sequence of tests and treatments) including contingencies (e.g. what will be done following a positive test) and the basis for comparing them (e.g. quality-adjusted life expectancy, five-year survival, and/or financial costs).

Structuring the problem

The next step is to structure the problem by constructing a decision model which may take one of several forms including a decision tree, influence diagram, Markov process, or simulation model. The choice of model reflects a compromise between clinical realism and available data and must be appropriate to the clinical setting. For example, the model must not use such a fine level of detail that the necessary probabilities cannot be supplied. Clinical problems with recurrent risk or for which the timing of events influences their utility cannot be represented adequately by simple decision trees and require Markov models or simulation models.[11]

A *simple tree* (Fig. 6.3) represents each choice as the branch of a decision node (filled square). The example shown is a choice between empiric therapy, (diagnostic) testing, and observation (no testing and no treatment). Chance nodes (open circles) represent sets of possible alternative events that are not subject to the control of the decision maker. In the example shown, the chance events are

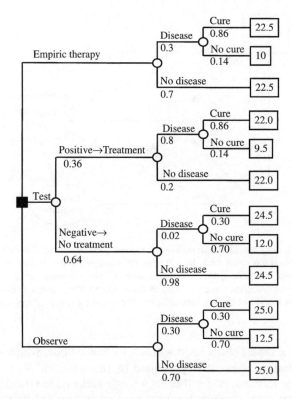

Fig. 6.3 Decision tree. The decision node is represented by a filled square, chance nodes by open circles, and terminal nodes by rectangles containing numbers which represent utilities. The name of each branch appears above it; the probability of each branch of a chance node appears below the branch.

the presence of disease and the occurrence of cure, which may be spontaneous. The branches of chance nodes must represent mutually exclusive outcomes which are collectively exhaustive; that is, they must cover the entire range of outcomes possible for a given event. Thus, the probabilities of the branches (appearing just below each branch in Fig. 6.3) must sum to unity. The terminal nodes (represented by rectangular boxes) represent final outcomes of interest, each comprising a unique combination of actions and chance outcomes. Each terminal node must be assigned a utility (in this case a quality-adjusted life expectancy, measured in years) which appears as an expression within the box. The determination of utilities will be discussed in detail, below.

Influence diagrams are an alternate graphical representation of decision models.[9] An influence diagram depicting the same model as in Fig. 6.3 is shown in Fig. 6.4. Influence diagrams contain decision nodes (represented by rectangles) and chance nodes (represented as ellipses) as in decision trees. However, there are no branches; alternative events are represented as a joint probability distribution

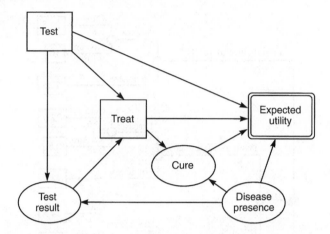

Fig. 6.4 Influence diagram. Decision nodes are represented by rectangular boxes, chance nodes by ellipses, and the value node by a double rounded rectangle. Arrows into decision nodes represent information available at the time the decision is made; arrows into chance nodes represent factors that influence the probability of the outcome of the chance node; arrows into the value node represent factors that influence the value (or utility) of the outcome.

(in the form of a table), associated with each chance node, which specifies every possible combination of events represented by the node and its predecessors. In place of multiple terminal nodes there is a single *value* node (the double rounded rectangle in Fig. 6.4) associated with a table that specifies its value for every combination of its predecessors. Arrows connecting nodes specify the flow of information in the model. Arrows leading into a decision node indicate information that is available at the time the decision is made. For example, in the diagram shown in Fig. 6.4, arrows into the decision node 'Treat' indicate that the test decision and the test result are known at the time the treatment decision is made. Arrows leading into chance nodes are influences on the probabilities of events represented by that node. In this case, the test decision (which test is performed) and the presence of disease influence the probability of each test result. The treatment decision and the presence of disease influence the probability of cure. All nodes, except the test result, influence the value node since the disease, the test, and the treatment may be associated with morbidity or cost.

It is important to realize that influence diagrams are semantically equivalent to decision trees.[12] A decision tree and the corresponding influence diagram will result in identical expected utilities; they are merely different representations. The advantages of influence diagrams are that they provide a more compact graphical representation, a more explicit representation of probabilistic dependencies, and freedom for the analyst to assess conditional probabilities in the most intuitive direction.[13] For example, in an influence diagram one can assess the probability of a given test result given the presence of disease, whereas in a decision tree the analyst may have to specify directly the probability of disease given the test result, which may be less intuitive or require calculations to apply Bayes' rule.[14] Evaluation of influence diagrams may be carried out using a number of computer based algorithms[12,15] which automatically perform the Bayesian inference required to convert probabilities to the form needed for the analysis. The major limitation of influence diagrams is the lack of a direct equivalent of Markov models (see below). They are thus best suited to models that can be represented as simple trees.

The simple tree has a number of limitations. First, the structure generally represents each clinical event only once whereas in many clinical situations (e.g. recurrent episodes of infection, myocardial infarction, or risk of stroke) events may happen more than once. The timing of the event may be variable, but representation of an event as the branch of a chance node requires choosing a single representative time. Also, the utility of an event may depend on timing, as for example when discounting is considered. Continuous risk and explicit timing of events can be represented by Markov models.[16]

Assignment of probabilities

Sources of probabilities include reports in the medical literature, mathematical models, and expert opinion. One of the greatest practical barriers to application of decision analysis is that the probabilities of the events of interest either are not available in the literature at all, or are not applicable to the patient at hand because the published figures apply to patients with different characteristics. Often, probabilities can be adapted to the patient for whom the analysis is done, by means of mathematical models of disease and survival, multivariate logistic regression analysis,[17,18] and Bayesian 'belief nets' which use a graphical representation of variables and their probabilistic interdependencies.[19-21] For some situations, particularly those highly dependent on individual patient characteristics, only expert opinion is available as an estimate of important probabilities.

While critics claim that the lack of highly accurate estimates of probabilities is a fatal flaw in applied decision analysis, it must be said that the same limitations apply to medical decision making using any other method. Practitioners of decision analysis must, however, avoid the pitfall of placing undue confidence on their probability estimates. Sensitivity analysis determines the effect of uncertainty in these estimates.

Assignment of utilities

The final step in the construction of the decision model is the assignment of values (utilities) to health states. The term 'utility' is somewhat misleading because the measure has nothing to do with the usefulness of a health state. Utility is a measure of *desirability* or *preference* and that distinguishes it from other types of health status measures.[22] Early applications of decision analysis in the medical literature relied on arbitrary utility scales (e.g. numbers from 0 to 100).[2,23] However, these quantities were hard to assign and to interpret and were quickly abandoned in favour of measures based on life expectancy.[24] Quality of life is often an important factor in medical decisions and may be incorporated into a utility measure by weighting each interval of survival according to its quality (a number between 0 and 1) yielding quality-adjusted life expectancy.[24] When financial costs are important to an analysis, they may also be incorporated into the model by creating a second 'utility structure'[25] based on costs. The model is evaluated twice; once using the health based utilities to yield the expected utility of each strategy and the second time using the financial costs to yield the expected cost of each strategy.

Utilities may be measured by means of one of several techniques.[22] The first technique, referred to as the *categorical* or *rating scale* (Fig. 6.5) uses a line with end-points marking the best and worst possible health states at the top and bottom of the scale, respectively. The subject is asked to place the health state for which the utility is being measured (the intermediate state) somewhere between these two extremes.

The second method, which is most true to decision theory, is the *standard gamble* (SG) or *reference lottery* technique (Fig. 6.6). The subject is presented with a hypothetical choice between the health state being assessed (the intermediate state), and a lottery (represented by the chance node with two branches on the right side of Fig. 6.6). The lottery provides a chance with a variable probability p of the best outcome (perfect health) and the complementary chance $(1-p)$ of the worst health outcome. The value of p for which the subject is indifferent to the choice is equal to the utility of the intermediate health state. The SG is analogous to asking 'What probability of dying from surgery would you accept if the surgery would be guaranteed to restore you to perfect health if you survived?'.

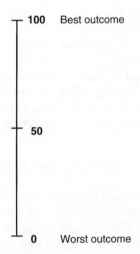

Fig. 6.5   Rating scale. The best possible outcome (usually perfect health) is arbitrarily assigned a value of 100; the worst possible outcome (usually death) is arbitrarily assigned a value of zero. Subjects mark the scale at a point corresponding to their estimated rating of a third state of health that is (by definition) intermediate to the best and worst states.

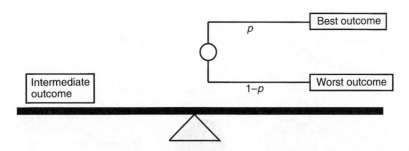

Fig. 6.6 Standard gamble. Also referred to as the 'reference lottery', offers a hypothetical choice between having a specific intermediate health state with certainty, represented by the rectangle on the left and a *lottery* which signifies that the patient has a chance of achieving the best health outcome with probability p and the worst outcome with probability $1-p$. The value of p for which the subject is indifferent to the choice is, by definition, the utility of the intermediate health state.

The worse the health state, the higher is the probability of dying from surgery that would be acceptable in order to restore health.

Figure 6.7 shows application of the SG to measure the utility of current health in a 60 year old man with class III angina. Angina is represented by shaded circles; perfect health by a white pie slice; and death by a black pie slice. The size of each slice is proportional to the probability of the corresponding outcome. Choices 1 and 2 are extreme and are presented primarily to serve as anchor points and to ensure that the subject understands the process. Choice 1 is between a certainty of angina (staying as he is) and a gamble with a 100 per cent chance of perfect health. Obviously, the patient would choose the gamble. Choice 2 is between angina and a gamble with a 100 per cent chance of immediate death. Unless the angina is worse than death, the patient would choose to stay as he is. Subsequent choices are presented until the patient is indifferent to the two alternatives.

Choice 3 is between angina and a gamble with a 95 per cent chance of perfect health and a 5 per cent chance of death. This is equivalent to accepting a 5 per cent chance of dying during coronary bypass graft surgery to correct the angina. Choosing the gamble here indicates that the utility of angina is less than 0.95. Choice 4 is the reverse of choice 3 and is between angina and a gamble with only a 5 per cent chance of perfect health. Choice 5 is between angina and a gamble with a 90 per cent chance of perfect health. If the patient is indifferent to this choice, then the utility of angina is about 0.9. If the patient definitely prefers angina, then the utility is somewhere between 0.9 and 0.95. The process of alternating high and low probabilities of the best outcomes is referred to as the 'ping pong' approach. It helps the subject by initially presenting extreme choices that are easy and then gradually approaching the indifference probability from both sides.

In the *time trade-off* (TTO),[26] the subject is presented with a choice between the intermediate health state with a fixed survival time and the best possible health for a shorter survival time t which is varied (Fig. 6.8). As for the SG, there is a value of t for which the subject would be indifferent to the choice. The percentage

Angina   Gamble

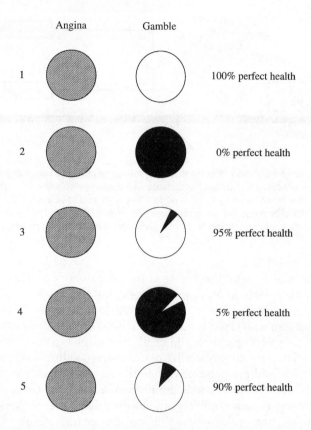

1   100% perfect health

2   0% perfect health

3   95% perfect health

4   5% perfect health

5   90% perfect health

Fig. 6.7 Illustration of the standard gamble. Five choices are presented to a subject in sequence. Each choice consists of a shaded circle representing the health state of angina. The gamble is represented by a pie chart in which the size of the white area is proportional to the probability of perfect health and the size of the black area is proportional to the probability of death.

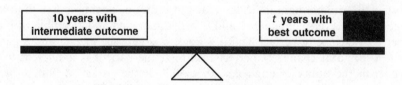

Fig. 6.8 Time trade-off. Analogous to the reference lottery, offers a hypothetical choice between having an intermediate health state with a normal life expectancy (10 years, in this example) represented by the rectangle on the left and having the best health outcome for a shorter period, designated as t. When the subject is indifferent to the choice, the fraction of normal life-expectancy represented by t is the utility of the intermediate health state.

of life expectancy represented by *t* is equal to the utility for the intermediate state. The TTO is analogous to asking subjects 'How much of your remaining life expectancy would you be willing to give up if you could be restored to perfect health?'. The worse the intermediate state, the more time a patient would be willing to forgo.

Figure 6.9 shows a detailed illustration of the TTO technique. Consider the same subject, a 60 year old man with class III angina. We estimate that the patient has

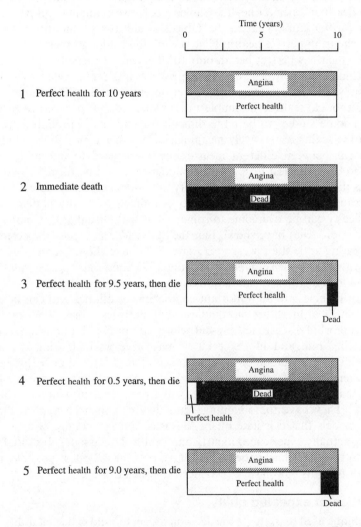

Fig. 6.9 Illustration of the time trade-off. Five choices are presented in sequence. Each consists of a pair of bars. The shaded bars represents the outcome of angina with a survival of 10 years. The other bar (filled or open) presents a shortened survival, but with perfect health. The length of the white bar is proportional to the length of survival in perfect health; the length of the black bar is proportional to the survival time forfeited by the trade-off.

a life expectancy of about 10 years. For the TTO, the subject is presented with a choice represented by two rectangular bars between angina (with a survival of 10 years) and perfect health, but with a varied survival time. As before, choices 1 and 2 are extreme. Choice 1 is between angina for 10 years and perfect health for 10 years. Obviously, the subject will choose perfect health. Choice 2 is between angina for 10 years and immediate death. Obviously, the subject would choose angina unless angina is considered worse than death. However, the previous ranking of states has already determined that Angina is an outcome intermediate between death and perfect health. Choice 3 is between angina and perfect health, but only for 9.5 years. That is, the subject would lose six months of life expectancy by choosing perfect health. If he prefers the trade-off, then he is faced with choice 4 which has perfect health only for 0.5 year. If the subject reaches choice 5, and is indifferent between angina and perfect health for 9.0 years, then the utility of Angina would be 0.9, the same answer obtained by the SG technique.

The categorical scale is the simplest to understand, but paradoxically, has been shown in some studies to be more difficult for patients,[27] probably because the units on the scale are relatively meaningless. Another major shortcoming is that comparisons between different measurements are hard to interpret. The TTO appears to be the easiest for patients to understand and perform.[27] By definition, the SG is the criterion standard for utility measurement but is more difficult than TTO because the concept of probability is difficult for many patients to grasp. This difficulty can be overcome to some extent with visual aids. Comparisons of the three approaches have shown that the SG yields the highest expected utilities and the rating scale the lowest.[28] SG and TTO have shown acceptable reproducibility with repeat measurements and the TTO shows acceptable validity when compared to the criterion standard SG.

Life expectancies are an important component of utilities and can be obtained from the medical literature or standard vital statistics tables.[29] When combinations of comorbid diseases are present which do not match published studies, the net mortality rate and life expectancy may be estimated using the declining exponential approximation of life expectancy (DEALE)[30,31] or by projecting the patient's remaining lifetime using a Markov[32] or simulation model.

Utility based health status measures have been used in a number of clinical trials.[33,34] They have the advantage that they can then be applied directly to decision models that calculate quality-adjusted life expectancy. Because patients who have actually experienced a particular health state assign substantially higher utilities to the state than patients who have not[35] it is best, if possible, to assess utilities of patients who have experienced that health state.

Calculation of expected utility

The technique used to evaluate the decision model to yield expected utility depends on the type of model but, in almost all cases, is carried out using computer software.[36] The result is an expected utility for each strategy for the health outcome component of the model and an expected cost of each strategy for the economic component. Simulation models may also yield estimated rates of events.

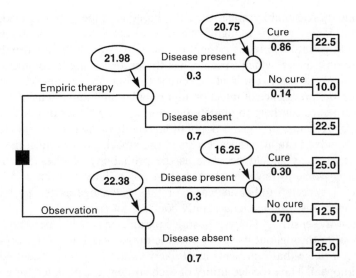

Fig. 6.10 Decision tree evaluation. Ellipses containing numbers represent the expected utilities of chance nodes. The expected utility of the chance node following the topmost branch labelled 'disease present' is equal to the sum of the products of the utility of each branch multiplied by the probability of the branch. In this case, the expected utility 20.75 is obtained from $(22.5 \times 0.86) + (10.0 \times 0.14)$.

Trees are evaluated by a process referred to as 'averaging out and folding back' or simply, 'folding back' a decision tree,[37] illustrated in Fig. 6.10. The expected utility of each terminal node is its associated utility. The expected utility of any branch is the expected utility of the node following the branch. The expected utility of a chance node is the sum of the products formed by multiplying the expected utility of each branch by the probability of the branch. Finally, the expected utility of a decision node is equal to that of the branch with the highest expected utility. For example, in Fig. 6.10, the expected utility of the decision node is equal to the expected utility of the 'observation' branch, since the expected utility is higher than that for the 'empiric therapy' branch. While 'folding back' requires nothing more than multiplication and addition, it can involve a large number of calculations and therefore cannot practically be done by hand for any but the smallest trees.

Sensitivity analysis

The original results of evaluating the decision model are often referred to as the 'baseline' or 'base case' analysis because all parameters in the model are set at their baseline values. In sensitivity analysis, the values of one or more parameters are varied systematically through a range and the expected utilities are calculated for each combination of values. The main purpose of sensitivity analysis is to determine the extent to which reasonable variations in the values of parameters affect the recommended decision. If a variable has no effect on a decision throughout its reasonable range, then the baseline value is not critical. On the other hand, if an analysis is highly sensitive to the value of a parameter, more effort should go into its precise estimation. Sensitivity analysis can also determine the conditions under which specific health strategies are recommended. For example, the cost-effectiveness of screening for human immunodeficiency virus depends on the prevalence of infection in a population[38] and a sensitivity analysis on the prevalence can help to guide a decision about whether or not to initiate a screening programme in a given population. The behaviour of the model during sensitivity analysis can also reveal errors in the model. For example, the expected utility of a strategy should decrease as the probability of disease is increased, because it is worse to have the disease than not to have it, even if it is treated optimally. If expected utility increases or fails to change as the probability of disease is increased, the model certainly contains an error.

In a one-way sensitivity analysis, a single parameter (the independent variable) is varied either throughout its entire possible range (e.g. 0 to 1 for a probability) or through a range that represents most likely values (e.g. 95 per cent confidence limits, if known). The expected utility of each strategy is calculated for each value of the independent variable. A one-way sensitivity analysis on the probability of disease for the decision tree from Fig. 6.3 is illustrated in Fig. 6.11. As expected, when the probability of disease is zero, 'observe' should have a higher expected utility than either 'test' or 'treat'. At intermediate probabilities the 'test' strategy is favoured. When the probability of disease is unity, 'treat' should have the

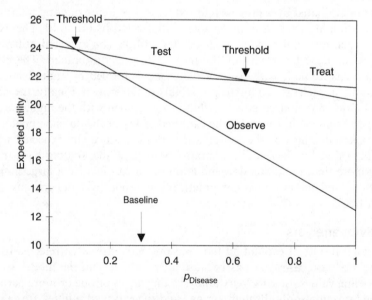

Fig. 6.11 One-way sensitivity analysis. Each line represents a plot of the expected utility (represented by the vertical axis) of one of three strategies while the probability of disease, $p_{Disease}$ (represented by the horizontal axis), is varied from zero to one. The point at which two of the lines cross is a *decision threshold*. The baseline value of $p_{Disease}$ is marked on the graph.

highest expected utility. The points at which two expected utility curves cross are referred to as a *decision thresholds*.[39]

In a two-way analysis, two variables are varied simultaneously. There are two ways in which the results can be expressed. One is simply to calculate the expected utility for each combination of values. The result can be summarized in a table. However, the graph of such an analysis would contain several series of lines and would be quite confusing. An alternative method calculates the threshold of one variable for each value of the second variable. This type of analysis can be plotted as a series of curves, each comparing only two strategies. When threshold lines are plotted for all combinations of two strategies, the plane of the graph will be divided into multiple regions as shown in Fig. 6.12, each corresponding to a preferred strategy. In Fig. 6.12 at the point corresponding to the baseline values of both parameters, 'Test' is the preferred strategy. This is a particularly convenient form for presenting the results of an analysis when two key parameters describe the population (e.g. age and prevalence of disease). A consumer of the analysis can simply find the point corresponding to a combination of interest and note the recommended strategy.

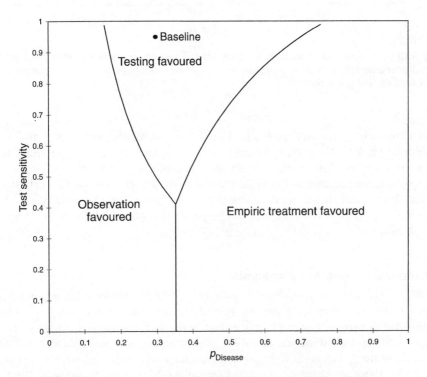

Fig. 6.12 Two-way sensitivity analysis. For each value of the probability of disease ($p_{Disease}$, represented by the horizontal axis) the threshold value of a second variable, test sensitivity (represented by the vertical axis), is plotted. The resulting lines divide the plane of the graph into three regions, each favouring one of the three strategies 'observation' 'testing', and 'empiric treatment'.

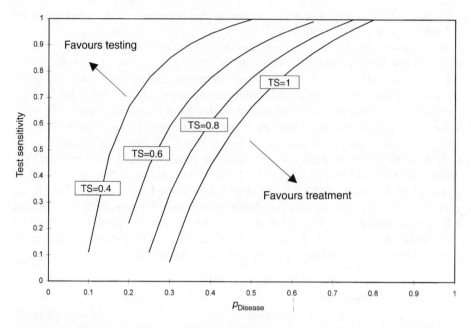

Fig. 6.13   Three-way sensitivity analysis. Each line is a two-way analysis indicating thresholds between 'test' and 'treat' at different values of $p_{Disease}$. Each line represents a different value of a third variable, test specificity (TS).

A three-way sensitivity analysis (Fig. 6.13) essentially performs a two-way threshold analysis for each of several values of a third variable. The result is a series of threshold lines which divide the plane of the graph differently for each value of a third parameter. Points above and to the left of each line favour testing; points below and to the right of the line favour treatment. Sensitivity analyses varying more than three variables can be performed but are difficult to represent graphically.

Monte Carlo sensitivity analysis

Monte Carlo sensitivity analysis[40] evaluates a decision model a large number of times (typically several thousand), permitting key variables to vary randomly within the constraints of probability distributions. Thus, each evaluation has a slightly different combination of values of parameters. The mean expected utility of each strategy will be exactly the same as for an ordinary sensitivity analysis. However, there are three main advantages of the Monte Carlo analysis. First, it permits quantifying the uncertainty in estimates of key parameters by representing them as probability distributions (e.g. with defined 95 per cent, confidence intervals) thus recognizing that not all values in the range used for sensitivity analysis are equally likely. Second, the analysis can vary all parameters in the model simultaneously, thus providing an 'all way' sensitivity analysis. Third, Monte Carlo analysis provides a distribution of the expected utilities (Fig. 6.14), thus quantifying the uncertainty in the difference in expected utilities between strategies and estimating the likelihood that the preferred strategy would actually yield a better outcome for a randomly selected patient.

There are several difficulties with Monte Carlo analysis. Except for unusual circumstances where values are based on primary data, the distributions representing parameters are not known and must be estimated using theoretical properties of distributions and estimates of confidence intervals.[40] Also, interpretation of the results of a Monte Carlo sensitivity analysis is not universally defined; there is no decision rule based on the expected utility distributions other than simply comparing their means.[41] Monte Carlo sensitivity analysis requires increased computation time compared to methods based on deterministic 'fold-back'.

Revision and refinement of the model

After the model is evaluated and sensitivity analysis is performed, the results are interpreted and the model is considered for refinement. For example, the sensitivity analysis may indicate an error, such as expected utility increasing with probability of disease. These errors must be identified and corrected and the model re-evaluated. Modifications may also involve adding increased detail at the suggestion of consultants who are experts in the clinical domain of the analysis. The process is repeated until the analyst is satisfied with the content of the model and confident that the behaviour of the model reflects clinical reality. This iterative refinement of the model is referred to as the *decision analysis cycle*.[9]

Other types of decision models

In practice, simple trees do not have enough expressive power to model complex clinical problems with sufficient realism. In a Markov model[42] events of interest are modelled as transitions among a finite number of health states occurring during fixed time intervals (Markov cycles). A simple Markov model with three states, 'well', 'disabled', and 'dead' is represented by a *Markov state transition diagram* in Fig. 6.15. The arrows connecting states indicate which transitions are allowed. The major advantage of the Markov model is that it permits a straightforward means of representing risk which is continuous over time and which may result in multiple occurrences of a given event. Because most medical applications require these features, most recent applications of medical decision analysis have used Markov models.

The major simplification required by the Markov model (the Markov property) is that all patients in a health state are considered identical. Thus, the Markov model does not consider the history of the patient prior to entering a given state.[16] When details of the history of the patient (e.g. number of prior episodes of illness or duration of therapy) are necessary to determine prognosis, the Markov property is too restrictive. A Markov model can represent these situations only by creating a set of states for each possible combination of historical factors. For even

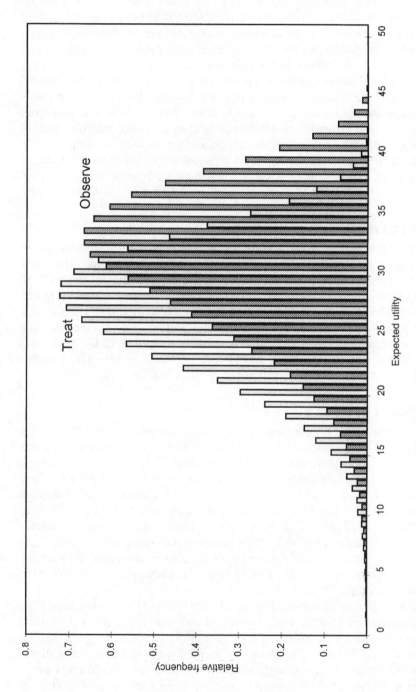

Fig. 6.14 Monte Carlo sensitivity analysis. The model is evaluated a large number of times with each evaluation drawing parameters of the model from probability distributions. The expected utility values for each strategy form a distribution with the expected utility value represented by the horizontal axis and the relative frequency of each value represented by the vertical axis. The mean value (not necessarily the peak of each distribution) is identical to the expected utility of each strategy calculated using the method illustrated in Fig. 6.8.

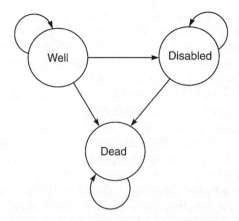

Fig. 6.15   Markov state transition diagram. Each circle represents a state of health. Arrows pointing from one state to another represent permitted transitions. An arrow from a state to itself means a patient can remain in a state for more than one cycle of the Markov process.

a moderately complex model, this can yield hundreds or even thousands of states, making the models unmanageable and computationally intractable. Traditional simulation modelling[43] can consider such effects with a computationally manageable model. Simulation modelling is more straightforward than Markov models when the details of the past history of the patient are important.[44] Simulation modelling is also preferred when the analysis involves a population of patients that is not closed, such as modelling the spread of an infectious disease in a population in which members are both entering and leaving.[43]

Health economic analyses

The challenge facing the health care system today is to reduce the costs of care while improving (or at least, not worsening) health outcomes by selecting the most 'cost-effective' interventions. However, the term 'cost-effective' is used in a variety of ways.[46] Cost-effectiveness is often equated with cost savings. However, few health interventions that improve health actually reduce costs. Such interventions are said to be *dominant* and may be adopted without further economic analysis.[47] However, more typically, a health intervention provides additional benefit at some additional cost compared with no action or a less expensive intervention. Analyses required to make these comparisons are referred to collectively as health economic analyses. Several excellent reviews of health economic analyses are available in the medical literature.[47-50]

In *cost-effectiveness analysis* (CEA) the health and financial outcomes are calculated separately as alternative utilities of a decision model. The results of such an analysis are expressed as the ratio of incremental cost to incremental benefit (the incremental or marginal cost-effectiveness (CE) ratio) when a more expensive strategy is compared to a less expensive one. Marginal CE ratios do not provide a clear decision rule because the best policy depends on willingness to pay, on the available resources, and on the specifics of competing programmes. The greatest health benefit will result from giving highest priority to funding programmes with the lowest marginal CE ratios.[47]

Cost–utility analysis (CUA) is similar to CEA, but the measure of health outcome may incorporate multiple considerations (e.g. duration of survival and quality of life) expressed in terms of a measure that reflects patients' *preference* for the outcome. As for cost-effectiveness analysis, the result of a cost–utility analysis is expressed in terms of the marginal cost–utility (CU) ratio, which is the ratio of incremental cost to incremental utility. Utilities in CUA are often expressed in quality-adjusted life-years (QALYs).[24] The major advantage of QALYs is providing a common measure of outcome which incorporates both quantity and quality of life and can be used to compare programmes that address different health problems. Increasingly, clinical trials are including measurements of both costs and utility based measures of outcomes so that QALYs can be determined empirically.

Information derived from a decision analysis

Decision analysis is useful in determining the role of *strategies* of health care defined as sequences of tests and treatments. Although certain elements of these strategies may have been tested in prospective clinical trials (for example the choice of a particular drug in asthma) it is unlikely that an entire strategy has been evaluated in precisely the same configuration in which it will be applied. Decision analysis can predict what will happen when the elements are combined in new ways. Moreover, decision models can estimate the effects of treatments and tests whose general characteristics are known from observational studies but for which clinical trial data is completely lacking. An example of this is a decision analysis of screening for prostate cancer using prostate-specific antigen (PSA) testing. Although the performance characteristics of PSA are well established, the effects of screening programmes are not yet known from clinical trials. The impact of a screening programme may be inferred by constructing models using the limited data that are available.[51]

Another important application of decision analysis is the ability to project the effects of a clinical strategy in a specific patient population that may differ in important ways from the population in which the manoeuvre has been evaluated. For example, a population in a managed care setting may include a higher or lower proportion of high risk individuals, which would affect the anticipated benefits of a screening procedure, or may be older or younger than the reference population, which would affect the risks of treatment or the magnitude of anticipated benefits. By incorporating patient-specific factors into the analysis, the target population can be subdivided into subsets, each with a different best choice.

Another area in which decision analysis provides unique advantages is when patient preferences drive an analysis. An example is treatment of benign prostatic hypertrophy (BPH). Innovative work done by the prostate disease patient outcomes research team (PORT) has shown the value of incorporating a formal assessment of patient preferences for various health states into an overall clinical protocol.[52] This assessment can identify patients who are troubled only minimally by their illness and who will therefore do well with minimally invasive or no treatment. On the other hand, the technique can identify patients for whom the complications of invasive treatment (e.g. surgical prostatectomy) would be associated with unacceptably low quality of life. Decision models can also estimate the magnitude of the benefits provided by following a given protocol; when the benefits are likely to be very small (a 'toss up'[53]) any one of several actions may be reasonable. This can give clinicians and patients an added measure of flexibility in clinical care.

Although health economic analysis can be carried out using a simple tabulation of costs and outcomes, or various mathematical models, the use of a formal decision model offers distinct advantages in performing cost-effectiveness and cost–utility analysis. The decision model provides a natural representation of the multiple clinical events that comprise the outcomes of a strategy, thus facilitating clinical realism. Moreover, the decision model links the tabulation of costs to the clinical events that generate them, thus ensuring a match between costs and outcomes. Iterative models such as Markov processes and simulations provide a natural means of applying discounting to future costs and benefits. The decision model provides a framework that makes the underlying assumptions explicit and facilitates explanation of the results. The explicit framework also permits updating of the analysis when new data are available.

Sensitivity analysis permits preparation of 'what if' scenarios to allow clinicians to determine which strategy is best for a given patient or which subpopulations of patients would benefit most from a strategy.

Future challenges in decision analysis

It is well documented that advice given to clinicians is most acceptable when it is explained.[54] By providing an explicit framework for reasoning, formal decision models provide a basis by which explanations may be determined automatically. Research to generate such explanations has produced natural language explanations of decision analytic results.[55]

Determining the necessary probability and cost data to support detailed decision models continues to be a challenge. Only a small fraction of specific probabilities has been determined with sufficient statistical certainty. Thus, analysts must make estimates based on available data, or rely on expert opinion. Formal collections of clinical trial results and meta-analyses such as the Cochrane collaboration[56] promise to make the highest quality data more widely available. In the future, the increasing use of routinely collected clinical outcomes databases promises to provide estimates of data not supplied by research.

Costs of care continue to be difficult to obtain and, at present, are determined primarily through administrative data sets that are designed more for reimbursement than for cost-accounting. However, with the increasing prevalence of competitive managed care, health provider organizations are finding it necessary to determine the true costs of providing services. As with clinical outcomes databases, cost databases collected prospectively promise to provide more reliable estimates of the cost of care.

Constructing formal decision models is highly labour intensive and requires special skills. Therefore, it is best if models are constructed that can be applied to a large number of patients, using appropriate means to adapt the analysis to characteristics of individual patients or specific patient populations. Intelligent decision systems[57,58] hold the promise of constructing and reformulating decision models automatically in response to new research data.

In summary, decision analysis is a formal process that permits comparison of specific management alternatives with respect to clinical outcomes and costs. It can serve as the basis for cost-effectiveness and cost–utility analysis, which are essential to the most efficient allocation of scarce health care resources. Decision analytic models can be used to determine the optimal combination of clinical options to be applied for each subpopulation, thus supporting the development of clinical guidelines and protocols. The incorporation of utilities, which are patient-specified measures of health state *preference*, ensures that the decisions will maximize benefit to patients in terms that matter most to them.

References

1. Kassirer, J.P. The principles of clinical decision making: an introduction to decision analysis. *Yale J. Bio. Med.*, 1976; **49**: 149–64.
2. Pauker, S.G. and Kassirer, J.P. Clinical application of decision analysis: a detailed illustration. *Seminars in Nuclear Medicine*, 1978; **8**: 324–35.
3. Pauker, S.G. and Kassirer, J.P. Decision analysis (medical progress). *New Engl. J. Med.*, 1987; **316**: 250–8.
4. Kassirer, J.P., Moskowitz, A.J., Lau, J., and Pauker, S.G. Decision analysis: a progress report. *Ann. Intern. Med.*, 1987; **106**: 275–91.
5. Ledley, R.S. and Lusted, L.B. Reasoning foundations of medical diagnosis. *Science*, 1959; **130**: 9–21.
6. Physicians for the twenty-first century. *The GPEP report*. Washington, DC: Association of American Medical Colleges, 1984. [Reprinted in *J. Med. Educ.*, 1984; **59** (11, pt 2).]
7. Sox, H.C. Decision analysis: a basic clinical skill? *New Engl. J. Med.*, 1987; **316**: 271–2.
8. Plante, D.A., Kassirer, J.P., Zarin, D.A., and Pauker, S.G. Clinical decision consultation service. *Am. J. Med.*, 1986; **80**: 1169–76.
9. Howard, R.A. and Matheson, J.E. (eds). Influence diagrams. In *The principles and applications of decision analysis, Vol. II: Professional collection*. Menlo Park: Strategic Decisions Group, 1984.
10. Raiffa, H. *Decision analysis: introductory lectures on choices under uncertainty*. Reading, MA: Addison-Wesley, 1968.

11. Sonnenberg, F.A., Roberts, M.S., Tsevat, J., Wong, J.B., Barry, M., and Kent, D. Toward a peer review process for medical decision analysis models. *Medical Care*, 1994; **32**: JS52–64.

12. Shachter, R.D. Evaluating influence diagrams. *Operations Research*, 1986; **34**: 871–82.

13. Shachter, R.D. and Heckerman, D. Thinking backward for knowledge acquisition. *AI Magazine*, 1987; **8**: 55–62.

14. McNeil, B.J., Keeler, E., and Adelstein, S.J. Primer on certain elements of medical decision making. *New Engl. J. Med.*, 1975; **293**: 211–15.

15. Rege, A. and Agogino, A.M. Topological framework for representing and solving probabilistic inference problems in expert systems. *IEEE Transactions on Systems, Man and Cybernetics*, 1988; **18** (3).

16. Beck, J.R. and Pauker, S.G. The Markov process in medical prognosis. *Med. Decision Making*, 1983; **3**: 419–58.

17. Harrell, F.E., Lee, K.L., Matchar, D.B., and Relchert, T.A. Regression models for prognostic prediction: advantages, problems and suggested solutions. *Cancer Treatment Reports*, 1985; **69**: 1071–7.

18. Pozen, M.W., D'Agostino, R.B., Selker, H.P., *et al.* A predictive instrument to improve coronary care unit admission practices in acute ischemic heart disease. *New Engl. J. Med.*, 1984; **310**: 1273–8.

19. Pearl, J. *Probabilistic reasoning in intelligent systems: networks of plausible inference.* San Mateo: Morgan Kaufmann, 1988.

20. Breese, J.S. Construction of belief and decision networks. *Computational Intelligence*, 1992; **8**: 624–47.

21. Howard, R.A. From influence to relevance to knowledge. In *Influence diagrams, belief nets and decision analysis*, (ed. R.M. Oliver and J.Q. Smith), pp. 3–24. Chichester: John Wiley, 1990.

22. Torrance, G.W. Utility approach to measuring health-related quality of life. *J. Chron. Dis.*, 1987; **40**: 593–600.

23. Barza, M. and Pauker, S.G. The decision to biopsy, treat, or wait in suspected herpes encephalitis. *Ann. Intern. Med.*, 1980; **92**: 641–9.

24. Pliskin, J.S., Shepard, D.S., and Weinstein, M.C. Utility functions for life years and health status. *Oper. Res.*, 1980; **28**: 206–24.

25. Torrance, G.W. Measurement of health state utilities for economic appraisal. A review. *J. Health Economics*, 1986; **5**: 1–30.

26. Torrance, G.W., Boyle, M.H., and Horwood, S.P. Application of multi-attribute utility theory to measure social preferences for health states. *Oper. Res.*, 1982; **30**: 1043–69.

27. Torrance, G.W. Social preferences for health states: an empirical evaluation of three measurement techniques. *Socio-Econ. Plan. Sci.*, 1976; **10**: 129–36.

28. Read, J.L., Quinn, R.J., Berwick, D.M., Fineberg, H.V., and Weinstein, M.C. Preferences for health outcomes: comparison of assessment methods. *Med. Decision Making*, 1984; **4**: 315–29.

29. National Center for Health Statistics. *Vital statistics of the United States, 1988, Vol. II, Mortality*, Part A, Section 6. Washington, DC: Public Health Service, 1991.

30. Beck, J.R., Kassirer, J.P., and Pauker, S.G. A convenient approximation of life expectancy (the 'DEALE'). I. Validation of the Method. *Am. J. Med.*, 1982; **73**: 883–8.

31. Beck, J.R., Pauker, S.G., Gottlieb, J.E., Klein, K., and Kassirer, J.P. A convenient approximation of life expectancy (the 'DEALE'). II. Use in medical decision making. *Am. J. Med.*, 1982; **73**: 883–8.

32. Sonnenberg, F.A. and Wong, J.B. Fine-tuning life-expectancy calculations using Markov processes. *Med. Decision Making*, 1993; **13**: 170–2.

33. Bombardier, C., Ware, J., Russell, I.J., Larson, M., Chalmers, A., Read, J.L., and the Auranofin Cooperating Group. Auranofin therapy and quality of life in patients with rheumatoid arthritis. Results of a multicenter trial. *Am. J. Med.*, 1986; **81**: 656–78.

34. Feeny, D.H., Torrance, G.W. Incorporating utility-based quality-of-life assessment measures in clinical trials: two examples. *Medical Care*, 1989; **27** (Suppl.): S190–204.

35. Boyd, N.F., Sutherland, H.J., Heasman, K.Z., Tritchler, D.L., and Cummings, B.J. Whose utilities for decision analysis? *Med. Decision Making*, 1990; **10**: 58–67.

36. Pauker, S.G. and Kassirer, J.P. Clinical decision analysis by personal computer. *Arch. Intern. Med.*, 1981; **141**: 1831–7.

37. Weinstein, M.C., Fineberg, H.V., Elstein, A.S., *et al. Clinical decision analysis.* Philadelphia: W.B. Saunders, 1980.

38. McCarthy, B.D., Wong, J.B., and Sonnenberg, F.A. Who should be screened for HIV infection? A cost effectiveness analysis. *Arch. Intern. Med.*, 1993; **153**: 1107–16.

39. Pauker, S.G. and Kassirer, J.P. The threshold approach to clinical decision making. *New. Engl. J. Med.*, 1980; **302**: 1109.

40. Doubilet, P.M. and Begg, C.A. Fundamentals of Monte Carlo analysis. *Med. Decision Making*, 1985; **5**: 157.

41. Fleming, C. and Pauker, S.G. An assessment of the performance of confidence measures obtained from probabilistic sensitivity analysis. *Med. Decision Making*, 1987; **7**: 281. (Abstract.)

42. Beck, J.R. and Pauker, S.G. The Markov process in medical prognosis. *Med. Decision Making*, 1983; **3**: 419–58.

43. Roberts, S.D. and Klein, R.W. The simulation of logical networks (SLN). *Simulation*, **43**: 224.

44. Roberts, M.S. Simulating complex disease: Monte-Carlo models with memory. *Med. Decision Making*, 1989; **4**: 325. (Abstract.)

45. Doubilet, P., Weinstein, M.C., and McNeil, B.J. Use and misuse of the term 'Cost-effective' in Medicine. *New Engl. J. Med.*, 1986; **296**: 253–6.

46. Detsky, A.S. and Naglie, I.G. A clinician's guide to cost-effectiveness analysis. *Ann. Intern. Med.*, 1990; **113**: 147–54.

47. Eisenberg, J.M. Clinical economics: a guide to the economical analysis of clinical practices. *Journal of the American Medical Association*, 1989; **262**: 2879–86.

48. Weinstein, M.C. and Stason, W.B. Foundations of cost-effectiveness analysis for health and medical practices. *New Engl. J. Med.*, 1977; **296**: 716.

49. Freund, D.A. and Dittus, R.S. Principles of pharmacoeconomic analysis of drug therapy. *PharmacoEconomics*, 1992; **1**: 20–32.

50. Krahn, M.D., Mahoney, J.E., Eckman, M.H., Trachtenberg, J., Pauker, S.G., and Detsky, A.S. Screening for prostate cancer: a decision analytic view. *Journal of the American Medical Association*, 1994; **272**: 773–80.

51. Wagner, E.H., Barrett, P., Barry, M.J., Barlow, W., and Fowler, F.J. Jr. The effect of a shared decision making program on rates of surgery for benign prostatic hyperplasia. Pilot results. *Med. Care*, 1995; **33**: 765–70.
52. Kassirer, J.P. and Pauker, S.G. The toss-up. *New Engl. J. Med.*, 1981; **305**: 1467–9.
53. Shortliffe, E.H. Computer programs to support clinical decision making. *Journal of the American Medical Association*, 1987; **258**: 61–6.
54. Langlotz, C.P., Shortliffe, E.H., and Fagan, L.M. A methodology for generating computer-based explanations of decision-theoretic advice. *Med. Decision Making*, 1988; **8**: 290–303.
55. Bero, L. and Rennie, D. The Cochrane collaboration. Preparing, maintaining, and disseminating systematic reviews of the effects of health care. *Journal of the American Medical Association*, 1995; **274**: 1935–8.
56. Holtzman, S. *Intelligent decision systems*. Reading: Addison-Wesley, 1989.
57. Sonnenberg, F.A., Hagerty, C.G., and Kulikowski, C.A. An architecture for knowledge based construction of decision models. *Med. Decision Making*, 1994; **14**: 27–39.

7 Using decision theory in clinical research: applications of quality-adjusted life-years

Carolyn E. Schwartz and Elissa A. Laitin

Introduction

The development of decision theory has provided medical researchers with important tools for dealing with uncertainty in group and individual treatment outcomes. These tools have included methods for generating utilities and preferences, yielding a unit of analysis such as the quality-adjusted life-year (QALY), which summarizes the treatment outcome in terms of time spent in a better health state. The application of these tools to the analysis and interpretation of clinical research is a critical step in disseminating decision theory to the patients and policy makers. This chapter will describe some of the issues which must be considered in applying QALYs to clinical research. We will begin by outlining the advantages and controversies concerning QALYs. We will then describe the application of QALYs to the later phases of clinical research (i.e. phase III and IV trials) and to preventive clinical research. Finally, we will discuss some of the emerging issues which arise in the application of QALYs to clinical research with regard to comparing QALYs across studies, considering the disease context in evaluating treatment trade-offs and resource allocation, and implications of inter- and intra-individual shifts in values over time.

The goal of any clinical research endeavour is to answer questions to facilitate an understanding of treatment effectiveness. In addition to the uncertainty inherent in investigating the unknown, there is the added uncertainty of treatment trade-offs which may mitigate the efficacy and feasibility of a treatment regimen. The advantage of applying decision theory to clinical research is to provide rational tools for dealing with the probabilistic nature of treatment benefits and risks. By applying analytic tools (i.e. utilities or preferences) borrowed from economists, decision analysis can facilitate the identification of the preferred treatment, given that treatment's benefits and risks.

The language of clinical trials

The preference based methods of utility assessment are relatively recent additions to the biostatistical repertoire for clinical trials. Given their reliance on additional data (i.e. utilities or preferences) which involve complex cognitive tasks, one might ask what these techniques bring to clinical research that is not already served by basic survival analytic techniques.

As Kant[1] and other philosophers of science have noted,[2] language is our bridge to the objective world. Indeed, let us consider the possible influence of the language of survival analytic methods. In such methods, the outcome of treatment is a dichotomous variable, where a value of zero usually indicates 'treatment failure' and a value of one represents a 'treatment responder'. In the fast-paced hospital environment of clinical trials, one is likely to hear clinicians reporting on a patient for whom a treatment is not effective as a 'treatment failure'. Hence, the statistical label becomes the shorthand way of expressing the fact that the treatment did not work for that particular patient. Whereas it is ironic that the statistical method determines the clinical language, it becomes unfortunate if such use of language begins to influence the relationship between doctor and patient. Indeed, one documented complaint of patients in clinical trials is the feeling that the process of clinical trials does not highlight their individual experience.[3] The addition of utility- and preference-based methods to the data analytic repertoire is a way of emphasizing the patient's perspective, and of considering treatment trade-offs in evaluating treatments.

The relevance of the quality-adjusted life-year

It is well recognized that the illness experience is multidimensional, affecting both physical and emotional well-being. A seminal step to measuring health was taken in 1948, when the World Health Organization[4] defined health as '... a state of complete physical, mental and social well-being and not merely the absence of infirmity'. This definition provides the basis for most measures of health outcome. Since the definition has three components, investigators have often used separate methods for measuring the three separate constructs.

For the thoughtful clinical investigator, distinguishing physical, mental, and social well-being may be a double-edged sword. That is, as helpful as it may be to have separate scores for each of these important components of health, the Gestalt of the illness experience may be lost by separating its parts from the whole. Treatment evaluations which use such profile measures may lead to a piecemeal understanding of the impact of an intervention if one subscale seems to change in a beneficial direction whereas others stay the same or deteriorate. Consequently, health researchers are faced with the need for methods which can combine multidimensional information in theoretically and psychometrically appropriate ways. Methods that yield QALYs respond to this need, and may validly reflect the illness experience. Further, QALYs can provide a common metric to compare different treatments with one another, to compare treatment side-effects versus benefits, or to compare the output of different sectors in health care.

Ware and Sherbourne[5] have emphasized that since mental health and physical health constitute different constructs, any attempt to measure them using a uniform measurement strategy is like comparing apples to oranges. Indeed, for some individuals the QALY concept does not seem meaningful or interpretable because it combines divergent components into a single index which is labeled 'time', which says little about the specifics of a patient's illness experience. However, a common outcome metric can allow for direct comparisons of treatment effectiveness among health care providers from diverse disciplines.[6]

The QALY concept can also be useful in an economic context which focuses on the social costs of illness. If the focus is on the social impact of illness, then it does not matter whether a complaint is physical or mental.[7] For example, a person may report a cough while another person reports depression. If the cough is severe, it may keep the person at home. If it is very severe, then it may require hospitalization. Similarly, depression may be mild or it may cause disruption of daily activities to the point where it keeps the person at home. In severe cases, depression may require hospitalization. Thus, quantifying the impact of illness with a metric which combines physical and mental symptoms would make sense from a social cost perspective.

QALY estimation

In the interest of balancing the forces of objectivity and subjectivity, investigators have developed utility based methods which attempt to integrate the patients' perspective. Utility based methods assign a value to a specific health state. This value is intended to reflect the global impact of that state on the patient's overall quality of life. Borrowed from the field of economics, the concept of a utility originally referred to the level of satisfaction or enjoyment experienced by the consumer of the good or service.[8] Economists generally do not attempt to measure utility directly, but rather infer it by examining how consumers trade off different bundles of goods and services in response to prices. In applying the utility concept to health economics, Torrance and colleagues developed a family of methods which attempted to lead the patient through a complex series of probabilities to define the value of a given health state.[9] For example, the standard gamble method asks individuals to decide upon acceptable levels of risk in exchange for given probabilities of cure for a range of health states. Since decision analysis requires respecting specific axioms and assumptions, the analytic tools must have the properties of interval scaling and independence.[8] Decision analysis thereby facilitates the identification of the preferred treatment, given that treatment's risks and benefits.

Some of these methods generate 'utilities' which are defined as having interval properties (i.e. a given interval reflects the same quality of life difference at all ranges of the scale), whereas others generate 'preferences', which are not interval scales but are alternative measures of the value of the health state. These types of methods are plagued by problems such as their cognitive complexity, their questionable validity in assessing the value of specific health states, and their lack of comparability. Consequently, relevant considerations in utility elicitation include both how and from whom they are derived.

Do utilities truly reflect health state value?

Common approaches for eliciting utilities include the standard gamble,[9] time trade-off,[10] and willingness-to-pay[11] methods. Rating scale[12] methods use a visual analogue scale which is simpler to understand but does not necessarily have interval properties. The latter will thus be discussed subsequently as a 'preference'.

Numerous studies have documented that values derived for the same health state using standard gamble, time trade-off, and rating scale approaches are not highly correlated[13] and have different ranges and means.[14-16] Since the correlations between utility measures and measures of health status have generally been modest,[13,14,17] some investigators have concluded that utilities do not reflect health status but actually reflect the value patients place on life, their risk aversion, or their attitudes toward certain types of medical intervention.[11,13,18] For example, willingness-to-pay methods are influenced by the respondent's income and assets and the value he or she attaches to money, as well as his or her preferences for health states. Similarly, time trade-offs assess preference concerning time as well as preferences related to health states. Standard gambles are influenced by how a respondent feels about risk. For example, individuals assign a higher utility to a given state of health than do risk-seeking individuals, all else being equal. Further, utilities are generally lower for hypothetical health states than when one rates an actual health state,[19] suggesting that patients may be reporting on a dispositional way of looking at the world rather than a state-specific evaluation. Since lower levels of functional status are not necessarily related to lower levels of satisfaction, people may be changing their expectations and aspirations as their circumstances change.[20]

Whose utility?

One of the central issues in using methods which generate QALYs is deciding whose utility is most relevant. One consideration in determining the most appropriate source of the utilities used to weight the treatment outcomes is accountability. For example, some investigators suggest that for cost-effectiveness analyses one should use utilities from the general population since health care expenses are supported by society.[21] Inferring utilities for health care expenditures based on rating hypothetical contexts may be problematic because it assumes that consumers would have the same values whether they are healthy or sick. Other investigators suggest that providers would be a reasonable source for utilities since they would have ample clinical experience and be well aware of toxicities and other indirect costs of treatment.[21]

This dilemma hinges on the assumption that health states have a gold standard score which does not vary across persons, contexts, or fluctuating experiences. However, research from the medical and social sciences suggests that there is substantial variation in utilities for similar health states depending on whether the person has experienced that state, and how disparate it is from their current health.[15] Further, sociodemographic factors such as age and education level[22] have been found to moderate utilities. Thus, using non-patient populations to estimate utilities may be problematic if one hopes to generalize the results for use in medical decision making.

Involving patients in medical decision making may become increasingly important as cost containment restricts the availability of health care resources. It would seem reasonable to judge treatments in a clinical trial using data and values from those people who are experiencing the study treatment and outcome. However, involving patients requires and assumes that patient-derived utilities are stable and consistent between patients with the same illness and severity,[23] and within patients over the course of acute health state changes.[19]

Further, it assumes that patient decision making is a based on adequate information. Since people generally rely on advice from a health care professional to make decisions,[24] a crucial consideration is how framing influences what patients prefer and choose. Indeed, the way a question is framed can have a salient effect on patient choices. For example, McNeil and colleagues[25] found that when informed consent forms gave mortality risk information rather than 'risk of living', patients were more likely to choose surgery rather than radiation therapy. Similarly, patients' choices may also change, depending on how risk-averse each person is. When the standard gamble method is used to calculate QALYs, risk neutrality is assumed. However, O'Connor et al.[26] found that different utilities resulted when patients undergoing chemotherapy were presented with riskless versus risky treatment choice approaches. Consequently, to infer utilities of patients from behaviour that is not solely determined by them may be unreliable.[24] Further, since most patients have access to third-party payment (health insurance) and thus do not bear fully the monetary cost of their treatment, it is unlikely that utilities can be inferred directly from expenditures.[24]

The issue is further complicated when the target population of the study is unable to provide utilities due to developmental or cognitive impairments (e.g. children or Alzheimer's disease). Such trials may require collection of utilities from proxy respondents, such as parents or spouses.[27] Providers might also be appropriate proxies for rating treatment toxicity and gain.

Preferences: an alternative to utilities

Whereas utilities are required to have interval scale properties, other approaches for weighting health states rely on a related category of measures which have relaxed that assumption. These measures elicit preferences, which are more akin to measuring the importance and value a person explicitly places on a health state or quality-of-life dimension. Such methods may use a visual analogue scale (e.g. a feeling thermometer), paired adjective checklists, or other methods. Preference methods can be advantageous because they are simple to understand (i.e. face valid), are more clearly linked to patient-reported values (i.e. construct valid), are less time consuming to collect, and thus less costly. Further, methods are available for testing whether the derived values have an interval scale (e.g. Anderson's functional measurement theory[28]), attenuating the problem of QALY estimation using methods without interval scaling.

Although preferences may be simpler approaches to addressing the importance and value of various dimensions of health status, they may share selected measurement caveats with utilities. For example, preferences have been found to remain stable despite important fluctuation in health status,[20] suggesting that some methods for eliciting preferences may be highlighting the dispositional aspects as opposed to the health-state-specific aspects.

Adjusting QALYs for future values

Since one enjoys more options if one receives a benefit earlier or incurs a cost later, most health economists believe that QALYs should be discounted to reflect this time preference.[29] For example, in estimating the benefit of a preventive intervention which requires more of a financial outlay early on with the promise of a cost saving later on, one might discount future costs to present values. The concept of discounting may be particularly relevant when dealing with utility methods such as time trade-off since the value of a given amount of time has been found to vary depending on one's life expectancy and on how far away the trade-off is based.[30] In contrast, decision analysis based on more psychometric measures of preferences (e.g. rating scale measures of importance) may not need to discount because the context of the assessment is unlikely to be influenced by time preference.

Caveats of QALYs

Despite its comprehensiveness, even the QALY approach does not include all relevant factors. For example, it addresses only part of the issue of equity (27). At the individual level, equity is defined in the model as treating each person's QALY gained equally, regardless of the individual's age, sex, race, occupation, or other characteristics. Using QALYs as a measure of value gained by health care may be discriminatory against chronically ill or permanently disabled populations when they are compared to non-disabled populations because the former two populations are put at an additional disadvantage.[31] 'Double jeopardy' might occur under the circumstances where the additional length of life after treatment is the same, but the quality of this life is different. For instance, if two people need an operation that would extend their life for 10 years, but one already has a disability, then the QALY approach counts the gain made by the operation as much greater in the person without the disability.[31] When making decisions to allocate health care resources, care should be taken not to penalize systematically those whose prior health state puts them at a disadvantage. A policy of maximizing QALYs does not automatically limit health care for a person with a severe disability or illness, especially if one directs resources to those groups of patients where the greatest QALY *gains* can be expected. This is not necessarily the patients who will have the highest QALY levels at the end of the treatment.[31]

An additional shortcoming of the QALY is the potential for neglecting the social welfare factors with which policy makers are concerned. Health interventions may have outcomes other than change in duration or quality of life, and it is unclear how indirect effects such as future production or welfare costs should be handled.[32] For instance, the person who suffers from a condition or receives treatment is not the only person affected. Quality of life for other family members can be positively or negatively affected if health improves or death occurs, and treatment with no measurable effect on the individual may still have a positive effect on care givers and others.[33] Despite these weaknesses, the principles underlying QALYs have gained widespread support.

Finally, the QALY model may not capture the political feasibility of rationing choices based on QALYs. For example, the Oregon cost effectiveness list[34] applied QALYs using the Quality of Well-Being index[35] to rate a variety of health care procedures according to quantity and quality of life to be gained by such procedures. The committee ended up abandoning the idea of rationing services based on cost-effectiveness because they felt that cost-effectiveness had failed to capture people's values regarding how to ration health care.[36,37] Indeed, Ubel and colleagues[38] found that compared with the rationing choices, all three utility elicitation methods placed less value on the importance of saving lives and treating more severely ill people compared with less severely ill ones. Hadorn[39] noted that any such list would fail because cost-effectiveness underestimates people's desires to rescue those whose lives are endangered or who are seriously ill. Eddy[40] and Nord[41] felt that cost-effectiveness could work as long as utilities were elicited in a manner which considered values and contexts. Thus, an alternative that is slightly weaker on cost-per-QALY-gained may be more attractive overall because of political factors that make it more acceptable.[27]

An alternative to QALYs? – the Healthy-Year Equivalent

The Healthy-Year Equivalent (HYE) was proposed in 1989 as an alternative to the QALY. In introducing this concept, Mehrez and Gafni's[42,43] goal was to express individuals' preferences in units that are more meaningful, as HYEs are defined as the number of years in full health instead of utilities. Mehrez and Gafni proposed a two-stage procedure to measure HYEs. In the first stage, the standard gamble is used to measure the utility of all potential lifetime health profiles and calculate the expected utility for each treatment option. In the second stage, the utilities of the treatment options are converted to the number of years in full health, using the standard gamble. The HYE was purported not to require the same assumptions as QALYs, i.e. (1) constant proportional risk posture with respect to time in all health states for risk-averse QALYs; and (2) additive independence of quality in different periods required for both risk-neutral and risk-averse QALYs.

Weinstein and Pliskin, however, argue that the HYE measurement procedure is equivalent to a one-stage time trade-off, and does not reflect attitudes towards risk.[44] While the QALY requires risk neutrality with respect to time in all health states, the HYE requires risk neutrality with respect to healthy years of life.[45] The number of HYEs has to be measured for every possible duration of time in a health state, whereas only one measurement of the QALY weight is carried out that is assumed to be valid for any duration of time in the health state. The HYE thus adds flexibility to the risk-neutral form of the QALY by permitting the rate of trade-off between life-years and quality of life to depend on the life span, albeit at the cost of eliciting numerous additional time trade-off assessments.[45] While the advantages and the disadvantages of the QALY and the HYE have been debated in the literature for the past several years, the HYE remains a theoretical concept. The feasibility of measuring and computing HYEs has yet to be shown; in the mean time, we hope that this dialogue will lead to improvements in the QALY and outcome measurement in general.

Applying QALYs to clinical research

With increasing costs and competition in the health care setting, a new medical technology often must pass stringent criteria before being adopted. Eddy[46] proposes that the criteria for adoption of a new technology should be that

(1) it improves the health outcomes about which patients care (e.g. pain, anxiety, disfigurement, disability, death);

(2) the benefits outweigh the harms;

(3) the health effects are worth the costs; and

(4) it deserves priority over other technologies if resources are limited.

As clinical investigators seek to implement research which is increasingly patient-centered, the application of QALYs becomes more standard and diversified. Decision analysis facilitates a systematic approach for integrating quality of life and cost data under conditions of uncertainty.[47] Direct and indirect costs are combined to calculate QALYs, which can then be used as outcome measures to compare directly the effectiveness and cost–utility of interventions. In the following section, we will provide examples of studies that have applied QALY-based approaches in evaluating randomized controlled trials, preventive care, and in the post-marketing phase of clinical research. An exhaustive review is beyond the scope of the present chapter, as our intent is to provide selected examples of extant QALY applications and to suggest other applications of QALYs to clinical research.

Randomized controlled trials

In the context of randomized trials, establishing the value of an intervention may involve not only demonstrating an impact on clinical parameters (primary end-point), but also showing the impact on quality of life (secondary end-point). Since QALY approaches can be used to develop relatively comprehensive outcomes which accurately reflect the illness experience, they may be a useful indicator of the effectiveness of the intervention. Applying decision analysis to randomized trials may involve data from one trial as well as meta-analyses of several trials. These methods may also be useful for evaluating the cost-effectiveness of a treatment based on empirical data or projecting the cost-effectiveness over the short- and long-term future. Two studies will be described below to illustrate the use of

QALYs in cost–utility analysis, an approach which quantifies cost-effectiveness in terms of clinical gain adjusted for quality-of-life effects.

One example of such an analysis is a study of interferon-α_{2b} for patients with chronic hepatitis B virus (HBV) infection by Wong et al.[48] Using a decision-analytic model, Wong et al. implemented a meta-analysis of nine randomized controlled trials which compared interferon-α_{2b} to standard care alone in the treatment of cirrhosis-related signs of HBV infection. This meta-analysis aimed to evaluate the cost-effectiveness of this treatment based on the projected clinical and economic outcomes resulting from changes in serologic markers of HBV replication. HBV infection causes significant morbidity and mortality, induces substantial costs, can lead to cirrhosis, and leads to a 300-fold increased risk of hepatocellular carcinoma.[49] Consequently, a comprehensive approach to outcomes assessment would be appropriate.

Direct medical costs were estimated, and assumptions about outcome and prognosis were based on published literature. Utilities were estimated by a panel of clinicians using an average of the standard reference gamble and the time trade-off technique for hypothetical health states.

Results of the cost-effectiveness analysis suggested that using interferon should prolong survival and diminish lifetime costs. The marginal cost-effectiveness for interferon was estimated based on varying several outcome parameters using a sensitivity analysis, and suggested that the cost-effectiveness ratio did not exceed $12 000 per gain in QALY. Restricting the analysis to a 10 year time frame showed a cost of $3600 per discounted QALY gained.

This study demonstrates the feasibility of using decision analysis and QALYs as tools to project results from completed studies to answer questions about future outcomes. Their analyses were based on projections of the effects of interferon on serologic markers and did not represent trials showing benefits on hard clinical end-points.[49] When long-term trials are not possible or are ongoing, these types of analyses can be helpful for patients and clinicians who need to make decisions in the present day. One limitation of the study was that indirect costs were not included in the cost-effectiveness analysis. Given the substantial indirect costs of hepatitis B infection,[50,51] it is likely that interferon therapy would have been found to be even more cost-effective if work productivity, side-effects, and care-giver time had been considered in the analysis. The cost-effectiveness of treatments in other contexts may be less apparent when a drug or other intervention has high toxicities or does not cure a disease. In these cases, the subtleties of quality of life must be measured with responsive measures to maximize the information gained by a formal decision-analytic approach to clinical trials evaluation.

Another example of a cost–utility analysis is an evaluation of the maintenance therapies for recurrent depression done by Kamlet and colleagues.[52] In this trial, patients were randomized to one of five maintenance treatments:

(1) interpersonal therapy (IPT) alone;

(2) IPT plus placebo drug;

(3) imipramine drug therapy (drug) alone;

(4) IPT plus drug; or

(5) placebo alone for three years or until they experienced a recurrence of illness.[52]

Results were then projected to estimate health over a lifetime.

Time until recurrence was evaluated for all groups using survival analysis, and direct medical costs were calculated. The mean daily utility for depression was based on preferences from the general public and from depressed patients, as documented in the literature. Because this intervention also influenced patients' social functioning, work, and leisure, the monetary equivalent of leisure time devoted to treatment was measured using a willingness-to-pay method. Indirect costs of the illness were inferred from quality-of-life measures, and were included in the denominator of the cost-effectiveness ratio.

Using a Markovian state transition model and Monte Carlo analysis, the drug maintenance protocol improved expected lifetime health and reduced direct medical costs compared to placebo, even when severe side-effects were considered. Interpersonal therapy alone and with drug treatment improved expected lifetime health compared to placebo, although direct medical costs were not reduced in either case. Imipramine alone was found to be cost-effective compared to interpersonal therapy, as it improved expected lifetime quality of life and reduced direct costs. Similarly, drug plus interpersonal therapy was cost-effective compared to therapy alone, despite a moderate increase in direct costs. The costs of the resulting health improvements were estimated to be under $3000 per QALY for therapy and under $5000 per QALY for therapy plus imipramine. Both of these cost–utility ratios are well below the $50 000 per QALY threshold typically invoked in the literature to determine whether a health care intervention is an appropriate use of health care resources.[53] Thus, this study used available clinical, economic, and quality-of-life data to reveal that maintenance treatments primarily enhance the quality, not the quantity, of life. When treatments are anticipated to have a stronger impact on the quality rather than the quantity of life, cost–utility applications of QALYs can be an important evaluation tool.[52]

These two examples thus illustrate how QALYs can be applied to randomized trials to elucidate the comprehensive impact of treatments in terms of the quality of life, direct costs, and indirect costs of treatment. Whereas cost-effectiveness analyses do not necessarily require utility-based QALYs, they can be used in such analyses. In contrast, cost–utility analyses involve explicit consideration of costs using utilities and thus require values based on standard utility methods so that such analyses are comparable across cost–utility studies.

Preventive clinical research

Analysis of projected direct and indirect costs over a lifetime can also be used in cost-effectiveness and cost–utility evaluations of screening interventions. The challenge of applying QALYs to screening is related to the numerous other factors which must be considered when evaluating a screening intervention. These factors include the statistical validity of the screening intervention, such as the sensitivity and specificity of the screening test, as well as the probability (i.e. estimated base rate) of disease in the population being tested, a parameter which influences the false positive rate of screening tests.[54]

Although applying QALYs to screening interventions has not been done often, Danese and colleagues[55] do provide one example of a cost-effectiveness analysis of periodic screening for mild thyroid failure by measurement of serum thyroid stimulating hormone (TSH) concentration. Based on an analysis of a hypothetical cohort of women and men screened every five years after age 35, Danese *et al.* evaluated the addition of the TSH assay to total serum cholesterol screening in comparison to cholesterol screening alone. Mild thyroid failure is relatively common and increases with age. The argument for screening is based on potential health benefits such as prevention of progression to overt hypothyroidism, reducing serum cholesterol levels, and decreasing symptoms which have an impact on quality of life. However, most physician organizations have not recommended screening the general population due to a low risk of overt disease.[56]

Probabilities for events were derived from the literature, and direct medical costs were calculated. Indirect medical costs and non-utility based estimates of quality of life were not included. Health utilities were either based on reports from prior studies[57,58] or estimated by the authors in relation to these utilities. In the base–case analysis, the cost-utility of adding a serum TSH measurement to the total cholesterol measurement was $9223 per QALY for women and $22 595 per QALY for men. In the sensitivity analysis, the cost of the TSH assay was the most influential variable in the model. A limitation of this study was that author estimates of utilities based on prior studies were used rather than tracking the indirect costs and quality-of-life effects of the screening intervention on the individuals studied. Considering the comprehensive impact of the screening test might have yielded a lower cost per QALY.

Incorporating quality-of-life issues into medical decision making allows the investigator to gauge the long-term benefits of screening beyond the face-value benefits of cost savings alone. A further consideration in screening tests is the potential for effectively intervening on the condition which is being screened. For example, it may ultimately be destructive to identify a high-risk status for a condition which is life threatening and for which there is no treatment. If the condition which is identified by a screening test does have treatment options, then relevant considerations would be the treatments' effectiveness, the side-effect profile, and the relative accessibility of treatment for those who test positive. Given the comprehensive nature of these considerations, applications of QALYs for screening interventions would be eminently appropriate.

Other applications: post-marketing studies and quality of care assessment

In an age of cost cutting and managed care, competition among drug companies has increased, and drugs must be marketed in a more competitive manner to show the relative advantages of their product.[59] QALY-based quality-of-life assessment can provide relevant information to providers and patients. When a drug is more effective and more costly than a comparative agent, cost-effectiveness analysis estimates the incremental gain in the therapeutic benefit per unit cost.[60] The use of quality-of-life measures allows a more focused assessment on parameters that are perceived to be important to patients.

However, incorporating quality-of-life measures into the evaluation of health care technologies does not end the controversy over which treatments should be prescribed. Demonstration of cost-effectiveness does not necessarily mean that the therapy is affordable. For example, the recent success of protease inhibitors in treating HIV-positive patients does not ensure that insurance companies will cover this extremely expensive treatment. With limited resources, a health care system must make choices even among cost-effective therapies, and the cost impact on others in the system can influence decision making.[61] The appropriateness of an allocation rule will depend on the societal values. Further, multiple guidelines are needed to accommodate diverse allocation strategies for life-threatening and symptomatic drug therapies.[61]

Since QALYs capture the illness experience and provide an opportunity to integrate values and severity of various health states, it would seem appropriate to apply decision-analytic methods based on QALYs to evaluate outcomes in the context of studies of quality of care. If such studies were done longitudinally, one could thus evaluate the impact of diverse systems of care not only in terms the structure and process of care, but also in valid and responsive outcomes of care.[62]

The next step: integrating key perspectives

Thus far, we have reviewed the issues and controversies regarding QALYs and their application to various clinical research designs. In the interest of highlighting how such measures can facilitate treatment evaluation, we will now describe a preference-based method which was developed by Schwartz and colleagues[63-65] to integrate the perspectives of the patient, the provider, and social cost in a single analysis. In lieu of assuming stability and comparability of subjective values across and within patients, Schwartz and colleagues consider this variability in patient preferences to be informative and essential to understanding treatment trade-offs.[63-65] The Extended Q-TWiST represents an extension of the Quality-Adjusted Time Without Symptoms and Toxicity (Q-TWiST) method, a quality-adjusted survival analysis designed to integrate quality-of-life considerations into the comparison of treatments being evaluated in randomized clinical trials for AIDS and cancer (see Chapter 15). The standard Q-TWiST method was not immediately applicable to the chronic disease setting because of the difficulty in defining dichotomous health states for the analysis: health states may follow a transition along a continuum in chronic illness, whereas in terminal illness they may be more discrete and mutually exclusive.[63] The Extended Q-TWiST also differs from the standard Q-TWiST by extending the definition of health to include not only clinical parameters, but also psychological, social, or functional status aspects of health as per the WHO definition,[4] as well as the indirect or social costs of impaired health states. Finally, the Extended Q-TWiST integrates the perspectives of the patient, the provider, and social cost in a single analysis by using data from patient- and provider-report and by allowing preferences to be collected from patients, providers, payers, care givers, or others whose perspectives might be relevant to treatment evaluation. Despite these differences, the standard and Extended Q-TWiST are both concerned with the trade-off between treatment costs and improved response. The success of any therapy relies on its efficacy as well as on the patients' ability to adhere to the therapeutic regimen. If the treatment costs are high and/or not fully covered by health insurance, patients are unlikely to continue in therapy.[66]

Implementing an Extended Q-TWiST analysis requires definition of quality-of-life dimensions which highlight specific aspects of the disease and treatments under study, and which consider the indirect costs of illness and psychosocial morbidity. The data required for an Extended Q-TWiST analysis include provider-reported clinical parameters, treatment-related toxicities as reported by providers and/or patients, and patient-reported quality of life, social costs, and preferences (Fig. 7.1). Appropriate time intervals for data collection and analysis should be selected so that any major changes in the patients' quality of life affected by the treatment can be captured in the analysis.

The resulting assessment data and importance weights are used to compute a Q-TWiST score for each treatment. This is done by first computing a weighted assessment score for each time interval. This weighted assessment score is analogous to a global utility value for each time interval. In the Extended Q-TWiST

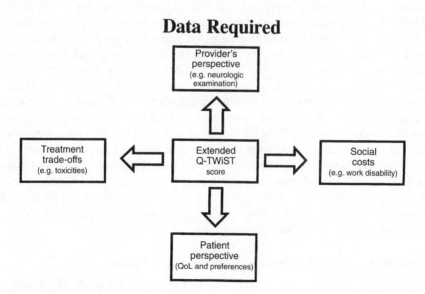

Fig. 7.1 *Data required for an Extended Q-TWiST analysis.* These include provider-reported clinical parameters, treatment-related toxicities as reported by providers and/or patients, and patient-reported quality of life, social costs, and preferences.

method, these weighted assessment scores represent severity of symptoms for each dimension measured, weighted by preference values for each dimension measured. Each individual assessment is weighted by its patient-derived preference value, which is collected from individual patients at each data collection time point using various methods of preference assessment. (See Schwartz *et al.*[63-65] for complete descriptions of the method.) The statistical analysis proceeds by computing parameter estimates separately for each treatment group in QALYs.

One might also collect preferences from other perspectives (e.g. the provider, the payer, the care giver). An examination of these juxtaposed perspectives might then yield a more comprehensive evaluation of treatment costs and benefits. Health policy decisions based on the information gleaned from this juxtaposition might be more likely to reflect the diverse priorities of individual patients, providers, payers, and care givers. This information can be used to demonstrate the value of treatment programmes in ways that consider dimensions of consequence to managed care, third-party payers, and legislative representatives for health appropriations. By using statistically efficient methods, preference-based approaches provide a vehicle that is more than statistically significant. It is clinically meaningful.

Emerging issues

Considering disease context in determining a 'good' outcome

An important consideration in evaluating treatments is determining a 'good' outcome by considering explicitly the patient population. An example from rehabilitation might be contrasting treatment for patients with a permanent disability of acute onset (e.g. head trauma, myocardial infarction) with those who have a chronic progressive disease. Whereas the former may realistically seek to enhance functional status to a stable and higher level of function from treatment initiation, the latter may seek to extend baseline function[67] (Fig. 7.2). Thus, in comparison to the control group, optimal rehabilitation in the first scenario would seek improvement in functional outcomes over time, whereas it would seek reduced deterioration over time in the latter group. Similarly, for terminally ill cancer patients, outcome goals for palliative care may not include prevention of progression and may rather focus on reduced pain, enhanced functional status, and improved mood and appetite as compared to controls. Thus, QALYs may be applied to various patient populations and treatment goal scenarios and the included dimensions used to derive the QALYs should be tailored to focus on salient and reasonable treatment outcomes.

Prioritizing outcomes when not all can be achieved

One of the distinct benefits of applying decision-analytic tools which rely on preference assessment is that the values of the referent population can be considered explicitly in treatment evaluation. Consequently, outcomes can be prioritized based on what patients or other relevant parties determine to be of most

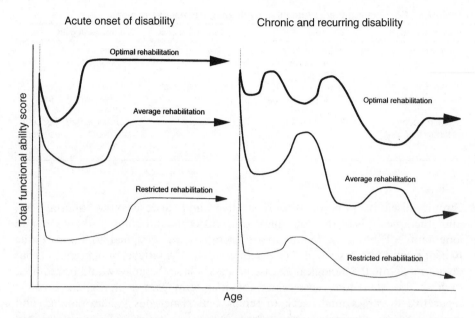

Fig. 7.2 *Determining a 'good' outcome by considering explicitly the patient population.* A desirable outcome for patients with a permanent disability of acute onset (e.g. head trauma, myocardial infarction) might seek realistically to enhance functional status to a stable and higher level of function from treatment initiation (left-hand side). In contrast, rehabilitation for those who have a chronic progressive disease might seek to extend baseline function (right-hand side). Reprinted with permission from NICHD.

importance. This prioritization might be based on a consideration of different perspectives. For example, patients can decide on what is important to them, providers might decide upon what makes the most sense for long-term gain, and care givers might decide on what dimensions are relevant for reducing disease burden. Decision-analytic methods which allow one to consider diverse perspectives explicitly would facilitate such treatment evaluations.

Considering therapy goals in evaluating treatment trade-offs

With the addition of utility and preference based methods to the analytic repertoire for randomized controlled trials, one has the advantage of comparing treatments in terms of a patient-centred metric that evaluates the quality-adjusted time resulting from the experimental treatment regimens. Although this approach has some obvious advantages, it would be important to consider treatment outcomes in the context of acceptable treatment trade-offs given the anticipated range of treatment benefits over time.

For example, patients may be more willing to tolerate treatment-related toxicities and reduced quality of life in the short-term if the long-term gain seems worthwhile (Table 7.1). For example, there may be three types of therapy for

Table 7.1 Considering therapy goals in evaluating treatment trade-offs

Type of therapy	Example	Short-term cost	Long-term gain
Symptomatic	Anti-spasticity, anti-fatigue, anti-depressant	Low	None
Reparative	Remyelination for multiple sclerosis	Moderate cost	Large potential but unknown at present time
Disease-course altering therapies	Immunotherapies	High cost	Documented moderate impact on preserved function

chronic diseases: symptomatic, reparative, and disease-course altering immunotherapies. These therapies have different costs and gains in the short and long term (Table 7.1). Symptomatic therapies are designed to improve the patient's day-to-day experience (e.g. reduce spasticity, fatigue, or depression), but do not moderate the biological disease process. These therapies would be required to have few short-term costs since the long-term gain is negligible. Possible reparative therapies might seek to repair central nervous system damage and would tend to have bigger short-term costs (i.e. bothersome toxicities) but represent a substantial potential gain in the long term. Finally, disease-course altering immunotherapies might have a bigger short-term cost but may result in preserved function in the long term. Conceptualizing treatment trade-offs should consider the context of the type of therapy so that the relationship between short- and long-term costs and gains are presented clearly.

A related challenge of applying QALY-based methods to clinical research is interpreting the results for the specific audience. For example, patients may find a small objective treatment gain due to subjective factors not considered in the analysis.[2] Similarly, a very small treatment gain may be deemed salient by providers who are working with a disease with which medical technology has had little success in mitigating. Thus, the interpretation of QALYs gained should be presented with the specific disease context and treatment goals in mind.

Ethics in outcomes research: how and when should treatment be allocated?

Decision analysis has been applied to health contexts to facilitate treatment allocation in the face of uncertainty. Some crucial considerations in such allocation include deciding when a treatment is too costly and how durable a treatment should be to merit use. A standard guideline for treatment cost-effectiveness, which most investigators have adopted is a cut-off point of $50 000 per QALY gained.[29] Given the various contexts under which decision-analytic treatment evaluations may occur, guidelines for the desired durability of treatments would be useful. Such guidelines would help to prevent the wasting of valuable resources. For example, 10–12 per cent of all health care expenditures and 27 per cent of all

Medicare (health insurance) expenditures[68] are currently spent on interventions in the last year of life which do not extend the quantity and may even reduce the quality of life.[69] Consequently, investigators who seek to apply decision-analytic tools to clinical research should begin by defining a reasonable duration of treatment gain. QALYs and decision-analytic methods would easily be amenable to such determination, and may facilitate cost containment and enhanced quality of life in the last year of life.

Comparing QALYs across studies

As preference based methods are increasingly used to summarize treatment outcomes in terms of QALYs, one is tempted by the enhanced feasibility of comparing treatment outcomes across studies using these QALYs. Rather than relying on complex meta-analytic techniques,[70] one might simply list QALY gains across studies. However, if the preference based methods are integrating diverse quality-of-life dimensions, then the resulting QALYs may not be comparable.

One possible solution to such a problem would be for the published studies to report the mean preferences and severity levels for all dimensions at each data collection time point. Secondary meta-analytic endeavours could then compute their own QALYs based on similar dimensions collected across the studies. This effort would be enhanced if future clinical researchers were to ensure that they collected data on quality-of-life parameters which reflected the WHO definition of health, as well as social cost and clinical outcome data.

Response shift phenomenon

An emerging area of interest and work by researchers from a broad range of disciplines is focused on understanding the response shift phenomenon. This term refers to the idea that individuals facing a significant health challenge may experience a change in their internal standards of expectations for optimal functioning.[71-73] As both Heraclitus and Ahphonse Karr noted long ago, change is a constant in life; yet there is an underlying and undeniable structure to personality.[74] Quality-of-life investigators have documented a type of inconsistency in self-reported health outcomes which is likely to have important implications for utility and preference based methods.

Acute health-state changes may have an impact on psychological morbidity, followed by accommodation and adaptation to the functional limitations imposed by the illness. This shift explains how an individual's life satisfaction may not be related directly to their functional status. Bach and Tilton[75] found, for example, that individuals with tetraplegia who were dependent on a ventilator reported higher life satisfaction than tetraplegics who were able to breathe independently. Individuals facing a significant health challenge may scale down their expectations of health, may be more appreciative of the social resources which support their daily living activities, and may be making significant adjustments in the importance of life domains.[75]

These individual values may also play an important role in determining the complex inter-relationships underlying quality of life. For example, satisfaction with one's functional status has been found to be related to psychological well-being only among those individuals who viewed the abilities being evaluated as very important.[76] Interventions which improve social support may affect patient values, priorities, and appreciation of the resources they have. These social support interventions may allow them to maximize their quality of life despite important physical set-backs. Thus, it may be hard to differentiate change due to active interventions and truly improved functional status from change due to patient accommodation to level of function.

Response shift represents a challenge to health researchers. It lies under the surface of measurement, camouflaged by an apparent lack of change in treatment outcomes. Intra-individual shifts in referents and priorities may mediate both well-being and functional status. Understanding the predictive significance of this intra-individual variability is at the heart of meaningful outcomes measurement, and has the potential to lead to a paradigm shift in the many fields of investigation that rely on patient self-report.

Summary

We have provided an overview of the application of QALYs to clinical research. Although QALYs have distinct advantages, there is some controversy about the methods used to derive them, who should be the referent population for preferences, and how to ensure that they actually reflect the value of a given health state. It may not be useful or informative to assume that utilities or preferences for a given health state should have one 'gold standard' score across people, contexts, or experiences. In fact, this variability may reveal important differences in values, priorities, and adjustment to illness, all of which may be worth considering in outcomes assessment. It would thus seem to be the case that QALY-analytic methods should allow the comparison and integration of patient, provider, and societal values in evaluating treatments. Their application to clinical research was illustrated in published examples of QALY outcomes assessment in randomized trials of experimental treatments (i.e. phase III), screening or preventive care, and post-marketing studies (i.e. phase IV). Some emerging issues were discussed which are important considerations for medical researchers, including consideration of the disease context in evaluating treatment trade-offs and resource allocation, and implications of inter- and intra-individual shifts in values over time.

Acknowledgements

This project was supported by grant number RO1 HSO8582-01A1 from the Agency for Health Care Policy and Research to Dr Schwartz. The authors would like to thank Scott B. Cantor PhD, Frank Sonnenberg MD, and Paul Cleary PhD, for their helpful suggestions on earlier drafts of the manuscript.

References

1. Kant, I. *Critique of pure reason* (Transl. J.M.D. Meiklejohn). London: J.M. Dent, 1781.
2. Hundert, E.M. *Philosophy, psychiatry, and neuroscience: three approaches to the mind.* Oxford: Clarendon Press, 1989.
3. Wynne, A. Is it any good? The evaluation of therapy by participants in a clinical trial. *Soc. Sci. Med.*, 1989; **29**: 1289–97.
4. World Health Organization. *The World Health Organization Constitution.* Geneva: WHO, 1947.
5. Ware, J.E. and Sherbourne, C.D. The MOS 36-item short-form health survey (SF-36): conceptual framework and items selection. *Med. Care*, 1992; **30**: 473–83.
6. Sturm, R. and Wells, K.B. How can care for depression become more cost-effective? *J. Am. Med. Assoc.*, 1995; **273**: 51–8.
7. Kaplan, R.M. Health-related quality of life outcomes in mental health services evaluation. In *Cost-effectiveness of psychotherapy: A guide for practitioners, researchers, and health policy makers.* (ed. N.E. Miller and K.M. Magruder). New York: John Wiley & sons, (In press).
8. von Neumann, J. and Morganstern, O. *Theory of games and economic behavior.* Princeton: Princeton University Press, 1944.
9. Torrance, G.W. Measurement of health state utilities for economic appraisal. *J. Health Econ.*, 1986; **5**: 1–30.
10. Torrance, G.W., Thomas, W.H., and Sackett, D.L. A utility maximization model for evaluation of health care programs. *Health Serv. Res.*, 1972; **7**: 118–33.
11. Tsevat, J., Weeks, J.C., Guadagnoli, E., *et al.* Using health-related quality-of-life information: clinical encounters, clinical trials, and health policy. *J. Gen. Intern. Med.*, 1994; **9**: 576–82.
12. Froberg, D.G. and Kane, R.L. Methodology for measuring health state preferences II: Scaling methods. *J. Clin. Epidemiol.*, 1989; **42**: 459–71.
13. Tsevat, J., Goldman, L., Soukup, J.R., *et al.* Stability of time-tradeoff utilities in survivors of myocardial infarction. *Med. Decis. Making*, 1993; **13**: 161–5.
14. Revicki, D.A. Relationship between health utility and psychometric health status measures. *Med. Care*, 1992; **30** (Suppl.): MS274–82.
15. Boyd, N.F., Sutherland, H.J., Heasman, K.Z., *et al.* Whose utilities for decision analysis? *Med. Decis. Making*, 1990; **10**: 58–67.
16. Bass, E.B., Steinberg, E.P., Pitt, H.A., *et al.* Comparison of the rating scale and the standard gamble in measuring patient preferences for outcomes of gallstone disease. *Med. Decis. Making*, 1994; **14**: 307–14.
17. Laupacis, A., Wong, C., and Churchill, D. The use of generic and specific quality-of-life measures in hemodialysis patients treated with erythropoietin. *Control Clin. Trials*, 1991; **27**: 27–43.
18. Fowler, F.J. Jr, Cleary, P.D., Massagli, M.P., Weissman, J., and Epstein, A. The role of reluctance to give up life in the measurement of the values of health states. *Med. Decis. Making*, 1995; **15**: 195–200.
19. Christensen-Szalanski, J.J. Discount functions and the measurements of patients' values: women's decisions during childbirth. *Med. Decis. Making*, 1984; **4**: 47–58.

20. Wilson, I.B. and Cleary, P.D. Linking clinical variables with health-related quality of life. *J. Am. Med. Assoc.*, 1995; **273**: 59–65.
21. Smith, T.J. and Hillner, B.E. Decision analysis: a practical example. *Oncology*, 1995; **9** (Suppl.): 37–45.
22. Dolan, P. and Kind, P. Inconsistency and health state valuations. *Soc. Sci. Med.*, 1996; **42**: 609–15.
23. Nease, R.F., Kneeland, T., O'Connor, G.T., *et al.* Variation in patient utilities for outcomes of the management of chronic stable angina. *J. Am. Med. Assoc.*, 1995; **273**: 1185–90.
24. Feeny, D., Labelle, R., and Torrance, G.W. Integrating economic evaluations and quality of life assessments. In *Quality of life assessments in clinical trials*, (2nd edn), (ed. B. Spilker). Philadelphia: Lippincott-Raven, 1996; pp. 85–95.
25. McNeil, B.J., Pauker, S.G., Sox, H.C., and Tversky, A. On the elicitation of preferences for alternative therapies. *New Engl. J. Med.*, 1982; **306**: 1259–62.
26. O'Connor, A.M.C, Boyd, N.F, Warde, P., Stolback, L., and Till, J.E. Eliciting preferences for alternative drug therapies in oncology: influence of treatment outcome description, elicitation technique and treatment experience on preferences. *J. Chron. Dis.*, 1987; **40**: 811–18.
27. Torrance, G.W. and Feeny, D. Utilities and quality-adjusted life years. *Intl. J. Technol. Assessment in Health Care*, 1989; **5**: 559–75.
28. Anderson, N.H. and Zalinski, J. Functional measurement approach to self-estimation in multiattribute evaluation. *J. Behav. Decis. Making*, 1988; **1**: 191–221.
29. Drummond, M.F., Stoddart, G.L., and Torrance, G.W. *Methods for the economic evaluation of health care programmes.* Oxford: Oxford University Press, 1987.
30. Johannesson, M., Pliskin, J.S., and Weinstein, M.C. A note on QALYs, time tradeoff, and discounting. *Med. Decis. Making*, 1994; **14**: 188–93.
31. Singer, P., McKie, J., Kuhse, H. and Richardson, J. Double jeopardy and the use of QALYs in health care allocation. *J. Medical Ethics*, 1995; **21**: 144–50.
32. Kerridge, R.K., Glasziou, P.P., and Hillman, K.M. The use of 'quality-adjusted life years' (QALYs) to evaluate treatment in intensive care. *Anaesth. Intens. Care*, 1995; **23**: 322–31.
33. Loomes, G. and McKenzie, L. The use of QALYs in health care decision making. *Soc. Sci. Med.* 1989; **28**: 299–308.
34. Klevit, H.D., Bates, A.C., Castanares, T., Kirk, E.P., Sipes-Metzler, P.R., and Wopat, R. Prioritization of health care services: a progress report by the Oregon Health Services Commission. *Arch. Intern. Med.*, 1991; **151**: 912–16.
35. Kaplan, R.M. A quality-of-life approach to health resource allocation. In *Rationing America's medical care: the Oregon plan and beyond*, (ed. M.A. Strosberg, J.M. Wiener, R. Baker, and I.A. Fein). Washington DC: Brookings Institution, 1992; pp. 60–77.
36. Codman, E.A. The product of a hospital. *Surg. Gynecol. Obstet.*, 1914; **18**: 491–6.
37. Karnofsky, D.A. and Buchenal, J.H. The clinical evaluation of chemotherapeutic drugs. In *Evaluation of chemotherapeutic agents*, (ed. C.M. Macleod). New York: Columbia University Press, 1949; pp. 191–4.

38. Ubel, P.A., Loewenstein, G., Scanlon, D., and Kamlet, M. Individual utilities are inconsistent with rationing choices: a partial explanation of why Oregon's cost-effectiveness list failed. *Med. Decis. Making*, 1996; **16**: 108–16.

39. Hadorn, D.C. Setting health care priorities in Oregon: cost-effectiveness meets the rule of rescue. *J. Am. Med. Assoc.*, 1991; **265**: 2218–25.

40. Eddy, D.M. Oregon's methods: did cost-effectiveness fail? *J. Am. Med. Assoc.*, 1991; **266**: 2135–41.

41. Nord, E. Unjustified use of the quality of well-being scale in priority setting in Oregon. *Health Policy*, 1993; **24**: 45–53.

42. Mehrez, A. and Gafni, A. Quality-adjusted life years, utility theory and healthy-years equivalents. *Med. Decis. Making*, 1989; **9**: 142–9.

43. Mehrez, A. and Gafni, A. Healthy-years equivalents versus quality-adjusted life years: in pursuit of progress. *Med. Decis. Making*, 1993; **13**: 287–92.

44. Weinstein, M.C. and Pliskin, J.S. Perspectives on healthy-years equivalents. HYEs: What are the issues? *Med. Decis. Making*, 1996; **16**: 205–6.

45. Johannesson, M., Pliskin, J.S., and Weinstein M.C. Are healthy-years equivalents an improvement over quality-adjusted life years? *Med. Decis. Making*, 1993; **13**: 281–6.

46. Eddy, D.M. Rules for evaluating medical technologies. In *Quality of life and pharmacoeconomics in clinical trials*, (ed. B. Spilker). Philadelphia: Lippincott-Raven, 1996; pp. 761–71.

47. Weinstein, M.C., Fineburg, H.C., Elstein, A.S., *et al. Clinical decision analysis*. Philadelphia: W.B. Saunders, 1980.

48. Wong, J.B., Koff, R.S., Tine, F, and Pauker, S.G. Cost-effectiveness of interferon-α_{2b} treatment for hepatitis B and antigen-positive chronic hepatitis B. *Ann. Intern. Med.* 1995; **122**: 664–75.

49. Alward, W.L., McMahon, B.J., Hall, D.B., Hey Ward, W.L., Francis, D.P., and Bender, T.R. The long-term serological course of asymptomatic hepatitis B virus carriers and the development of primary hepatocellular carcinoma. *J. Infect. Dis.*, 1985; **151**: 604–9.

50. Perrillo, R.P. and Aach, R.D. The clinical course and chronic sequelae of hepatitis B virus infection. *Semin. Liver Dis.*, 1981; **1**: 15–25.

51. Lange, W. and Masihi, K.N. Epidemiology and economic importance of hepatitis B in the Federal Republic of Germany. *Postgrad. Med. J.*, 1987; **63** (Suppl.): 21–6.

52. Kamlet, M.S., Paul, N., Greenhouse, J., Kupfer, D., Frank, E., and Wade, M. Cost utility analysis of maintenance treatment for recurrent depression. *Controlled Clin. Trials*, 1995; **16**: 17–40.

53. Fryback, D.G. and Thornbury, J.R. The efficacy of diagnostic imaging. *Med. Decis. Making.* 1991; **11**: 88–94.

54. Cleary, P.D., Barry, M.J., Mayer, K.H., Brandt, A.M., Gostin, L, and Fineburg, H.V. Compulsory premarital screening for the human immunodeficiency virus. Technical and public health considerations. *J. Am. Med. Assoc.*, 1987; **258**: 1757–62.

55. Danese, M.D., Powe, N.R., Sawin, C.T., and Ladenson, P.W. Screening for mild thyroid failure at the periodic health examination. A decision and cost-effectiveness analysis. *J. Am. Med. Assoc.*, 1996; **276**: 285–92.

56. US Preventive Services Task Force. *Guide to clinical preventive services*, (2nd edn). Baltimore: Williams & Wilkins, 1996.

57. Epstein, K.A., Schneiderman, L.J., Bush, J.W., and Zettner, A. The 'abnormal' screening serum thyroxine (T_4): analysis of physician response, outcome, cost and health effectiveness. *J. Chronic. Dis.*, 1981; **34**: 175–90.

58. Tsevat, J., Goldman, L., Soukup, J.R., *et al.* Stability of time tradeoff utilities in survivors of myocardial infarction. *Med. Decis. Making*, 1993; **13**: 161–5.

59. Morris, L.A., Beckett, T.K., and Lechter, K.J. A marketing perspective: theoretical underpinnings. In *Quality of life and pharmacoeconomics in clinical trials*, (ed. B. Spilker). Philadelphia: Lippincott-Raven, 1996; 541–8.

60. Testa, M.A. and Nackley, J.F. Methods for quality-of-life studies. *Ann. Rev. Public Health*, 1994; **15**: 535–9.

61. Schondelmeyer, S.W. Uses of pharmacoeconomic data by policy makers and pharmaceutical benefit managers. In *Quality of life and pharmacoeconomics in clinical trials*, (ed. B. Spilker). Philadelphia: Lippincott-Raven, 1996; 1153–64.

62. Brook, R.H., McGlynn, E.A., and Cleary, P.D. Quality of health care Part 2: Measuring quality of care. *New Engl. J. Med.*, 1996; **335**: 966–70.

63. Schwartz, C.E., Cole, B.F., and Gelber, R.D. Measuring patient-centered outcomes in neurologic disease: extending the Q-TWiST methodology. *Arch. Neurol.*, 1995; **52**: 754–62.

64. Schwartz, C.E., Cole, B, Vickrey, B, and Gelber, R. The Q-TWiST approach for assessing health-related quality of life in epilepsy. *Quality of Life Research*, 1995; **4**: 135–41.

65. Schwartz, C.E., Genderson, M.W., and Lee, H. Patient-centered outcomes in psychosomatic medicine: applications of the Extended Q-TWiST to cost-effectiveness research. **Mind/Body Medicine**, 1997; (In press).

66. King, R.B. Non-provider factors that impact health care cost and access. *Arch. Neurol.*, 1995; **52**: 17–20.

67. National Institutes of Health. *Research plan for the National Center for Medical Rehabilitation Research*. Bethesda, MD: NIH Publication No 93-3509, 1993.

68. Lubitz, J.D. and Riley, G.F. Trends in Medicare payments in the last year of life. *New Engl. J. Med.*, 1993; **328**: 1092–6.

69. Callahan, D. *Setting limits: medical goals in an aging society*. New York: Simon & Schuster, 1987.

70. Wolf, F.M. *Meta-analysis: quantitative methods for research synthesis*. Beverly Hills: Sage Publications, 1986.

71. Breetvelt, I.S. and VanDam, F.S.A.M. Underreporting by cancer patients: the case of response-shift. *Soc. Sci. Med.*, 1991; **32**: 981–7.

72. Sprangers, M.A.G, Rozemuller, N., Vanden Berk, M.B.P, Boven, S.V., and VanDam, F.S.A.M. Response shift bias in longitudinal quality of life research. (Abstract.) *Quality of Life Research*, 1994; **3**: 49.

73. Sprangers, M., Broerson, J., Lodder, L., Wever, L., Smets, E., and VanDam, F. The need to control for response shift bias in longitudinal quality of life research. (Abstract.) *Quality of Life Research*, 1995; **4**: 488.

74. Funder, D.C. and Colvin, C.R. Explorations in personal consistency: properties of persons, situations, and behaviors. *J. Pers. Soc. Psychology*, 1991; **60**: 773–94.
75. Bach, J.R. and Tilton, M.C. Life satisfaction and well-being measures in ventilator assisted individuals with traumatic tetraplegia. *Arch. Phys. Med. Rehabil.*, 1994; **75**: 626–32.
76. Blalock, S.J., DeVillis, B.M., DeVellis, R.F., *et al.* Psychological well-being among people with recently diagnosed arthritis: do self-perceptions of abilities make a difference? *Arth. Rheum.* 1993; **35**: 1267–72.

8 *Possibilities for summarizing health-related quality of life when using a profile instrument*

Ron D. Hays, Jordi Alonso, and Stephen Joel Coons

Introduction

Health-related quality of life (HRQoL) refers to how well a person functions in daily life, and to his or her perceived well-being. HRQoL measures have assumed an increasingly important role in medical outcome studies. The 36-item health survey (SF-36) is one of the most widely used HRQoL measures in medical outcome studies today and has been included in over 500 clinical trials (Ware and Sherbourne 1992; Hays *et al.* 1993; Ware *et al.* 1995). The SF-36 is classified as a profile HRQoL measure because it yields scores for multiple domains of HRQoL: physical functioning, role limitations caused by physical health problems, pain, general health perceptions, emotional well-being, role limitations caused by emotional problems, social functioning, and energy/fatigue.

Profile measures such as the SF-36 provide fairly detailed information about multiple domains of HRQoL. This breadth of information is useful for specifying the pattern of functioning and well-being characterizing the individuals being studied. However, if a study shows improvements in some HRQoL scales and decrements in others, it is difficult to make an overall conclusion about HRQoL (Kaplan and Coons 1992). For example, Fig. 8.1 provides an illustration in which physical functioning is better for those in group X than those in group O, pain and emotional well-being are slightly better for those in group O, and social functioning is equivalent for both groups. Is HRQoL better for those in group X or those in group O? To make global conclusions such as this, it is necessary to have some method of summarizing the multiple scale scores.

Attrition of participants in a study over time due to mortality creates a noteworthy problem in applying profile measures. If those who die are dropped from the analysis, results can be biased; for example, if people in a study who are equivalent in HRQoL at baseline differ with respect to their access to medical care (high versus low access). At a follow-up assessment, one might find the results shown in Table 8.1. If one only looks at people who provided data at follow-up, persons with low access appear to have better HRQoL than those with high access (means of 75 and 50, respectively). However, this is a biased assessment of the

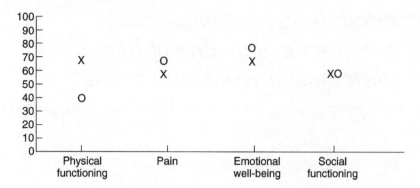

Fig. 8.1 Is HRQoL better for group X or group O?

Table 8.1 Baseline access and follow-up HRQoL

Person	Baseline access	Follow-up HRQoL (0–100 score or dead)
1	Low	Dead = missing data
2	Low	Dead = missing data
3	Low	50
4	Low	75
5	Low	100
6	High	0
7	High	25
8	High	50
9	High	75
10	High	100

data because 40 per cent of the people in the low access group died during the study. Some approaches to summarizing HRQoL are designed to deal with attrition due to mortality, while others are not.

Methods of summarizing profile measures

Factor scores

To help summarize the overall HRQoL impact, summary scores have been developed for some profile measures. For example, physical and mental health composite scores for the SF-36 scales are available (Hays *et al*. 1993; Ware *et al*. 1995). Factor analyses of the SF-36 provide strong support for a two-factor model of health, with physical health reflected primarily by measures of physical functioning, pain, and role limitations caused by physical health problems; and mental health reflected primarily by measures of emotional well-being and role limitations caused by emotional problems (Hays *et al*. 1993; Hays *et al*. 1994*a*). General health perceptions, energy/fatigue scales, and social functioning reflect both health dimensions.

Physical health measures best distinguished groups differing in severity of chronic medical illness whereas mental health measures best distinguished groups differing in the presence and severity of psychiatric disorders (McHorney *et al.* 1993). Reliability estimates for the physical and mental health composites exceed 0.90 (Ware *et al.* 1995).

The physical and mental health factors derived by Ware *et al.* (1995) in the Medical Outcomes Study (MOS) were forced to be uncorrelated (orthogonal) whereas those derived by Hays *et al.* (1993) were allowed to correlate (oblique), because correlations between physical and mental health factors at each of three years (baseline, two years post-baseline, and four years post-baseline) in the MOS ranged from 0.32 to 0.41 (see factor loadings in Table 8.2). In addition, oblique rotations often yield a more realistic representation of the factors than do orthogonal rotations (Rummel 1970) and 'it is more sensible to rotate the factors obliquely and then determine the tenability of the orthogonality assumption' (Ford *et al.* 1986).

Having both information about specific SF-36 scale scores and the composite scores can provide more information than the scales or composite scores alone. A longitudinal study of chiropractic patient adherence to treatment recommendations provides an example of the unique information from SF-36 scale and composite scores (Hays *et al.* 1995; Coulter *et al.* 1996). In this study, patients sampled in chiropractors' offices completed a slightly modified version of the SF-36 health survey. Change in the eight SF-36 scale scores and two factor scores were regressed on patient adherence to the chiropractor's recommendation to reduce stress and use relaxation techniques. The significance of the main effect of adherence on the SF-36 score was evaluated and predicted change scores (follow-up value − baseline value) were estimated for those with low adherence (1 SD below the mean) versus high adherence (1 SD above the mean).

As shown in Table 8.3, adherence was consistently related to more improvement in the SF-36 scales over time and significant effects of adherence were observed on one of the SF-36 scales (energy/fatigue) and on the physical and mental health composite scores. The effects of adherence on the two role limitations scales approached significance ($p = 0.052$ and 0.053). The composites reveal overall

Table 8.2 Loadings of SF-36 scales on physical (PH) and mental health (MH) factors in the medical outcomes study

	Baseline		Year 2		Year 4	
	PH	MH	PH	MH	PH	MH
Physical functioning	0.80	–	0.83	–	0.81	–
Role limitations – physical	0.80	–	0.80	–	0.78	–
Pain	0.73	0.08	0.72	0.08	0.72	0.08
General health perceptions	0.58	0.25	0.55	0.24	0.58	0.26
Emotional well-being	–	0.86	–	0.88	–	0.89
Role limitations – emotional	–	0.70	–	0.71	–	0.70
Social functioning	0.38	0.56	0.36	0.54	0.36	0.54
Energy/fatigue	0.50	0.45	0.51	0.46	0.50	0.46

Note: Data above were reported in Hays *et al.* (1994a).

Table 8.3 Predicted change in health-related quality of life by low versus high adherence to chiropractic recommendations

	Low adherence	High adherence	Difference*	p
Physical functioning	6.65	11.98	5.32	NS
Role limitations – physical health	14.49	33.05	18.56	0.053
Freedom from pain	16.12	21.38	5.25	NS
General health perceptions	1.08	2.35	1.27	NS
Physical health composite	8.68	16.61	7.93	0.016
Emotional well-being	7.31	10.62	3.31	NS
Role limitations – emotional problems	3.58	24.52	20.94	0.052
Social functioning	12.76	17.88	5.11	NS
Energy/fatigue	1.97	11.71	9.74	0.008
Mental health composite	6.67	16.36	9.69	0.025

Note: $N = 102$ patients and 45 chiropractors.
NS = not significant.
*Estimated change (follow-up – baseline) in health-related quality of life scores for those scoring one standard deviation below (low adherence) and one standard deviation above (high adherence) the adherence scale mean.

beneficial effects, but the specific scales suggest that the effects are concentrated in energy and role functioning.

Regression-weighted summary score

Regression weighting methods have been employed to derive a single overall HRQoL score for profile measures (Bozzette *et al*. 1994; Diehr *et al*. 1995). In this approach, weights are derived by regressing a criterion measure (e.g. current health perceptions, 0–10 visual analogue, probability of being in excellent, very good, or good health in the future, probability of being dead in the future) on HRQoL scales. These weights reflect the relative importance of the scales in predicting the criterion. The reliability of one summary HRQoL measure derived using a regression method was 0.93 (Bozzette *et al*. 1994).

A few proposals for imputing HRQoL scores for the dead have been entertained (Diehr *et al*. 1995). For example, it has been suggested that the lowest possible HRQoL score be assigned to those who have died. Unfortunately, none of these approaches are entirely satisfactory due to the inherent arbitrariness of the assigned value.

The use of utility and preference measures such as the standard gamble and time trade-off (TTO) as criteria for regression weighting has also been considered, but profile measures such as the SF-36 have been shown to account for a relatively small amount of variance (less than 30 per cent) in these criteria (Revicki and Kaplan 1993; Bosch and Hunink 1996).

Bult and Hunink (1995) noted that this was due to the fact that the regression model assumes similar preferences for different people. They used latent class analysis to identify four more homogeneous categories of respondents for which different regression weights were allowed. They regressed TTO scores on SF-36 scale scores, dummy variables for latent class, and interaction terms between the dummy variables and SF-36 scale scores. This model explained over 50 per cent of the variance in TTO scores. A similar amount of variance was accounted for in an analysis of the association of SF-36 scores with the standard gamble among 68 patients with symptomatic peripheral arterial disease (Bult *et al*. 1996). To be most useful, it will be necessary to identify characteristics of people in the latent classes so that different predictive weights can be applied using known characteristics when preference data are unavailable.

Multi-attribute utility measures

Another possibility for summarizing HRQoL is represented by measures derived using multi-attribute utility theory. Included in this category are the health utilities index (Feeny *et al*. 1995; Torrance *et al*. 1995), the EuroQoL or EQ-5D instrument (EuroQoL Group 1990; Nord 1991; Kind and Dolan 1995), and the quality of well-being scale (Kaplan and Bush 1982; Kaplan and Anderson 1988). In each of these examples, societal preferences are obtained for the range of possible health states and used to provide a 0–1 summary score for every possible health state assessed by the instrument.

One limitation of multi-attribute systems is the coarseness of health states they include in order to restrict the scope of possibilities to a manageable number. Limiting the number of possible states is necessary to implement the societal preference judgement task. An unknown (but potentially substantial) error in HRQoL assessment is introduced as a consequence. To illustrate this problem, assume a multi-attribute system with two dimensions, physical and mental health; and three levels within each dimension, low, medium, and high. Nine health states (not including death) can be defined by the combination of these two dimensions. Assume that judges were asked to provide ratings of the desirability of these health states and an additive, linear model was found to fit these ratings:

$$HRQoL = 1 - 0.20 * Medium\ physical - 0.50 * Low\ physical$$
$$- 0.30 * Medium\ mental - 0.40 * Low\ mental$$

where the hold-out group is high physical/high mental, and dummy variables are used to define the medium and low levels of both dimensions.

Preference values for each of the nine health states are shown in Fig. 8.2, which shows that the nine multi-attribute health states correspond to nine actual health states (denoted by 'x'). However, there are a number of actual health states (denoted by 'y') that are not represented in the multi-attribute scheme. These states are collapsed into the existing set of multi-attribute combinations, introducing an unknown element of error in the end result (preference scores).

The 15D-measure of HRQoL (Sintonen 1995) is a multi-attribute system that is less subject to the collapsing problem noted above, because it includes so many health states. However, the 15D weighting system assumes additivity in ratings and Nord (1996) has noted a 'floor problem'.

Chancellor *et al*. (1995) described a method for applying the multi-attribute utility method to data previously collected, which may be a better alternative for those using the SF-36. Factor analysis was used to identify the major dimensions

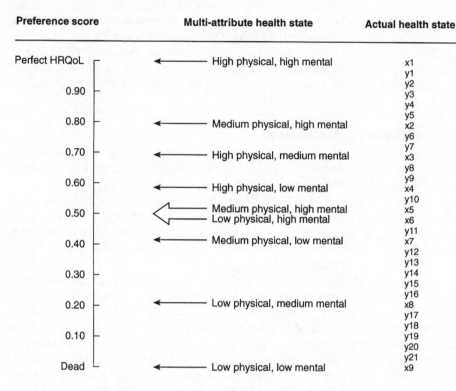

Fig. 8.2 Preference values for nine health states.

underlying the Rotterdam symptom checklist and the Hospital Anxiety and Depression scale (five factors were identified). Then a subset of items was selected from each factor (based on item–scale correlations) so that a manageable number of health states could be embedded in a multi-attribute scenario for preference judgements. Twelve-item subsets of the SF-36 which explain a substantial amount of variance in the physical and mental health composite scores have been selected (Radosevich and Pruitt 1995; Ware *et al.* 1995) and could be used to obtain preference ratings. However, if each level of the 12 items is used in defining a health state, the number of possible states is still very large (approximately four million).

Single-item overall rating

Another option is to use a single item to elicit a direct overall assessment of HRQoL. For example, respondents can be asked to rate their current health on a 0 to 10 scale, with 0 being worst possible health (as bad as being dead) and 10 being perfect health (Hays *et al.* 1994*b*) or 0 being worst imaginable health state and 100 best imaginable health state (Kind and Dolan 1995). The former anchor set makes the scoring of death straightforward (i.e. those who died are assigned a score of 0), but it does not allow for the possibility of health states worse than death (Patrick *et al*. 1994). The latter allows for that possibility, but leaves the location of death on the 0–100 scale unknown. These single item summary ratings are similar to the idea of the Karnofsky performance status scale (Karnofsky and Burchenal 1949; Grieco and Long 1984), but the rating is obtained directly from the patient. Although the single-item category rating is easy for respondents, it may not provide cardinal utility values. Nonetheless, category ratings have been used in several of the multi-attribute utility instruments to derive societal preferences, and then these values have been used to estimate utilities. In addition, recent work has confirmed earlier evidence that a power function can be used to transform group mean, visual analogue scale-derived health state values to TTO values (Stiggelbout *et al*. 1996).

Utilities

The standard gamble (SG) is the classical method of obtaining utilities. In this approach, one is asked to choose between a certain outcome (e.g. paralysis) and a gamble (e.g. x probability of complete mobility and $1-x$ probability of death). Varying the value of x, the preference value is defined as the point at which one is indifferent between the choices. The SG is based on the axioms of utility theory and is consistent with Von Neumann and Morgenstern's (1944) characterization of decision making when uncertain outcomes are involved. However, application of the SG is limited by the fact that it is not intuitive and therefore difficult for many respondents to do (Froberg and Kane 1989; Kaplan *et al*. 1993). Refusal rates of 10 per cent or higher for the SG are typically reported (Bult *et al*. 1996).

The TTO method presents the person a choice between two certain outcomes. The respondent is presented with a current health state (e.g. paralysis with a life expectancy of 10 years), and asked to trade the rest of his or her life (x years) in his or her current state of health against y ($y \leq x$) years of life in perfect health. When the respondent is indifferent between the two outcomes, the ratio y/x gives his or her utility for the current state of health relative to perfect health.

The TTO is not a utility measure in the strictest sense of the term, but it is a practical and popular alternative to the standard gamble (Torrance 1976; Bennett and Torrance 1996). An important assumption of TTO technique is indifference between equivalent gain due to life extension or improvement in quality of life (Richardson 1994).

Logistic problems in using the TTO have been discussed for a number of years (e.g. Sackett and Torrance 1978; Mohide *et al*. 1988). A recent study found that about 40 per cent of symptomatic cancer patients refused to do the TTO (Stigglebout *et al*. 1995). In another study, it was found that when survival was less than five years, some people were unwilling to trade any years of life to avoid losing their normal speech (McNeil *et al*. 1981). Similarly, Tsevat *et al*. (1995) reported that 35 per cent of seriously ill patients were unwilling to trade any time in their current state of health for shorter time in excellent health. The extent to which people are unwilling to trade years of life (reluctance to give up life) has been shown to vary across individuals independently of health status

(Fowler *et al*. 1995). Other methods that have been used for the valuation of health states include magnitude estimation and person trade-off (Coons and Kaplan 1996). These methods are much less common and will not be discussed here.

North American experts' input about different summary approaches

As noted in Chapter 10, a sample of seven North American experts was asked to rate various approaches to summarizing HRQoL on a 0–100 scale, with 0 representing the most inadequate and 100 the most adequate approach. They were also asked to rank order the different approaches from most (1) to least preferred (8). Results revealed that the TTO, Health Utilities Index, and the Quality of Well-Being scale received the highest overall ratings and best rankings of the different methods proposed. Factor analytic and regression weighting were rated lowest by the experts. The categorical rating/visual analogue approach received intermediate ratings/rankings (see Table 8.4). The EuroQoL (EQ-5D) was rated slightly lower than the categorical rating/visual analogue approach, but it is important to keep in mind that Europeans were not included in this sample of preference experts.

Conclusion

When using a HRQoL profile measure, we recommend that the multiple scale scores be supplemented with summary scores such as physical and mental health composite scores and/or an overall summary score. Whenever possible, a single item overall rating and a preference measure such as the HUI, QWB, or TTO should be administered. This combination of assessments will provide both comprehensive information about specific domains of HRQoL as well as a basis for summarizing this wealth of information into an overall assessment.

Table 8.4   Mean ratings and rankings of methods for summarizing HRQoL by seven North American experts

Method	Rating			Ranking	
	Mean	Median	Range	Mean	Median
Standard gamble	53.57	50	0–95	3.86	4
Time trade-off	65.00	70	0–100	2.86	2
Health utilities index	68.71	85	25–100	3.00	3
EuroQoL	27.83	30	5–52	5.57	6
Quality of well-being scale	71.43	80	50–100	3.00	3
Categorical rating	45.00	40	5–100	4.43	5
Factor-analytic	17.29	10	0–70	6.29	7
Regression-weighting	16.57	1	0–90	7.00	8

Note: Rating is on a 0–100 scale, with 0 representing the most inadequate method and 100 representing the most adequate method of deriving an overall HRQoL score for HCSUS.
Rank is on a 1–8 scale, from most (1) to least preferred (8).

Further research is needed to shed light on the variety of ways to summarize HRQoL and help point to those methods that are the most valuable for different applications.

References

Bennett, K.J. and Torrance, G.W. (1996). Measuring health state preferences and utilities: rating scale, time trade-off, and standard gamble techniques. In *Quality of life and pharmacoeconomics in clinical trials*, (2nd edn), (ed. B. Spilker), pp. 253–65. Lippincott-Raven, Philadelphia.

Bosch, J.L. and Hunink, M.G.M. (1996). The relationship between descriptive and valuational quality of life measures in patients with intermittent claudication. *Medical Decision Making*, **16**, 217–25.

Bozzette, S.A., Hays, R.D., Berry, S., and Kanouse, D. (1994). A perceived health index for use in persons with advanced HIV disease: derivation, reliability, and validity. *Medical Care*, **32**, 716–31.

Brazier, J.E., Harper, R., Jones, N.M.B., O'Cathain, A., Thomas, K.J., Usherwood, T., and Westlake, L. (1992). Validating the SF-36 health survey questionnaire: new outcome measure for primary care. *British Medical Journal*, **305**, 160–4.

Bult, J.R. and Hunink, M.G.M. (1995). Heterogeneity in the relationship between the time trade-off and short form-36 for HIV-infected and primary care patients. Paper presented at the meeting of the International Society of Technology Assessment in Health Care, Stockholm, Sweden, June 1995.

Bult, J.R., Bosch, J.L., and Hunink, M.G.M. (1996). Heterogeneity in the relationship between the standard gamble utility measure and health status dimensions. *Medical Decision Making*, **16**, 221–33.

Chancellor, J., Coyle, D., and Drummond, M. (1995). Health state preferences in lung cancer. Paper presented at the meeting of the International Society of Technology Assessment in Health Care, Stockholm, Sweden, June 1995.

Coons, S.J. and Kaplan, R.M. (1996). Cost–utility analysis. In *Principles of pharmacoeconomics*, (2nd edn), (ed. J.L. Bootman, R.J. Townsend, and W.F. McGhan), pp. 103–26. Harvey Whitney Books, Cincinnati, OH.

Coulter, I.D., Hays, R.D., and Danielson, C.D. (1996). The role of the chiropractor in the changing health care system: from marginal to mainstream. *Research in the Sociology of Health Care*, **13a**, 95–117.

Diehr, P., Patrick, D., Hedrick, S., Rothman, M., Grembowski, D., Raghunathan, T.E., and Beresford, S. (1995). Including deaths when measuring health status over time. *Medical Care*, **33**, AS164–72.

EuroQoL Group (1990). EuroQoL—a new facility for the measurement of health-related quality of life. *Health Policy*, **16**, 199–208.

Feeny, D., Furlong, W., Boyle, M., and Torrance, G.W. (1995). Multi-attribute health status classification systems: health utilities index. *PharmacoEconomics*, **7**, 490–502.

Ford, J.K., MacCallum, R.C., and Tait, M. (1986). The application of exploratory factor analysis in applied psychology: a critical review and analysis. *Personnel Psychology*, **39**, 291–314.

Fowler, F.J., Cleary, P.D., Massagli, M.P., Weissman, J., and Epstein, A. (1995). The role of reluctance to give up life in the measurement of the value of health states. *Medical Decision Making*, **15**, 195–200.

Froberg, D.G. and Kane, R.L. (1989). Methodology for measuring health-state preferences: II: Scaling methods. *Journal of Clinical Epidemiology*, **43**, 459–71.

Grieco, A. and Long, C.J. (1984). Investigation of the Karnofsky performance status as a measure of quality of life. *Health Psychology*, **3**, 129–42.

Hays, R.D., Sherbourne, C.D., and Mazel, R.M. (1993). The RAND 36-item health survey 1.0. *Health Economics*, **2**, 217–27.

Hays, R.D., Marshall, G.N., Wang, E.Y.I., and Sherbourne, C.D. (1994*a*). Four-year cross-lagged associations between physical and mental health in the Medical Outcomes Study. *Journal of Consulting and Clinical Psychology*, **62**, 441–9.

Hays, R.D., Kallich, J.D., Mapes, D.L., Coons, S.J., and Carter, W.B. (1994*b*). Development of the kidney disease quality of life (KDQOL™) instrument. *Quality of Life Research*, **3**, 329–38.

Hays, R.D., Anderson, R., and Revicki, D.A. (1995). Psychometric evaluation and interpretation of health-related quality of life data. In *The international assessment of health-related quality of life: Theory, translation, measurement and analysis*, (ed. S. Shumaker and R. Berzon), pp. 103–14. Rapid Communications, Oxford.

Kaplan, R.M. and Anderson, J.P. (1988). A general health policy model: update and applications. *Health Services Research*, **23**, 203–35.

Kaplan, R.M. and Bush, J.W. (1982). Health-related quality of life measurement for evaluation research and policy analysis. *Health Psychology*, **1**, 61–80.

Kaplan, R.M. and Coons, S.J. (1992). Relative importance of dimensions of health-related quality of life for patients with hypertension. *Progress in Cardiovascular Nursing*, **7**, 29–36.

Kaplan, R.M., Feeny, D., and Revicki, D.A. (1993). Methods for assessing relative importance in preference based outcome measures. *Quality of Life Research*, **2**, 467–75.

Karnofsky, D.A. and Burchenal, J.H. (1949). The clinical evaluation of chemotherapeutic agents in cancer. In *Evaluation of chemotherapeutic agents* (ed. C.M. MacLeod), pp. 191–205. Columbia Press, New York.

Kind, P. and Dolan, P. (1995). The effect of past and present illness experience on the valuations of health states. *Medical Care*, **33**, AS255–63.

McHorney, C.A., Ware, J.E., and Raczek, A.E. (1993). The MOS 36-item short-form health survey (SF-36): II. Psychometric and clinical tests of validity in measuring physical and mental health constructs. *Medical Care*, **31**, 247–63.

McNeil, B.J., Weischselbaum, R., and Pauker, S.G. (1981). Speech and survival: trade-offs between quality and quantity of life in laryngeal cancer. *New England Journal of Medicine*, **305**, 982–7.

Mohide, E.A., Torrance, G.W., Streiner, D.L., Pringle, D.M., and Gilbert, R. (1988). Measuring the well-being of family (are given) using the time trade-off technique. *Journal of Clinical Epidemiology*, **41**, 475–482.

Nord, E. (1991). EuroQoL: Health-related quality of life measurement: valuations of health states by the general public in Norway. *Health Policy*, **18**, 25–36.

Nord, E. (1996). Health status index models for use in resource allocation decisions: a critical review in the light of observed preferences for social choice. *International Journal of Technology Assessment in Health care*, **12**, 31–44.

Patrick, D.L., Starks, H.E., Cain, K.C., Uhlmann, R.F., and Pearlman, R.A. (1994). Measuring preferences for health states worse than death. *Medical Decision Making*, **14**, 9–18.

Radosevich, D. and Pruitt, M. (1995). *The 12-item Health Status Questionnaire (HSQ-12): Version 2.0*. Health outcomes Institute, Bloomington, MN.

Revicki, D.A. and Kaplan, R.M. (1993). Relationship between psychometric and utility-based approaches to the measurement of health-related quality of life. *Quality of Life Research*, **2**, 477–87.

Richardson, J. (1994). Cost–utility analysis: what should be measured? *Social Science and Medicine*, **39**, 7–21.

Rummel, R.J. (1970). *Applied factor analysis*. Northwestern University Press, Evanston, Illinois.

Sackett, D.L. and Torrance, G.W. (1978). The utility of different health states as perceived by the general public. *Journal of Chronic Disease*, **31**, 697–704.

Sintonen, H. (1995). The 15D-measure of health-related quality of life: properties, standards and applications. Paper presented at the meeting of the International Society of Technology Assessment in Health Care, Stockholm, Sweden, June 1995.

Stiggelbout, A.M., Kiebert, G.M., Kievit, J., Leer, J.W., Habbema, J.D., and de Haes, J.C. (1995). The 'utility' of the time trade-off method in cancer patients: feasibility and proportional trade-off. *Journal of Clinical Epidemiology*, **48**, 1207–14.

Stiggelbout, A.M., Eijkemans, M.J.C., Kiebert, G.M., Kievit, J., Leer, J.W., and de Haes, H.J. (1996). The 'utility' of the visual analog scale in medical decision making and technology assessment: is it an alternative to the time trade-off? *International Journal of Technology Assessment in Health Care*, **12**, 291–8.

Torrance, G.W. (1976). Social preferences for health states: an empirical evolution of three measurement techniques. *Socioeconomic Planning Science*, **10**, 129–36.

Torrance, G.W., Furlong, W., Feeny, D., and Boyle, M. (1995). Multi-attribute preference functions: health utilities index. *PharmacoEconomics*, **7**, 503–20.

Tsevat, J., Cook, F., Green, M.L., Matchar, D.B., Dawson, N.V., Broste, S.K., *et al.* (1995). Health values of the seriously ill. *Annals of Internal Medicine*, **122**, 514–20.

Von Neumann, J. and Morgenstern, O. (1944). *Theory of games and economic behavior*. Princeton University Press, Princeton, NJ.

Ware, J.E. and Sherbourne, C.D. (1992). The MOS 36-item short-form health survey (SF-36): I. Conceptual framework and item selection. *Medical Care*, **30**, 473–483.

Ware, J.E., Kosinski, M., Bayliss, M.S., McHorney, C.A., Rogers, W.H., and Raczek, A. (1995). Comparison of methods for the scoring and statistical analysis of SF-36 health profile and summary measures: summary of results from the medical outcomes study. *Medical Care*, **33**, AS264–79.

IV

Psychometry

9 *Questionnaire scaling: models and issues*

Dennis A. Revicki and Nancy Kline Leidy

Introduction

The theory and practice of psychological measurement and scaling methods have been developed over more than 100 years (Guilford 1954). These theoretical developments and the research accumulated over the past 50 to 60 years provide the foundation for the measurement of health status and health-related quality of life (HRQoL). Nunnally and Bernstein (1994) described measurement as 'rules for assigning symbols to objects so as to (1) represent quantities of attributes numerically (scaling)...' (Nunnally and Bernstein 1994; p. 3). Objects or persons, *per se*, are not directly measured. Rather, we measure attributes (characteristics or traits) of a given person, such as height or weight, or, in the case of HRQoL, level of physical functioning, mental well-being, or social functioning. Different dimensions of HRQoL thus reflect different attributes of health and life quality.

Scaling rules form the basis of standardized measurement, enabling different users of a given instrument to obtain similar results under similar conditions (Nunnally and Bernstein 1994). The quantification and scaling of HRQoL and other health outcomes allow for continued scientific development and evaluation of the impact of disease progression, treatment, sociodemographic characteristics, and different health care delivery systems on patient health outcomes.

This chapter reviews the different methods for scaling HRQoL data, using a classical psychometric approach, and addresses some of the practical issues related to the scaling process and associated analytical considerations. Examples are drawn from the HRQoL and clinical literature in order to illustrate the structure underlying the various scaling models and how they might be used in practice. In this discussion, we concentrate on psychometric-based scaling procedures. Preference-based utility measurement, such as standard gamble, time trade-off, and Q-TWiST, are addressed briefly in our discussion of levels of measurement. The theoretical underpinnings and scale structure of these approaches are addressed in Chapters 5, 6 and 15.

Levels of measurement

It is useful to think about scaling within the context of the four traditional classes or levels of measurement: nominal, ordinal, interval, and ratio, defined by the manner in which numerical values or labels are assigned to a given attribute (Stevens 1951). Nominal level measurement is represented by groupings of patients or objects with qualitative similarities on the specified attribute, with no quantitative ordering across group. The clustering of patients by medical diagnosis is an example of nominal level measurement. Patients within each group share the qualitative attribute of disease, but there is no quantitative ordering. Numbers assigned to each category simply represent membership, for example, diabetes = 3, emphysema = 2, and leukaemia = 1. Diabetes is not greater or less than leukaemia.

Nominal scales can be used to measure trial outcomes directly, such as clinical improvement/no improvement or dead/alive, or to stratify outcomes, such as evaluating HRQoL score by disease, gender, or ethnic group. This method can also be used for scaling individual items in HRQoL measures. The yes/no response scale to the question 'Are you able to climb one flight of stairs?' can be considered nominal and is often used as the underlying structure for scalogram analysis (see below) and the Rasch measurement model (see Chapter 11). Nominal scales, in the form of improved HRQoL/not improved HRQoL, are rarely used as outcomes in clinical trials.

Ordinal, interval and ratio scales are commonly used levels of measurement in quality of life research. Ordinal scales provide a relative ranking of subjects on a specific attribute, that is, from least to most, low to high. For ordinal scales, no information is available about the magnitude of the attribute or how far apart the subjects are with respect to the attribute. All that is known, for example, is that subject A is more independent than subject B, subject A has more energy than subject B, or subject A feels more strongly than subject B about a given experience or statement.

The Likert scale, frequently used to structure items comprising HRQoL measures, is an example of an ordinal scale. Subjects are asked to respond to a given statement by indicating, for example, whether they strongly agree, agree, are neutral or undecided, disagree, or strongly disagree. Their responses are assigned scores, from one to five, to reflect the magnitude of the appraisal. Similarly, questions on vitality in the medical outcomes study short-form 36 (SF-36) health survey are rated on a six-point scale from 'all of the time' to 'none of the time' (Ware et al. 1993).

The visual analogue scale (VAS) is another example of an ordinal level format, although many suggest it also meets the criteria of an interval or ratio level scale (Maxwell 1978; Price et al. 1983; Wewers and Lowe 1990). A VAS is a line, generally 10 cm in length, bounded on each end by the extreme limits of the dimension being measured (Pfennings et al. 1995). The subject is asked to place a mark along the line which best describes his or her feelings or experience with the attribute under consideration. The distance from the minimal end-point to the mark, on a pre-specified measurement interval, represents the scale score (McCormack et al. 1988). Although scores can range from 1 to 5 or 1 to 200, a 100-point scale based on millimetres is generally used.

Although construction of a VAS appears to be simple, attention to detail is required in order to maximize data quality. The sensation or response under consideration must be defined carefully. The words or phrases appearing at the end-points must clearly represent the extremes. A standardized question or stem must be selected or created and tested, and the measurement intervals must be specified (Scott and Huskisson 1976). Horizontal presentation is preferred over vertical, due to a lower failure rate (Scott and Huskisson 1976). Lines shorter than 10 cm tend to produce greater error variance (Revill *et al*. 1976). Right angle stops are placed at each end to reduce the likelihood of marks placed beyond the scale itself, and anchor phrases are placed beyond the stops, rather than above or below (McCormack *et al*. 1988). To avoid clustering of scores, intermediate points along the continuum should not be defined (Aitken 1969; Scott and Huskisson 1976). A variation of the VAS, the graphic rating scale (GRS), includes descriptors at intervals along the line. While the descriptors are intended to assist subjects in scoring, they generally lead to response clustering and response distributions that mirror a Likert-type scaling approach (Wewers and Lowe 1990).

The VAS technique is often used in the evaluation of clinical symptoms (particularly pain and shortness of breath), affective state (mood, anxiety), sleep, functional performance, and behaviour (Morrison 1983; Wewers and Lowe 1990; Olsen *et al*. 1992). The VAS is also used in HRQoL measures (Priestman and Baum 1976; Coates *et al*. 1983). The 'feeling thermometer' is a VAS method for assessing patient preferences and has been used as a simple warm-up exercise in studies to derive utility estimates for the calculation of quality-adjusted life-years (Bennett and Torrance 1996). Although the VAS is often equated with a single-item measure of a given construct, multiple items can and are used, in an attempt to improve precision and data quality. Several measures of HRQoL in patients with cancer have used this approach (Presant *et al*. 1981; Padilla *et al*. 1983).

Dichotomous response options can be considered ordinal when the assigned value of 1 is considered greater than 0, rather than a numerical representation of a classification. The Nottingham health profile comprises items with dichotomous response options (McEwen and McKenna 1996).

An interval scale is one which reflects a rank ordering of objects (subjects/patients) on an attribute and where numerically equal distances on the scale represent equal distances on the attribute. The absolute magnitude of the attribute for the object is either not meaningful or unknown. Likert and dichotomous item scores described above can be aggregated across items to derive what many believe conforms to an interval-level total score. The difference between a physical function score of 60 and 65 on the SF-36, for example, is equal to the difference between scores of 90 and 95. The method for aggregating individual Likert scores, known as the method of summative rating, is described in detail below.

Ratio scaling is the final and 'highest' level of measurement. Ratio scales share all of the properties of interval scales with the addition of a known absolute magnitude on the attribute of interest; that is, the distance from a rational zero point is known. A value of zero on a ratio scale means that the person has none of the attribute being measured. Numbers on the scale indicate the actual amounts of the attribute being measured. Borg's combined category–ratio scales for the measurement of perceived exertion is an example of ratio scaling (Borg 1962, 1982).

The Borg scale assesses an individual's perception of their amount of physical performance and capacity.

Issues

One of the most frequently asked questions concerning the use of Likert-type ordinal scales for individual questionnaire items is the optimal scoring interval. Unfortunately, there is no definitive answer. Measures of pain intensity vary from four levels to as many as 101 levels, motivated by the assumption that 'more is better'. In practice, research indicates that 10- to 21-point scales possess sufficient discriminatory capabilities (Jensen et al. 1994). Most Likert-type items used in HRQoL measures offer between four and seven options, generally a reflection of the trade-off between ease of administration and item variance. Theoretically, the greater the number of options, the larger the expected variance, the more accurate and responsive the item and hence the measure. Clearly a point must be reached where the gain in variance no longer warrants the increase in scale complexity. In fact, the complexity may lead to respondent confusion and a reduction in response rate. Furthermore, variance is a function not only of the number of response options, but the quality of the item stem (wording, clarity) and the characteristics of the sample. A poorly worded item with a seven-point Likert scale can have less variance than a well-constructed item with a four-point scale. The number of items in the measure also plays a role in the accuracy and responsiveness of a measure, suggesting that an instrument with few items should employ a wider range of response options to achieve reasonable reliability.

The VAS has been viewed as an alternative to the Likert scale and as a solution to the scoring interval debate. Proponents of this method, which gained widespread use in the 1970s, suggest that the VAS is a better reflection of the continuous nature of feelings or attitudes and is thus a more valid and sensitive scaling method (Aitken 1969; Aitken and Zealley 1970). There are disadvantages to the approach, however, which may account for its limited use in studies of HRQoL. Although some respondents express a preference for this assessment technique due to its simplicity, others favour the Likert scale format for the same reason (McCormack et al. 1988). Psychometric studies of the VAS have found a tri-modal distribution of scores in some samples, suggesting many respondents do not view the scale as a continuum and are responding only in terms of high, medium, and low (McCormack et al. 1988). The fact that little is known about the influence of education or diagnostic group (e.g. psychiatric or medical patients) on VAS response characteristics is a concern. The scoring system for a VAS is somewhat arbitrary, and the interpretation of group differences and change can be difficult. Is a 1 mm change along a 100 mm scale clinically significant? Finally, scoring itself can be somewhat cumbersome in large, multicentre clinical trials. As studies become more computer intensive with direct data entry, this problem may be eliminated. Evidence that a VAS approach to HRQoL measurement may be more responsive than a Likert-type format suggests that it may be beneficial to subject this technique to further testing and standardization (Pfennings et al. 1995).

Another issue in questionnaire scaling around which there are questions and debate concerns the statistical analyses appropriate to each level of measurement. Theoretically, as one moves up the scaling hierarchy, analytical options move from simple frequencies (nominal) to non-parametric procedures (ordinal level; rank order statistics), and ultimately to parametric statistics (interval and ratio) (Nunnally and Bernstein 1994). Arguments supporting and refuting this position appeared in the literature almost 40 years ago (Luce 1959). Although many mathematicians and statisticians have moved away from the hierarchical approach, some continue to hold this view (Davison and Sharma 1990). Nunnally and Bernstein (1994) present a cogent summary of the major issues underlying this debate, from a general measurement and statistical perspective. The challenge is to consider these issues and their implications within the context of HRQoL measurement.

Most individual HRQoL items are scaled ordinally. Subscale and total scale scores, aggregated across items, are treated as interval scales. Although some critics argue that the underlying scale properties of a measure must be demonstrated before applying certain analytic methods, it is not clear what kinds of evidence would justify unequivocally the assumptions of a particular type of scale (Nunnally and Bernstein 1994). Furthermore, like most physical and psychological measurements, HRQoL measures are based on correlates of the underlying attributes rather than the attributes themselves. Reliance on evaluation of visualizable characteristics for determining measurement scales renders many scientific measurements no more than ordinal.

We can evaluate scale characteristics using different scaling models for the construction of measures. A scaling model is a plan or set of rules for establishing the convention about the scaling of an attribute, that is, for establishing the scale's properties. These models are based on a number of assumptions concerning the behaviour of empirically derived data. Since psychological and HRQoL attributes cannot be observed directly, we must test the fit of the data to the standards of a model to determine whether a ratio, interval, or ordinal scale holds. If the data generated from the application of a measure fit the assumptions of the scaling model under consideration then the measure has the scale properties specified by the model. If the measure is established as a ratio scale, the zero point can be taken seriously and the intervals can be treated as equal for any statistical analysis. If the measure is found to be an interval scale, the intervals can be treated as equal in all forms of analysis.

Price et al.'s (1983) study of the data characteristics of the VAS provides a useful example of this approach. In this controlled experiment, healthy subjects were asked to record their pain experiences on a VAS of pain intensity as they were exposed to graded changes in noxious thermal stimuli. The investigators found that variation in VAS score was proportional to change in stimuli, suggesting the VAS possessed the properties of a ratio scale. While this form of validation is useful for sensations that can be controlled experimentally, it is virtually impossible to use for HRQoL measures. An alternative approach is a *post hoc* examination of data quality, such as McHorney et al.'s (1994) study of the SF-36. This evaluation will be described in greater detail in the following section on scaling models.

In practical terms, scaling models can be evaluated according to the 'good sense' criteria (Nunnally and Bernstein 1994).

1. Does the model possess intuitive appeal, that is, is there reason to believe that specific operations will yield a useful measurement approach?

2. Is the model consistent with what is known about other, similar data?

3. Are there any preliminary data upon which the effect of alternative operations can be tested?

4. How much measurement error is associated with the scale?

The latter criterion has a great deal to do with a measure's utility in science, that is, its capacity to explain phenomena and accurately characterize treatment outcomes. Ultimately, we are concerned with the extent to which the model produces the most accurate estimate of the underlying attribute, accurate in terms of measurement error (reliability) and validity. Basically, the true test is whether the scaling procedure produces a scale or measure which works well in practice. However, we can never be entirely certain about whether the scaling model provides the best estimate of the targeted attribute.

More than one scaling model may fit the data. In these cases, evidence needs to be accumulated about which scale best fits the observed data. However, competing scaling approaches are often monotonically related to each other; both measures will demonstrate similar relationships with other variables. Monotonicity refers to situations where the relationship between two variables can be reflected in either an increasing or decreasing mathematical function. In situations in which the measure is used as a dependent variable in a data analysis, it will make relatively little difference which of two monotonically related scales is used. This is because transformations of the scale of a dependent measure make little difference in the results of statistical analyses. Once again, the true test is whether the scaling model fits the observed data and whether the specific scaling of the attribute of interest is useful in the examination of relationships between the attribute and other variables.

Scaling models

Unidimensional scaling models address rules for aggregating a set of data items which theoretically and empirically correspond to a single common dimension. Multidimensional scaling (MDS) permits multiple dimensions to underlie a set of items or measures. MDS is a useful method of understanding data structure, uncovering relationships among variables, developing or refining theory, and generating empirically based hypotheses and instruments. Factor analysis (described in Chapter 12) is related to MDS and plays an important role in instrument development and evaluation. Because MDS is generally not useful in HRQoL assessment in clinical trials, however, the following discussion is restricted to unidimensional scaling methods. Readers interested in learning more about MDS are referred to the works of Carroll, Kruskal, and Wish (Kruskal 1964; Carroll and Wish 1974; Carroll 1976; Wish 1976; Kruskal and Wish 1978).

A number of different scaling models have been used to create measures, that is, to aggregate data across a set of related individual scales or items to represent a single, unidimensional construct. Three classic models continue to dominate the psychometric literature and underlie the vast majority of HRQoL measures: the method of summated ratings (Likert 1932), method of equal-appearing intervals (Thurstone and Chave 1929), and scalogram analysis (Guttman 1944). (Readers are directed to books by Guilford (1954), Nunnally and Bernstein (1994), Torgerson (1958), and Edwards (1957) for more information about methods of scaling stimuli and persons.) The intent of each method is to represent the underlying construct as precisely as possible, optimizing validity, minimizing error, and maximizing the probability that data gathered through this method will meet the assumptions required for the application of the more powerful parametric statistical approaches.

Method of summated ratings

The method of summated ratings, more generally known as the Likert technique, is the most frequently used method for constructing health status and psychological scales (Likert 1932; Murphy and Likert 1937). In this technique, individuals are asked to respond to a set of questions on a five-level (or k-level) ordinal response scale, the Likert-type scale described previously. For each respondent, the total score on the scale is obtained by summing his or her scores on individual questions. Because each response to a question is considered a rating and because these are summated over all questions, the Likert method of scale construction is referred to as the method of summated ratings. Likert (1932; Murphy and Likert 1937) and others (Edwards and Kenney 1946) found that this approach was strongly correlated with other more complicated scaling methods, such as the method of equal-appearing intervals (Thurstone and Chave 1929).

Likert's technique is based upon two key assumptions: that the overall score is a good measure of the attribute, and that the aggregate is better than any one item alone. That is to say, the items, as a group, measure only one attribute; each item is monotonically related to the underlying attribute; and the summative model is used to minimize measurement error associated with any one item alone (McIver and Carmines 1981). These assumptions form the basis for the psychometric analyses performed when evaluating the quality of an instrument. Likert himself, for example, proposed a full examination of item response distributions, equivalence of item means and standard deviations, and internal consistencies of items within scales (Likert 1932). These techniques are discussed in greater detail in Chapter 10. It should be noted here, however, that these assumptions form the basis for multiple-item measures. Single item scales are frowned upon not only because they are more prone to random error, but because a single data point does not allow the investigator to estimate the measurement properties of the instrument, most importantly, the error (McIver and Carmines 1981). As the number of items in a scale increases, the contribution of each to the total variance decreases, resulting in a reduction in bias associated with each item (McIver and Carmines 1981). Thus, although the parsimony associated with single-item indicators is appealing, their use is ill advised and generally imprudent.

The medical outcomes study SF-36 is an example of the method of summative rating. McHorney et al. (1994) evaluated whether the eight subscales comprising the SF-36 satisfied the scaling assumptions for summated ratings. They evaluated the distribution of item responses, equivalence of item means and standard deviations, item internal consistency, and item-discriminant validity for each subscale using data from the MOS ($N = 3445$ patients with chronic medical and psychiatric conditions). They found that the scaling assumptions were consistently met for the total sample and subsamples grouped according to age, gender, ethnic group, education, poverty status, medical diagnosis, and disease severity (McHorney et al. 1994).

The method of summated ratings has been shown to fit Nunnally's criteria of 'good sense' scaling and works well in most instances. It should be noted that individual scores cannot be interpreted independently of the distribution of some defined group. This is because only the extreme scores have meaning. There is no evidence that the neutral point corresponds to the mid-point of the possible range of scores and no real zero point is known (Edwards 1957). This limitation of the Likert technique is not problematic for HRQoL studies in which the intent is to compare scale mean or mean change scores, as in comparative studies or clinical trials, or to evaluate the relationship between two or more variables, as in descriptive studies and causal models. The simplicity of the scaling technique and its usefulness has led to its widespread application in the measurement of HRQoL.

Method of equal-appearing intervals

The method of equal-appearing intervals was developed by Thurstone (Thurstone and Chave 1929) to construct attitude scales. Although this scaling method has been used infrequently in HRQoL measures *per se*, it has been used in the development of item weights. Weights for the Sickness Impact Profile, for example, were developed from equal-appearing interval scaling procedures (Carter et al. 1976; Bergner et al. 1981). This method requires a group of judges to rate statements (questions) into a specified number of intervals, usually 11. The two extreme and the neutral intervals are defined according to the dimension of interest. The median of the distribution of ratings for each statement is used as its scale value. Some investigators have adapted the scaling task to have the judges rate each statement on an 11-point scale. Early studies used more than 300 subjects to complete the rating task (Thurstone and Chave 1929). Research has demonstrated that small samples of judges may approximate the ratings of large samples (Edwards 1957). Equal-appearing interval scales have a theoretical zero point, that is, a neutral point from which values increase or decrease as one moves in either direction.

Scalogram analysis

Scalogram analysis is a procedure for evaluating existing scales to determine whether they meet the requirements of a Guttman scale (Guttman 1944). A set of items constitutes a Guttman scale when the items can be ordered hierarchically, such that a person responding positively to a given item also responds positively to each item that falls below it in the hierarchy. Thus, a subject with a higher score than another subject on a set of items also ranks (or scores) just as high or higher on every item compared to the other subject (Guttman 1950). This procedure can be used in situations in which there is an identifiable hierarchy to the items or questions, such as the performance of daily activities. An affirmative response to an item high on a performance scale, such as 'jogs one mile', will imply an affirmative response to all other questions involving lower levels of performance, such as 'walks one block'. When a group of items meets this requirement, the set of items reflects a unidimensional scale.

To construct a Guttman scale, the investigator first hypothesizes a hierarchical ordering to the selected set of questions along a unidimensional continuum. The set of questions is administered to a group of individuals and the responses are evaluated to determine whether the questions actually demonstrate a hierarchical and reproducible scale. Coefficients of reproducibility are used to evaluate the scaling, with values exceeding 0.90 considered supportive. The selection of items is critical and it is important to examine the item score distributions to avoid spuriously high coefficients of reproducibility (Edwards 1957).

The Guttman scaling technique is used most frequently in physical disability or functional status measures. The Physical Self-Maintenance Scale (Lawton and Brody 1969), Katz index of independence in Activities of Daily Living (Katz and Akpom 1976), and the Arthritis Impact Measurement Scale (AIMS), have each shown hierarchical characteristics, with reproducibility coefficients for the latter scale exceeding 0.90 (Meenan *et al*. 1980, 1982). Nortström and Thorslund's (1991) analysis of data from 421 Swedish elders suggests that their index of intermediate activities of daily living (IADL) meets the criteria for a Guttman scale. Activities were ordered according to level of dependence, as follows: bed-making, cooking, conducting business at the post office and bank, bathing, food shopping, laundry, and cleaning. Elders dependent in bed-making were likely to be dependent on all remaining activities. The Rasch measurement model, an outgrowth of Guttman's scalogram analysis, has also been useful in developing scales of functional performance, including ADL and IADL measures (McArthur *et al*. 1991; Fisher 1993). This model, together with item response theory, is addressed in Chapter 11.

Summary

In summary, questionnaire scaling involves the application of rules for quantifying attributes, forming the basis of standardized measurement. It is the foundation for reproducing empirical results across different investigators under similar conditions. Scaling models are useful for understanding the structure of individual items in a questionnaire, as well as methods used for aggregating data. There are four levels of measurement: nominal, ordinal, interval, and ratio. The most frequently used methods for scaling items in HRQoL questionnaires are dichotomous, considered nominal or ordinal depending upon the rule underlying the assignment of values, and Likert-type scales, considered ordinal or interval level. The visual analogue scale can also be used and has been a popular method for evaluating the symptomatic or emotional component of HRQoL. In order to improve measurement precision, data are aggregated across individual, related items. Three scaling models are generally used to aggregate data: the method of summated ratings (used to aggregate multiple Likert and VAS-derived responses), the method of equal-appearing intervals (commonly used in deriving weights), and scalogram analysis (used to evaluate Guttman scales, particularly in measures describing activity performance). The intent of any scaling method is to represent the underlying construct as precisely as possible, by optimizing validity, minimizing error and maximizing reproducibility.

References

Aitken, R.C.B. (1969). A growing edge of measurement of feelings. *Proceedings of the Royal Society of Medicine*, **62**, 989–996.

Aitken, R.C.B. and Zealley, A.K. (1970). Measurement of moods. *British Journal of Hospital Medicine*, **IV**, 215–225.

Bennett, K.J. and Torrance, G.W. (1996). Measuring health state preferences and utilities: rating scales, time trade-off, and standard gamble techniques. In *Quality of life and pharmacoeconomics in clinical trials*, (2nd edn), (ed. B. Spilker), pp. 253–66. Lippincott-Raven, New York.

Bergner, M., Bobbitt, R.A., Carter, W.B., and Gilson, B.S. (1981). The sickness impact profile: development and final revision of a health status measure. *Medical Care*, **19**, 787–805.

Borg, G. (1962). *Physical performance and perceived exertion*. Gleerup, Lund, Sweden.

Borg, G. (1982). A category scale with ratio properties for intermodal and interindividual comparisons. In *Psychophysical judgment and the process of perception*, (ed. H.G. Geissler and P. Petzold), pp. 25–34. VEB Deutscher, Berlin.

Carroll, J.D. (1976). Spatial, non-spatial and hybrid models for scaling. *Psychometrika*, **41**, 439–63.

Carroll, J.D. and Wish, M. (1974). Multidimensional perceptual models and measurement methods. In *Handbook of perception*, Vol. 2, (ed. E.C. Carterette and M.P. Friedman), pp. 391–447. Academic Press, New York.

Carter, W.B., Bobbitt, R.A., Bergner, M., and Gilson, B.S. (1976). Validation of an interval scaling: the sickness impact profile. *Health Services Research*, **14**, 57–67.

Coates, A., Dillenbeck, C.F., McNeil, D.R., Kate, S.B., Sims, K., Fox, R.M., *et al*. (1983). On the receiving end. II. Linear analogue self-assessment (LASA) in evaluation of aspects of the quality of life of cancer patients receiving therapy. *European Journal of Cancer and Clinical Oncology*, **19**, 1633–7.

Davison, M.L. and Sharma, A.R. (1990). Parametric statistics and levels of measurement: factorial designs and multiple regression. *Psychological Bulletin*, **107**, 394–400.

Edwards, A.L. (1957). *Techniques of attitude scale construction*. Prentice-Hall, Englewood Cliffs, New Jersey.

Edwards, A.L. and Kenney, K.C. (1946). A comparison of the Thurstone and Likert techniques of attitude scale construction. *Journal of Applied Psychology*, **30**, 72–83.

Fisher, A.G. (1993). The assessment of IADL motor skills: an application of many-faceted Rasch analysis. *American Journal of Occupational Therapy*, **47**, 319–29.

Guilford, J.P. (1954). *Psychometric methods*. McGraw-Hill, New York.

Guttman, L. (1944). A basis for scaling qualitative data. *American Sociological Review*, **9**, 139–50.

Guttman, L. (1950). The basis for scalogram analysis. In *Measurement and prediction*, (ed. S.A. Stouffer, *et al.*), Princeton University Press, New Jersey.

Jensen, M.P., Turner, J.A., and Romano, J.M. (1994). What is the maximum number of levels needed in pain intensity measurement? *Pain*, **58**, 387–92.

Katz, S. and Akpom, C.A. (1976). A measure of primary sociobiological functions. *International Journal of Health Service*, **6**, 493–507.

Kruskal, J.B. (1964). Nonmetric multidimensional scaling: a numerical method. *Psychometrika*, **29**, 115–29.

Kruskal, J.B. and Wish, M. (1978). *Multidimensional scaling*. Sage, Beverly Hills.

Lawton, M.P. and Brody, E.M. (1969). Assessment of older people: self-maintaining and instrumental activities of daily living. *Gerontologist*, **9**, 179–86.

Likert, R. (1932). A technique for the measurement of attitudes. *Archives of Psychology*, **140**, 1–55.

Luce, R.D. (1959). On the possible psychophysical laws. *Psychological Review*, **66**, 81–95.

Maxwell, C. (1978). Sensitivity and accuracy of the visual analogue scale: a psycho-physical classroom experiment. *British Journal of Clinical Pharmacology*, **6**, 15–24.

McArthur, D.L., Cohen, M.J., and Schandler, S.L. (1991). Rasch analysis of functional assessment scales: an example using pain behaviors. *Archives of Physical Medicine and Rehabilitation*, **72**, 296–304.

McCormack, H.M., Horne, D.J., and Sheather, S. (1988). Clinical applications of visual analogue scales: a critical review. *Psychological Medicine*, **88**, 1007–19.

McEwen, J. and McKenna, S.P. (1996). Nottingham health profile. In *Quality of life and pharmacoeconomics in clinical trials*, (2nd edn), (ed. B. Spilker), pp. 253–66. Lippincott-Raven, New York.

McHorney, C.A., Ware Jr, J.E., Lu, J.F.R., and Sherbourne, C.D. (1994). The MOS 36-item short-form health survey (SF-36): III. tests of data quality, scaling assumptions, and reliability across diverse patients groups. *Medical Care*, **32**, 40–66.

McIver, J.P. and Carmines, E.G. (1981). *Unidimensional scaling*. Sage, Newbury Park.

Meenan, R.F., Gertman, P.M., and Mason, J.H. (1980). Measuring health status in arthritis: the arthritis impact measurement scales. *Arthritis and Rheumatism*, **23**, 146–52.

Meenan, R.F., Gertman, P.M., Mason, J.H., and Dunaif, R. (1982). The arthritis impact measurement scales: further investigations of a health status measure. *Arthritis and Rheumatism*, **25**, 1048–53.

Morrison, D.P. (1983). The Crichton visual analogue scale for the assessment of behavior in the elderly. *Acta Psychiatrica Scandinavica*, **68**, 408–13.

Murphy, G. and Likert, R. (1937). *Public opinion and the individual*. Harper, New York.

Norström, T. and Thorslund, M. (1991). The structure of IADL and ADL measures: some findings from a swedish study. *Age and Ageing*, **20**, 23–8.

Nunnally, J.C. and Bernstein, I.H. (1994). *Psychometric theory*, (3rd edn). McGraw-Hill, New York.

Olsen, S., Nolan, M.F., and Kori, S. (1992). Pain measurement: an overview of two commonly used methods. *Anesthesiology Review*, **6**, 11–15.

Padilla, G.V., Presant, C., Grant, M.M., Metter, G., Lipsett, J., and Heide, F. (1983). Quality of life index for patients with cancer. *Research in Nursing and Health*, **6**, 117–26.

Pfennings, L., Cohen, L., and van der Ploeg, H. (1995). Preconditions for sensitivity in measuring change: visual analogue scales compared to rating scales in a Likert format. *Psychological Reports*, **77**, 475–80.

Presant, C.A., Klahr, C., and Hogan, L. (1981). Evaluating quality-of-life in oncology patients: pilot observations. *Oncology Nursing Forum*, **8**, 26–30.

Price, D.D., McGrath, P.A., Rafil, A., and Buckingham, B. (1983). The validation of visual analogue scale measures for chronic and experimental pain. *Pain*, **17**, 45–56.

Priestman, T.J. and Baum, M. (1976). Evaluation of quality of life in patients receiving treatment for advanced breast cancer. *Lancet*, **i**, 899–901.

Revill, S.I., Robinson, J.O., Rosen, M., and Hogg, M.I.J. (1976). The reliability of a linear analogue for evaluating pain. *Anesthesia*, **31**, 1191–8.

Scott, J. and Huskisson, E.C. (1976). Graphic representation of pain. *Pain*, **2**, 175–84.

Stevens, S.S. (1951). Mathematics, measurement, and psychophysics. In *Handbook of experimental psychology*, (ed. S.S. Stevens). Wiley, New York.

Thurstone, L.L. and Chave, E.J. (1929). *The measurement of attitude*. University of Chicago Press, Chicago.

Torgerson, W.S. (1958). *Theory and methods of scaling*. Wiley, New York.

Ware, J.E., Snow, K.K., Kosinski, M., and Gandek, B. (1993). *SF-36 health survey: manual and interpretation guide*. The Health Institute, New England Medical Center, Boston.

Wewers, M.E. and Lowe, N.K. (1990). A critical review of visual analogue scales in the measurement of clinical phenomena. *Research in Nursing and Health*, **13**, 227–36.

Wish, M. (1976). Comparisons among multidimensional structures of interpersonal relations. *Multivariate Behavioral Research*, **11**, 297–327.

10 *Assessing reliability and validity of measurement in clinical trials*

Ron D. Hays, Roger T. Anderson, and Dennis Revicki

Health-related quality of life instruments are often used to evaluate patient-centered outcomes in randomized clinical trials and other outcomes research studies. An understanding of the reliability and validity of measurement is needed to select HRQoL instruments for clinical studies and to interpret the findings of completed clinical trials. This chapter summarizes reliability and validity and the various techniques that have been used to evaluate the psychometric characteristics of HRQoL instruments.

Reliability

Reliability refers to the extent to which the measure yields the same number or score each time it is administered, all other things being equal (i.e. no true change in the attribute being measured has occurred). Classical test theory regards observed responses as consisting of the sum of true score and error. True score for an individual is assumed to be invariant on repeated measurements. However, two parallel measurements will yield non-identical observed scores as a result of random error of measurement. Because random errors are normally distributed, the true score will be located at the mean of the distribution of parallel measures. Observed HRQoL scores actually include a true score component, a systematic error component, and a random error component. If no random error is present, the reliability is 1.0. Reliability approaches zero as the relative amount of random error increases.

Both the true score component and systematic error contribute to the reliability of the measure because they drive the observed score for an individual towards a consistent value. However, systematic error leads to bias in measurement, because it causes the score to be consistently too high or too low relative to the true score. Systematic errors include social desirability responding (reporting in such a way as to minimize the presentation of undesirable and maximize the presentation of desirable characteristics), acquiescent responding (agreement with statements regardless of content), and observational bias (such as halo effects whereby a single positive feature colours the general impression and ratings of another).

Reliability assessment involves examining agreement between an individual's score on two or more measures of the same thing. There are four basic categories of reliability estimation, each reflecting somewhat different ways by which random error of measurement is estimated: inter-rater, equivalent forms, test–retest, and internal consistency reliability.

Inter-rater reliability

Inter-rater reliability refers to a comparison of scores assigned to the same target (either patient or other stimuli) by two or more raters (Marshall *et al.* 1994). Both rater selection and intra-individual response variability influence random error in this case.

The kappa statistic can be used if one is interested in estimating exact agreement between raters for a variable measured on a nominal, ordinal or interval-level scale (it is also possible to provide partial credit for non-exact agreement using a weighted kappa; Cohen 1968). Kappa is known a quality index, because it compares observed agreement with agreement expected by chance. The general formula for kappa is

$$\kappa = \frac{\text{observed proportion agreement} - \text{chance expected proportion agreement}}{1 - \text{chance expected proportion agreement}}.$$

Agreement expected by chance is determined by assuming each rater made their ratings randomly but with probabilities equal to the overall proportions or marginal frequencies. The chance proportion is the proportion of pairs that would be expected to end up by chance in the diagonal representing agreement between one rater and another in a two-way cross-tabulation of ratings. Rules of thumb for interpreting the magnitude of kappa have been provided by Fleiss (1981) and Landis and Koch (1977). The limitations and extent to which kappa depends on the degree of the balance and symmetry of marginals is discussed elsewhere (Feinstein and Cicchetti 1990; Cicchetti and Feinstein 1990). For nominal data, kappa is mathematically equivalent to the intraclass correlation. For ordinal and interval-level data, weighted kappa and the intraclass correlation are equivalent under certain conditions (Fleiss and Cohen 1973).

Data from ratings provided from seven North American experts provide an example of estimating inter-rater reliability for interval-level variables. The experts were told that HRQoL was to be assessed using a generic HRQoL profile measure (such as the SF-36) in a longitudinal study with the possibility of noteworthy attrition over time. In addition, they were told that the study team was interested in deriving an overall summary HRQoL score. In providing their ratings, they were instructed that the study was facing severe time constraints in assessing HRQoL because of competing study needs. Experts were asked to rate each of eight approaches for deriving an overall HRQoL score (standard gamble, time trade-off, Health Utilities Index, EuroQoL, Quality of Well-Being Scale, global categorical rating/visual analogue, factor analysis, regression weights) on a 0–100 scale, with 0 representing the most inadequate and 100 representing the most adequate approach. The ratings given by each of the seven raters for the eight different approaches are provided in Table 10.1 along with the mean and standard deviation for each approach. The dash for one entry in the table represents a missing data point.

An ANOVA table summarizing the sources of variance of these ratings is given in Table 10.2. Reliability and intraclass correlation estimates are provided in Table 10.3. The reliability coefficients in Table 10.3 estimate the reliability for the average of multiple assessments (seven ratings) whereas the intraclass correlations estimate the corresponding reliability for a single assessment (one rater). In inter-rater reliability evaluations such as this example, one is most probably interested in the reliability of multiple ratings. The intraclass correlation would be of interest if the reliability of a single rater was of concern.

The one-way model separates the targets being rated (the eight approaches in the example) as the between-group variance and the remaining variance is assigned to the within-error term (Shrout and Fleiss 1979). The estimated reliabilities for the average rating and single rating (intraclass correlation) under the one-way model are 0.78 and 0.34, respectively (see Table 10.3).

If the number of assessments (raters) is the same across respondents, it is also possible to estimate the main effect of raters (i.e. mean differences). The two-way mixed (fixed rater effect) effects model estimates the reliability of the average of the multiple assessments by subtracting the mean square error from the mean

Table 10.1 Ratings of eight approaches to summarizing health-related quality of life by seven North American experts

Approach	Rater							Mean	SD
	1	2	3	4	5	6	7		
1	90	00	50	95	30	60	50	53.57	33.00
2	90	00	70	100	60	55	80	65.00	32.79
3	90	51	40	90	25	100	85	68.71	29.44
4	30	52	05	30	–	10	40	27.93	17.78
5	80	50	80	60	80	50	100	71.43	18.64
6	30	100	05	50	50	40	40	45.00	28.72
7	20	70	00	20	10	00	01	17.29	24.86
8	20	90	00	00	05	00	01	16.57	33.18

Note: Ratings were made on a 0–100 possible scale.
– represents missing data

Table 10.2 Sources of variance in North American experts' ratings of eight approaches to summarizing health-related quality of life

Source	Degrees of freedom	Mean square	Label for mean square
Ratees (N − 1)	7	3608.69	BMS
Within	47	789.68	WMS
Raters (K − 1)	6	825.72	JMS
Raters × ratees	41	784.40	EMS
Total	54		

square between, then dividing by the mean square between. The mean square error is estimated by the interaction between respondents and the multiple assessments (the main effect of multiple assessments is excluded from the error term). For this example, the estimated reliabilities of the average rating and single rating under this model, respectively, are 0.78 and 0.34 (see Table 10.3).

The two-way random effects model assumes that the different assessments (e.g. raters) are randomly selected. In this model, the main effect of multiple assessments is incorporated into the estimate of total variability. For the example, the estimated reliabilities of the average rating and single rating under this model are 0.78 and 0.34, respectively (see Table 10.3).

Shrout and Fleiss (1979) note that the one-way model will tend to yield smaller values than the two-way models and the random effects model will tend to yield lower values than the fixed effects model. The fixed effects model is described as assessing consistency of raters because rater variance is ignored. The random effects model, in contrast, provides an estimate of agreement because it assesses whether raters are interchangeable. The formulae for each of these models are provided in Table 10.4.

The mean square within term in Table 10.2 is 789.68 and therefore the estimated common within-subject standard deviation is 28.10 (Bland and Altman 1996). This value is an estimate of the measurement error. We can check for the assumption that the error is not related to the magnitude of the ratings by correlating the means and standard deviations in Table 10.2. The Spearman rank order correlation between mean and standard deviation is not statistically significant (rho $= -0.17$, $p = 0.69$) for these data. The difference between the mean

Table 10.3   Reliability and intraclass correlation estimates for experts' ratings of eight approaches to summarizing health-related quality of life

Model	Reliability	Intraclass correlation
One way	0.781	0.338
Two-way		
Fixed effects	0.783	0.340
Random effects	0.782	0.338

Table 10.4   Intraclass correlation and reliability formulae

Model	Reliability	Intraclass correlation
One-way	$\dfrac{MS_{BMS} - MS_{WMS}}{MS_{BMS}}$	$\dfrac{MS_{BMS} - MS_{WMS}}{MS_{BMS} + (K-1)MS_{WMS}}$
Two-way, fixed	$\dfrac{MS_{BMS} - MS_{EMS}}{MS_{BMS}}$	$\dfrac{MS_{BMS} - MS_{EMS}}{MS_{BMS} + (K-1)MS_{EMS}}$
Two-way, random	$\dfrac{N(MS_{BMS} - MS_{EMS})}{NMS_{BMS} + MS_{JMS} - MS_{EMS}}$	$\dfrac{MS_{BMS} - MS_{EMS}}{MS_{BMS} + (K-1)MS_{EMS} + K(MS_{JMS} - MS_{EMS})/N}$

MS = mean square; N = number of ratees; K = number of replications (e.g. raters). Subscripts are defined in Table 10.2.

value for each approach and the true value is expected to be less than 1.96 times the measurement error 95 per cent of the time. The difference between two ratings for the same approach is expected to be less than 2.77 times the measurement error for 95 per cent of pairs of observations (2.77 times the measurement error is referred to as the repeatability).

Equivalent forms reliability

Equivalent forms reliability refers to the agreement between an individual's score on two or more measures designed to measure the same attribute. Both item selection and intra-individual response variability contribute to random error in this method of estimating reliability. If the forms are truly equivalent in terms of item content, then the correlation between scores provides a good estimate of their reliability. However, it is difficult to devise equivalent forms and intervening events or practice effects can distort the results from this method of reliability assessment. The same formulae used for inter-rater reliability can be used to estimate equivalent forms reliability, with the different forms substituted for multiple raters.

Test–retest reliability

Test–retest reliability is the relationship between scores obtained by the same person on two or more separate occasions. Intra-individual response variability is used to estimate random error in test–retest assessments. The approach described above for inter-rater reliability is the same one used for test–retest reliability, with multiple times of assessment substituted for multiple raters. Several factors may influence the reliability of a measure between test dates, such as the conditions of administration, testing effects, specific factors affecting the participants in their daily lives, or the length of time between administrations. The assessment of reliability is further complicated by the fact that changes in the attribute being measured may have occurred between administrations. For example, scores may change notably for patients assessed initially during a doctor's office visit (when they were symptomatic) and subsequently when their symptoms have gone away. A low test–retest correlation may therefore not accurately reflect the reliability of the test. Thus, test–retest assessments become less useful to the extent that real changes occur from the first to the second assessment of the attribute being measured.

Internal consistency reliability

Internal consistency reliability for a scale is a function of the number of items and their covariation. Random error due to item selection is modelled in this type of reliability estimate. Cronbach's (1951) alpha is the coefficient commonly used to estimate the reliability of instruments based on internal consistency. Cronbach's alpha is calculated using the two-way fixed effects model described for inter-rater reliability with items substituting for the rater effect. Generally, one is most interested in the reliability of the average of the items (rather than the intraclass correlation, or estimated reliability of a single item). Formulae for computing the significance of difference between alpha coefficients are provided elsewhere (Feldt *et al.* 1987).

For each reliability model, the intraclass correlation can be derived from the estimated reliability for multiple assessments using a variant of the Spearman–Brown prophecy formula (Clark 1935), where R_{ii}=intraclass correlation, R_{tt}= reliability of average assessment, and K=number of assessments per target,

$$R_{ii} = \frac{R_{tt}}{K + (1-K)R_{tt}}.$$

Likewise, the reliability of the multiple assessments can be obtained from the intraclass correlation using the formula

$$R_{tt} = \frac{KR_{ii}}{1 + (K-1)R_{ii}}.$$

Standards for reliability

For clinical trials, the standard for reliability of measures is less stringent than it is for individual assessment. Because different groups of people (e.g. HIV patients who receive or do not receive AZT treatment before the onset of AIDS) are compared rather than individuals, a 0.70 standard is appropriate for clinical trials (Nunnally 1978).

A reliability level of 0.90 was advocated by Nunnally (1978) as a minimum standard for measurement that is designed for interpretation of scores at the individual level. This recommendation stems from the fact that the standard error of measurement is about one-third of the measure's standard deviation if it has a reliability of 0.90 (standard error of measurement is estimated by the product of the measure's standard deviation and the square root of the difference between the reliability of the measure and 1.0). Confidence intervals around an individual's estimated true score are wide at reliabilities below this recommended cut-off point.

Despite the rationale for the 0.90 reliability standard for individual assessment, in practice it may be too stringent. To achieve this level of reliability requires several items per scale. Many highly regarded instruments fail to meet these standards. For example, only two of the eight subscales (physical functioning and emotional well-being) in the SF-36 satisfied the 0.90 reliability standard in the medical outcomes study (MOS) (Ware and Sherbourne 1992; Hays *et al.* 1993). Test–retest reliabilities (24 hour) for blood pressure did not meet this standard either (Prisant *et al.* 1992). Systolic blood pressure and diastolic blood pressure reliabilities were 0.87 and 0.67, respectively.

Even if measures fall short of the 0.90 reliability level, obtaining this information is preferred to not doing so. Although the confidence interval around an individual patient's score is wider than one might like, the interval is still tighter than that based on no information at all. Clinicians need to be aware of the extent of unreliability in all of their measures and interpret them with appropriate caution.

However, as noted above, reliabilities exceeding 0.70 are acceptable for group comparisons in randomized clinical trials and other clinical studies.

A Guttman scale is a special case of internal consistency

Large correlations among items in a multi-item scale contribute to internal consistency reliability. In HRQoL research, physical functioning scales have been shown frequently to exhibit a special type of internal consistency embodied in Guttman scales. Guttman scales consist of dichotomous items that adhere to a strict deterministic response model related to the prevalence of item endorsement. If observed data fit the Guttman scale model, then individuals with same total scale score also tend to exhibit the same pattern of responses to each item in the scale. Thus, by knowing a person's scale score it is possible to predict with good accuracy their answer to every item in a Guttman scale. In general, the number of possible response patterns is two raised to a power equal to the number of items, but the number of response patterns consistent with a Guttman scale equals the number of items plus one.

To determine if a scale is consistent with the Guttman model, observed patterns of responses are compared with the patterns predicted for a Guttman scale, examining the degree to which observed response patterns deviate from expected response patterns. The coefficient of reproducibility (CR) for Guttman scales is defined as the proportion of error (i.e. proportion of differences between observed and expected responses) subtracted from unity. A CR value of 0.90 or higher is considered acceptable (Menzel 1953). In addition, an index of reproducibility is typically computed by determining how well item modes reproduce the observed response patterns. Errors are counted as differences between each observed item response for an individual and the modal response for that item across all respondents (Goodenough 1944). This index, the minimum marginal reproducibility (MR), is used to calculate the coefficient of scalability (CS) defined as $(CR-MR)/(1-MR)$. A CS of 0.60 has been recommended as a minimum standard for acceptability (Menzel 1953). The standard error of reproducibility for Goodenough scoring can be estimated by the square root of $[(1+CR) (1-CR)/NK]$ (Ellickson *et al.* 1992). For a recent application of Guttman scalogram analysis with HRQoL data, see Cunningham *et al.* (1995). For recent methods of analysis that go beyond the traditional Guttman model, see Chapter 11 on item response theory.

Validity

Validity is the degree to which the measure reflects what it is supposed to measure rather than something else. The distinction between reliability and validity is important because a measure may be reliable (i.e. always yield the same score for the same patient), but it may be consistently measuring the wrong thing (i.e. not what it is supposed to measure).

Demonstrating reliability in measurement is essentially accumulating evidence indicative of the existence of a stable property over repeated measurement.

Validity, in contrast, is an estimation of the extent to which an instrument measures what it was intended to measure. Reliability is necessary, but not sufficient for valid measurement. If an HRQoL measure does not yield a similar or identical number when an individual has not changed in HRQoL, it must not be giving a valid reading of the individual (i.e. both of the inconsistent numbers cannot be correct). The process of validating measures involves accumulating evidence of many different types which indicate the degree to which the measures denote what they were intended to represent. The following kinds of evidence are generally used to infer validity of measurement.

Content validity

Content validity is the extent to which a measure samples a representative range of the content under study. In interpreting content validity, questions regarding item sufficiency and patient population should be addressed carefully. For example, the range of items needed adequately to assess physical functioning in arthritic patients may be too gross for application to many coronary heart disease samples. Also, some self-report depression questionnaires are dominated by one or two aspects of depression, such as organic concomitant or somatic complaints. A clear idea of what aspects of a concept are to be measured is essential in assessing content validity. Content validity evaluations tend to be fairly subjective, but ideally include systematic comparison of a measure with existing standards, well-accepted theoretical definitions, expert opinions, and interviews with individuals for whom the measure is targeted (Stewart *et al.* 1992). Often in the development of a new scale a content map is created and items are constructed to cover the dimensions of interest.

Construct validity

Construct validity is evaluated by hypothesizing how measures should 'behave' and confirming or disconfirming these hypotheses (Cronbach and Meehl 1955). Hypotheses are stated regarding the direction (and sometimes the strength) of relationships that might be expected, and validity is supported when the associations are consistent with hypotheses. Construct validation is iterative by its very nature with empirical results feeding into revision of measures, retesting, and further revisions, if necessary.

Convergent and discriminant validity are two fundamental aspects of construct validity. Convergent validity refers to the extent to which different ways of measuring the same trait intercorrelate with one another. Discriminant validity involves demonstrating that a measure does not correlate too strongly with measures that are intended to indicate different traits from it. When two or more constructs (traits) are assessed using more than one method of assessment, convergent and discriminant validity can be assessed using multitrait–multimethod (MTMM) analytic methods (Campbell and Fiske 1959).

Procedures for implementing the MTMM methodology have been developed based on zero-order correlations among measures (Hayashi and Hays 1987) and confirmatory factor analysis (Kenny and Kashy 1992). The zero-order correlation method is generally easier to implement than confirmatory factor analysis. Some HRQoL studies have employed this approach (Nelson *et al.* 1990; Hadorn and Hays 1991; Siu *et al.* 1993*a*). However, interpretation of MTMM data 'can be ambiguous and misleading' if only zero-order correlations are examined (Cole 1987). Confirmatory factor analysis allows for explicit separation of trait, method, and unique variance, but ill-defined solutions and interpretation of method effects are a source of concern (Marsh 1989).

Criterion validity can be viewed as a special case of construct validity in which stronger hypotheses are made possible by the availability of a criterion or 'gold standard' measure. For example, a thermometer might serve as a gold standard against which self-reported temperature might be compared. It is well-known that absolute gold standard measures do not exist for HRQoL measures, but it is often the case that 'quasi gold standard' criterian are available. For example, a performance based measure of walking might function as a quasi gold standard against which self-reported ability to walk a block might be evaluated (Siu *et al.* 1993*a*). Performance based measures of daily activities, such as fastening buttons and preparing and boiling a pot of water can be used to validate self-reported activities of daily living.

A quality of life measure developed to assess the impact of mild disease should discriminate a patient group from a general population sample. Evaluation of the extent to which this holds can be considered a variant of quasi gold standard validation. This 'know groups' strategy typically involves evaluating an instrument in relation to clinical measures of disease status (Stewart *et al.* 1992).

Relative validity calculations (between group ANOVA *F* ratios) can be used to evaluate the sensitivity of different HRQoL measures to known groups differences. Relative validities are determined by dividing the *F*-statistic for each measure by the *F* ratio of a designed reference measure. The relative validity of the reference measure is thereby set to 1, by definition (Liang *et al.* 1985). These relative validities are equivalent to the ratio of sample sizes that would be required to detect the known group difference using one measure versus the other.

When a dichotomous criterion is used, it is possible to perform standard contingency table analysis, examining sensitivity and specificity of the HRQoL measure at designated cut-off points. To minimize the effects of a specific cut-off point, receiver operator characteristic (ROC) methods can be employed. Hanley and McNeil (1982) reported a practical method of estimating the area under an ROC curve using the Wilcoxon statistic. They also developed a non-parametric method for comparing ROC curves from the same sample (Hanley and McNeil 1983). The areas under ROC curves, their standard errors, and the significance of difference between areas for different measures can be calculated.

Responsiveness

The validity of a measure may be supported by cross-sectional analyses; however, the measure may not perform well at detecting small, but meaningful, changes over time. A final indicator of validity which is important in clinical trials is responsiveness (Guyatt *et al.* 1987). Responsiveness refers to the ability of a measure to reflect underlying change (Hays and Hadorn 1992). Although reliability and cross-sectional validity studies have been conducted on the widely used HRQoL measures, there is very little information about their responsiveness.

Quality of life changes can be compared to change in clinical status, intervening health events, interventions of known or expected efficacy, and direct reports of change by patients or providers (MacKenzie et al. 1986; Chambers et al. 1987; Guyatt et al. 1987). Four statistics used to index responsiveness are

(1) effect size (Kazis et al. 1989);

(2) t-test comparisons (Liang et al. 1985);

(3) the standardized response mean (Liang, Fossel, and Larson 1990); and

(4) the responsiveness statistic (Guyatt et al. 1987).

The formula for these statistics are as follows, where D = raw score change on measure; SE = standard error of the difference; SD = standard deviation at time 1; SD* = standard deviation of D; SD# = standard deviation of D among stable subjects (those whose true status is constant over time):

$$\text{Paired } t\text{-statistic} = D/\text{SE}$$
$$\text{Effect size statistic} = D/\text{SD}$$
$$\text{Standardized response mean} = D/\text{SD*}$$
$$\text{Responsiveness statistic} = D/\text{SD\#}.$$

The paired t-statistic is best suited to pre–post assessments of interventions of known efficacy. Relative validity calculations (ratios of the squares of paired t-statistics – see earlier discussion) for alternative measures can be used to compare their responsiveness to the intervention. The effect size statistic relates change over time to the standard deviation of baseline scores. The standardized response mean compares change to the standard deviation of change. The responsiveness statistic looks at HRQoL change relative to variability for clinically stable respondents.

The effect size statistic ignores variation in change entirely, the t-statistic ignores information about variation in scores for clinically stable respondents, and the responsiveness statistic ignores information about variation in scores for clinically unstable respondents. When the results of a clinical trial comparing an intervention of known clinical efficacy with a control group are available, the most useful measure of responsiveness is a between group t-statistic for change scores (see below). This t-statistic allows for direct determination of the sample size needed to detect a given clinical effect for a particular HRQoL measure. So, for a between group t-statistic for change,

$$\text{score} = (D_1 - D_2)/\text{SE}$$

where D_1 = raw score change for intervention group; D_2 = raw score change for control group; SE = standard error of the difference between group means.

Although not enough attention was given to the responsiveness of HRQoL measures previously, investigators are increasingly providing this information. For example, responsiveness of a HRQoL battery was assessed using paired t-statistics in a sample of 12 patients who at the commencement of the study had either just received an initial diagnosis of major depression and were starting antidepressant therapy or they were beginning antidepressant therapy for a new episode of depression (Revicki *et al*. 1992). This study found significant ($p < 0.05$) t-statistics for measures of depression, life satisfaction, social behaviour, and cognitive function/distress. Siu *et al*. (1993*b*) provided three responsiveness statistics in an analysis of 120 older persons entering a residential care facility. They found that the physical function scale from the MOS 20-item short-form health survey was more sensitive to decrements in physical performance than were the COOP physical function chart, the Katz activities of daily living scale, and the Lawton–Brody instrumental activities of daily living scale. None of the measures were very sensitive to improvement in performance-based physical function. Recently, Beusterien *et al*. (1996) found that the introduction of recombinant human erythropoietin to dialysis patients increased scores on the SF-36 energy scale by 9.3 points (about one-half a standard deviation) from baseline to follow-up (average of 99 days). In addition, significant improvements were observed on physical functioning, social functioning, and emotional well-being.

Additional work is needed to calibrate the meaning of the responsiveness statistics themselves and how they relate to one another. If one statistic suggests one conclusion about relative scale performance and a second statistic suggests a different conclusion, which one is to be believed? For example, Smith (1997) has argued that the traditional indicators of responsiveness are inadequate and that a more appropriate indicator is the correlation between prospective changes and retrospective reports of change.

Summary

It is important to evaluate the reliability of a quality of life scale before widespread use in clinical trials and health outcome studies. A number of techniques are available for evaluating the inter-rater reliability, equivalent forms reliability, internal consistency reliability, and test–retest reliability of scales. The main methods for determining the reliability of a scale are introduced in this chapter. Reliability is a necessary measurement characteristic of a scale, and provides evidence of its stability over different repeated measurements. However, a scale may be reliable, but not valid, that is, it does not measure what it is intended to measure.

Validity of a scale reflects how well it measures what it is intended to measure. For the developer and users of a quality of life scale, the accumulation of evidence of the scale's validity is continuous. The key question for validity evidence is whether the scale is valid for a particular application in a specific population. The assessment of validity normally begins with an assessment of content validity and then evaluates the construct validity and responsiveness of the scale to clinically meaningful changes in HRQoL. Construct validity and responsiveness are key psychometric criteria for measures used in clinical trials. Ongoing accumulation of research evidence regarding a scale's validity is important for demonstrating the scale's usefulness in a wide variety of research applications and patient populations.

References

Beusterien, K.M., Nissenson, A.R., Port, F.K., Kelly, M., Steinwald, B., and Ware, J.E. (1996). The effects of recombinant human erythropoietin on functional health and well-being in chronic dialysis patients. *Journal of the American Society of Nephrology*, **7**, 763–73.

Bland, J.M. and Altman, D.G. (1996). Measurement error. *British Medical Journal*, **312**, 1654.

Campbell, D.T. and Fiske, D.W. (1959). Convergent and discriminant validation by the multitrait–multimethod matrix. *Psychological Bulletin*, **56**, 81–105.

Chambers, L.W., Haight, M., Norman, G., and MacDonald, L. (1987). Sensitivity to change and the effect of mode of administration on health status measurement. *Medical Care*, **25**, 470–80.

Cicchetti, D.V. and Feinstein, A.R. (1990). High agreement but low kappa: II. Resolving the paradoxes. *Journal of Clinical Epidemiology*, **43**, 551–8.

Clark, E.L. (1935). Spearman–Brown formula applied to ratings of personality traits. *Journal of Educational Psychology*, **26**, 552–5.

Cohen, J. (1968). Weighted kappa: nominal scale agreement with provision for scaled disagreement or partial credit. *Psychological Bulletin*, **70**, 213–20.

Cole, D.A. (1987). Utility of confirmatory factor analysis in test validation research. *Journal of Consulting and Clinical Psychology*, **55**, 584–94.

Cronbach, L.J. (1951). Coefficient alpha and the internal structure of tests. *Psychometrika*, **16**, 297–334.

Cronbach, L.J. and Meehl, P.E. (1955). Construct validity in psychological tests. *Psychological Bulletin*, **52**, 281–302.

Cunningham, W.E., Bozzette, S.A., Hays, R.D., Kanouse, D.E., and Shapiro, M.F. (1995). Comparison of health-related quality of life in clinical trial and non-clinical trial human immunodeficiency virus-infected cohorts. *Medical Care*, **33**, AS15–25.

Ellickson, P.L., Hays, R.D., and Bell, R.M. (1992). Stepping through the drug use sequence: longitudinal scalogram analysis of initiation and heavy use. *Journal of Abnormal Psychology*, **101**, 441–51.

Feinstein, A.R. and Cicchetti, D.V. (1990). High agreement but low kappa: I. The problems of two paradoxes. *Journal of Clinical Epidemiology*, **43**, 543–9.

Feldt, L.S., Woodruff, D.J., and Salih, F.A. (1987). Statistical inference for coefficient alpha. *Applied Psychological Measurement*, **11**, 93–103.

Fleiss, J.L. (1981). *Statistical methods for rates and proportions*,(2nd edn). Wiley, New York.

Fleiss, J.L. and Cohen, J. (1973). The equivalence of weighted kappa and the intraclass correlation coefficient as measures of reliability. *Educational and Psychological Measurement*, **33**, 613–19.

Goodenough, W.H. (1944). A technique for scale analysis. *Educational and Psychological Measurement*, **4**, 179–90.

Guyatt, G., Walter, S., and Norman, G. (1987). Measuring change over time: assessing the usefulness of evaluative instruments. *Journal of Chronic Disease*, **40**, 171–8.

Hadorn, D.C. and Hays, R.D. (1991). Multitrait–multimethod analysis of health-related quality of life preferences. *Medical Care*, **29**, 829–40.

Hanley, J.A. and McNeil, B.J. (1982). The meaning and use of the area under a receiver operating characteristic (ROC) curve. *Radiology*, **143**, 29–36.

Hanley, J.A. and McNeil, B.J. (1983). A method of comparing the areas under receiver operating characteristic curves derived from the same cases. *Radiology*, **148**, 839–43.

Hayashi, T. and Hays, R.D. (1987). A microcomputer program for analyzing multitrait–multimethod matrices. *Behavior Research Methods, Instruments, and Computers*, **19**, 345–8.

Hays, R. and Hadorn, D. (1992). Responsiveness to change: an aspect of validlty, not a separate dimension. *Quality of Life Research*, **1**, 73–5.

Hays, R.D., Sherbourne, C.D., and Mazel, R.M. (1993). The RAND 36-item health survey 1.0. *Health Economics*, **2**, 217–27.

Kazis, L.E., Anderson, J.J., and Meenan, R.F. (1989). Effect sizes for interpreting changes in health status. *Medical Care*, **27**, S178–89.

Kenny, D.A. and Kashy, D.A. (1992). Analysis of the multitrait–multimethod matrix by confirmatory factor analysis. *Psychological Bulletin*, **112**, 165–72.

Landis, J.R. and Koch, G.G. (1977). The measurement of observer agreement for categorical data. *Biometrics*, **33**, 159–74.

Liang, M.H., Larson, M.G., Cullen, K.E., and Schwartz, J.A. (1985). Comparative measurement efficiency and sensitivity of five health status instruments for arthritis research. *Arthritis and Rheumatology*, **28**, 545–7.

Liang, M.H., Fossel, A.H., and Larson, M.G. (1990). Comparisons of five health status instruments for orthopedic evaluation. *Medical Care*, **28**, 632–42.

MacKenzie, C.R., Charlson, M.E., DiGioia, D., and Kelley, K. (1986). Can the sickness impact profile measure change? An example of scale assessment. *Journal of Chronic Disease*, **39**, 429–38.

Marsh, H.W. (1989). Confirmatory factor analyses of multitrait–multimethod data: many problems and a few solutions. *Applied Psychological Measurement*, **13**, 335–61.

Marshall, G.N., Hays, R.D., and Nicholas, R. (1994). Evaluating agreement between clinical assessment methods. *International Journal of Methods in Psychiatric Research*, **4**, 249–57.

Menzel, H. (1953). A new coefficient for scalogram analysis. *Public Opinion Quarterly*, **17**, 268–80.

Nelson, E.C., Landgraf, J.M., Hays, R.D., Wasson. J.H., and Kirk, J.W. (1990). The functional status of patients: how can it be measured in physicians' offices? *Medical Care*, **28**, 1111–26.

Nunnally, J. (1978). *Psychometric theory*, (2nd edn). McGraw-Hill, New York.

Prisant, L.M., Carr, A.A., Bottini, P.B., Thompson, W.O., and Rhoades, R.B. (1992). Repeatability of automated ambulatory blood pressure measurements. *Journal of Family Practice*, **34**, 569–74.

Revicki, D.A., Turner, R., Brown, R., and Martindale, J.J. (1992). Reliability and validity of a health-related quality of life battery for evaluating outpatient antidepressant treatment. *Quality of Life Research*, **1**, 257–66.

Shrout, P.E. and Fleiss, J.L. (1979). Intraclass correlations: uses in assessing rater reliability. *Psychological Bulletin*, **86**, 420–8.

Siu, A.L., Hays, R.D., Ouslander, J.G., Osterweil, D., Krynski, M., and Gross, A. (1993*a*). Measuring functioning and health in the very old. *Journal of Gerontology: Medical Sciences*, **48**, M10–14.

Siu, A.L., Ouslander, J.G., Osterweil, D., Reuben, D.B., and Hays, R.D. (1993*b*). Change in self-reported functioning in older persons entering a residential care facility. *Journal of Clinical Epidemiology*, **46**, 1093–102.

Smith, K.W. (1997). Measuring responsiveness in quality of life research. Paper presented at the meeting of the Drug Information Association, Scottsdale, Arizona, 13 January 1997.

Stewart, A.L., Hays, R.D., and Ware, J. (1992). Methods of validating MOS health measures. In *Measuring functioning and well-being: The medical outcomes study approach*, (ed. A.L. Stewart and J.E. Ware). Duke University Press, Durham, NC.

Ware, J.E. and Sherbourne, C.D. (1992). The MOS 36-item short-form health survey (SF-36): I. Conceptual framework and item selection. *Medical Care*, **30**, 473–83.

11   *Item response theory models*

Ron D. Hays

Classical test theory methods

As noted in Chapter 10, classical test theory (CTT) methods partition observed responses into true score plus error. The probability of a particular item response is a function of the person to whom the item is administered and the nature of the item itself. For example, the SF-36 physical functioning scale (Haley *et al.* 1994) includes 10 items that assess the extent to which one is limited in a range of functional activities from very basic (bathing or dressing) to quite advanced (vigorous activities). The probability of an answer of 'no, not limited' depends on the type of item (item 'difficulty') and the underlying level of physical functioning of the person ('ability'). The item about bathing or dressing is considered to be a less difficult item than the vigorous activities item, because more people are able to perform the former than the latter without limitations. Similarly, an olympic athlete would be more likely to report being able to perform vigorous activities than a person living in a long-term care facility.

A fundamental limitation of the CTT method is that it is unable to estimate item difficulty and person ability characteristics separately (i.e. they are confounded). Another limitation of CTT is that it yields only a single reliability estimate (and corresponding standard error of measurement), but the precision of measurement varies by ability level. Because of these limitations, the CTT method is less than ideal for applications that require distinct estimates of item difficulty, person ability, and conditional standard error of measurement.

Item response theory methods

Item response theory (IRT) methods represent a departure from CTT. IRT methods model the association between a respondent's underlying level on a characteristic (latent variable) and the probability of a particular item response using a non-linear monotonic function (Reise *et al.* 1993). The relationship between observed response to an item and the underlying characteristic or 'ability' is known as the item-characteristic curve (Haley *et al.* 1994). Item responses are assumed to be unidimensional and locally independent in IRT models. Unidimensional means that the items assess a single underlying construct. Locally independent means that the items are uncorrelated with one another when the underlying ability level is controlled for or held constant.

There are different varieties of IRT models that are distinguished by the functional form specified for the relationship between underlying ability and item response probability (i.e. the item-characteristic curve). The simplest IRT model, the Rasch model (Rasch 1966), specifies a one-parameter logistic function. The Rasch model allows items to vary in their difficulty level (probability of endorsement or scoring high on the item), but assumes that all items are equally discriminating. If the assumptions of the Rasch model hold (unidimensionality of measurement, local independence), observed item scores can be described as a function of the respondent's ability (theta) and the difficulty of the item. The probability of 'passing' (endorsing) a dichotomous item, for example, is modelled as a logistic ogive:

Probability (given theta) = 1/[1 + exp(theta − item difficulty)].

The difficulty parameter indicates the level of ability (theta) necessary to have a 0.50 probability of responding in a particular category of an item. A dichotomous item, by definition, has only two possible responses. The response corresponding to more of the construct being measured is typically the one for which the probability is modelled for each item. A two-parameter IRT model goes beyond the one-parameter Rasch model by estimating item discrimination as well as item difficulty. The probability of response for the two-parameter model is modelled as:

Probability (given theta) = 1/{1 + exp[− discrimination(theta − difficulty)]}.

The discrimination parameter is similar to an item–total correlation in CTT; higher values of this parameter are associated with items that are better able to discriminate between contiguous ability levels and this is manifested as a steeper slope in the graph of the probability of a particular response (y axis) by underlying ability or theta (x axis). The three-parameter model adds a pseudo-guessing parameter to adjust for the fact that individuals may score higher than expected due to chance.

Regardless of the specific model, it is instructive to examine item-characteristic, item-information, test (scale) information, and conditional standard error of measure (SEM) curves (see Figs 11.1–11.4). The item-characteristic curve shows the non-linear regression of the probability of a particular response as a function of underlying ability (Fig. 11.1). The difficulty of an item is defined by the level of ability needed for the probability of response to be 50 per cent. Item 3 in Fig. 11.1 is the most difficult item of the three, because it requires a higher level of ability for a given response.

The item and scale information curves show the amount of information provided by an item or scale at different levels of underlying ability (Figs 11.2, 11.3). Information reflects the precision of the measure and is inversely related to the standard error of measurement. An item or scale provides the most information around its difficulty level. The peaks of each distribution in Figs 11.2 and 11.3

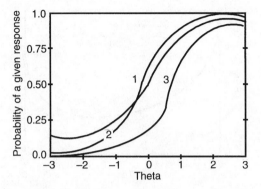

Fig. 11.1   Three item-characteristic curves.

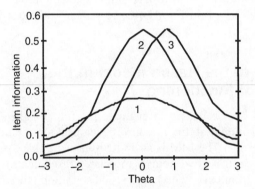

Fig. 11.2   Three item-information curves.

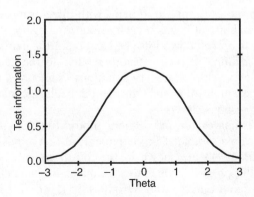

Fig. 11.3   Test information curve.

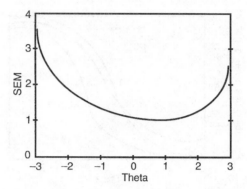

Fig. 11.4 Conditional SEM.

indicate where information is at a maximum. The conditional standard error of measurement curve shown in Fig. 11.4 corresponds to the test information curve in Fig. 11.3.

Applications of the Rasch model in the assessment of functioning

The Rasch model has been used to evaluate the functional independence measure (FIM), a functional status measure developed for inpatient rehabilitation (Hamilton *et al.* 1987). The FIM is an 18-item measure that assesses self-care (six items), sphincter control (two items), mobility (three items), locomotion (two items), communication (two items), and social cognition (three items). Each item is scored on a scale ranging from complete dependence (1) to complete independence (7). The first four domains of the FIM are combined into a 13-item motor function scale, and the last two domains are combined into a 5-item cognition scale.

When the Rasch model is applied to items with three or more ordinal response categories, the probability of being at each response category or level is modelled and item difficulty is broken down into the location of the item on the underlying attribute and the location of each category relative to the item location (Cella *et al.* 1996). In these multiple-category situations (sometimes referred to as the expanded Rasch measurement model), the item difficulty estimate is essentially an average across the response levels.

Item difficulty estimates for the 13-item motor function scale of the FIM gathered in 1990 from a sample of 14 799 patients at first admission to rehabilitation (Linacre *et al.* 1994) are shown in the fourth column of Table 11.1. The BIGSTEPS computer program, which uses an unconditional maximum likelihood method of estimation (Linacre and Wright 1995), was used to obtain these estimates. These difficulty estimates are reported as logits (log-odds) with the origin set at the centre of item difficulties.

Corresponding estimates for 1994 admission data for the neurological rehabilitation impairment category (RIC; see column one in Tablel 11.1), spinal cord RIC (column two), and brain dysfunction RIC (column three) are provided as well. These data were obtained from the uniform data system for medical rehabilitation (Carter, *et al*. 1996) and are used to assess the stability of the calibration of FIM item difficulties from the 1990 data shown in the fourth column. These data provide support for the stability of the item difficulty estimates. Intercorrelations between estimates for different subgroups ranged from 0.94 to 0.99. Similar estimates for the 5-item cognitive scale of the FIM are provided in Table 11.2. Intercorrelations among these different estimates ranged from 0.92 to 0.99.

Table 11.1   Item difficulty estimates for FIM motor items

1994 Data[†]			1990 Data*	
Neuro RIC (n=7211)	**Spinal cord** (n=4642)	**Brain dysfunction** (n=5187)		
−1.37	−1.77	−0.79	−1.19	Eating
−0.96	−1.13	−0.53	−0.78	Grooming
0.18	0.18	0.24	0.20	Bathing
−0.58	−0.57	−0.39	−0.48	Dressing–upper body
0.21	0.29	0.09	0.24	Dressing–lower body
0.11	0.23	0.06	0.05	Toileting
−0.43	−0.27	−0.42	−0.54	Bladder management
−0.73	−0.41	−0.58	−0.66	Bowel management
0.06	0.06	−0.19	0.00	Bed, chair, wheelchair
0.17	0.22	−0.01	0.14	Toilet
0.74	0.74	0.55	0.84	Tub, shower
0.64	0.50	0.51	0.44	Walk
1.96	1.91	1.45	1.73	Stairs

*Linacre *et al*. (1994) data were gathered in 1990 from a sample of 14 799 patients at first admission to rehabilitation. These difficulty estimates are reported as logits (log-odds) with the origin set at the centre of item difficulties.
[†]The 1994 data set includes approximately 139 000 patients in the uniform data system for medical rehabilitation (Carter *et al*. 1996).

Table 11.2   Item difficulty estimates for FIM cognitive items

1994 Data[†]			1990 Data*	
Neuro RIC (n=5466)	**Spinal cord** (n=2898)	**Brain dysfunction** (n=5145)		
−0.54	−0.48	−0.66	−0.41	Comprehension
−0.48	−0.74	−0.55	−0.39	Expression
−0.13	0.01	−0.27	−0.02	Social interaction
0.49	0.41	0.76	0.33	Memory
0.66	0.81	0.72	0.48	Problem solving

*Linacre *et al*. (1994) data were gathered in 1990 from a sample of 14 799 patients at first admission to rehabilitation. These difficulty estimates are reported as logits (log-odds) with the origin set at the centre of item difficulties.
[†]The 1994 data set includes approximately 139 000 patients in the uniform data system for medical rehabilitation (Carter *et al*. 1996).

Table 11.3   Conversion of raw scores to Rasch scores for motor scale (neurologic RIC)

Score	Measure	Score	Measure	Score	Measure
13	0	40	41	67	58
14	7	41	42	68	59
15	14	42	43	69	59
16	17	43	43	70	60
17	20	44	44	71	61
18	22	45	44	72	62
19	24	46	45	73	62
20	25	47	45	74	63
21	26	48	46	75	64
22	28	49	47	76	65
23	29	50	47	77	66
24	30	51	48	78	67
25	31	52	48	79	68
26	32	53	49	80	69
27	32	54	50	81	70
28	33	55	50	82	71
29	34	56	51	83	72
30	35	57	51	84	74
31	35	58	52	85	76
32	36	59	53	86	78
33	37	60	53	87	80
34	38	61	54	88	83
35	38	62	55	89	87
36	39	63	55	90	93
37	40	64	56	91	100
38	40	65	57		
39	41	66	57		

The estimates reported in Table 11.1 indicate that the least difficult motor item (the item for which the probability of being dependent is lowest) was eating and the most difficult item was climbing stairs. The more negative the score, the easier the item on the log-odds scale. The more positive the score, the harder the item. The estimates in Table 11.2 reveal that the easiest cognitive items are comprehension and expression. The hardest cognitive items are problem solving and memory. It is interesting that the memory item is hardest in the brain dysfunction RIC, but problem solving is hardest in the other groups shown in Table 11.2.

Table 11.3 provides the conversion of person raw scores to Rasch scores on the motor scale for those in the neurological RIC (1994 data) and Fig. 11.5 plots raw versus Rasch scores. As can be seen in Table 11.3 and Fig. 11.5, Rasch scores are a monotonic transformation of raw scores. Rasch scores are intended to transform the observed ordinal-level raw data into interval-level scores.

Concluding note

As the advantages of IRT models increase, their applications in quality of life assessment will rise. For example, IRT is likely to play a significant role in future

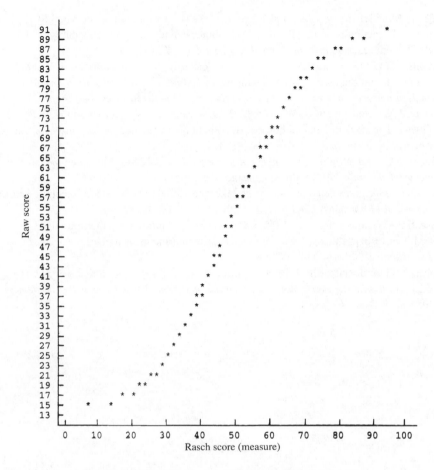

Fig. 11.5 Plot of raw versus Rasch scores for motor scale.

evaluations of the equivalence of measures among different subgroups, cultures, and countries (Cella *et al.* 1996). In addition, IRT methods are likely to prove to be essential for producing the most efficient quality of life measures in computer adaptive testing efforts (Waller and Reise 1989).

References

Carter, G.M., Relles, D.A., and Buchanan, J.L. (1996). A patient classification system for inpatient rehabilitation patients: a review and proposed revisions to the FIM-FRGs Report DRR-1450-HCFA. RAND, Santa Monica, CA.

Cella, D.F., Lloyd, S.R., and Wright, B.D. (1996). Cross-cultural instrument equating: current research and future directions. In *Quality of life and pharmacoeconomics in clinical trials*, (2nd edn), (ed. B. Spilker), pp. 707–15. Lippincott-Raven, Philadelphia.

Haley, S.M., McHorney, C.A., and Ware, J.E. (1994). Evaluation of the MOS SF-36 physical functioning scale (PF-10): I. Unidimensionality and reproducibility of the Rasch item scale. *Journal of Clinical Epidemiology*, **47**, 671–84.

Hamilton, B.G., Granger, C.V., Sherwin, F.S., Zielezny, M., and Tashman, J.S. (1987). A uniform national data system for medical rehabilitation. In *Rehabilitation outcomes: analysis and measurement*, (ed. M.J. Fuhrer), pp. 115–50. Brookes, Baltimore.

Linacre, J.M., Heinemann, A.W., Wright, B.D., Granger, C.V., and Hamilton, B.B. (1994). The structure and stability of the functional independence measure. *Archives of Physical Medicine and Rehabilitation*, **75**, 127–32.

Linacre, J.M. and Wright, B.D. (1995) *A user's guide to BIGSTEPS: Rasch-model computer program*. MESA Press, Chicago, IL.

Rasch, G. (1966). An item analysis which takes individual differences into account. *British Journal of Mathematical and Statistical Psychology*, **19**, 49–57.

Reise, S.P., Widaman, K.F., and Pugh, R.H. (1993). Confirmatory factor analysis and item response theory: two approaches for exploring measurement invariance. *Psychological Bulletin*, **114**, 552–66.

Waller, N.G. and Reise, S.P. (1989). Computerized adaptive personality assessment: an illustration with the absorption scale. *Journal of Personality and Social Psychology*, **57**, 1051–8.

12   *Factor analysis*

Peter M. Fayers and David Machin

Introduction

Factor analysis is one of the standard techniques that is used in scale validation; in fact, a search of the Medline bibliographic database reveals that over recent years about 15 papers per year contain the term 'factor analysis' in conjunction with 'quality of life'. The aim of this chapter, therefore, is to explain what factor analysis is, and the principles behind it. We illustrate factor analysis techniques with a detailed example of a scale widely used for assessing anxiety and depression; this example also serves to show the typical output that is obtained from most computer packages, and the way to interpret such output. We also discuss the reasons for using factor analysis in scale development and scale validation. Finally, we explain why and when it is a useful tool; why it is often over-used, misused, and abused; and describe some alternative methods.

Scale development

Sometimes quality of life (QoL) is regarded as a single concept, which can be assessed by asking the patient about their QoL status, and can be quantified as a quality of life score. However, most investigators agree that QoL is a multidimensional concept, and that it contains aspects that are best evaluated as distinct subscales, such as physical, psychological, and social well-being. Whichever view is taken, whether QoL is assumed to be a single scale or a collection of subscales, the concept is that there exists one or more underlying constructs that can be evaluated for individual patients by asking them questions. However, unlike measurements such as height, weight, and blood pressure, we cannot measure QoL scales or subscales objectively and directly; although we may postulate that 'quality of life' or, say, 'psychological well-being' really do exist as coherent constructs, they remain hypothetical. These unobservable constructs are often described as 'latent variables'.

How do we measure the latent variables? Sometimes, investigators attempt to use a single question. For example, the EORTC QLQ C-30[1] (QLQ C-30) contains a global question 'How would you rate your overall quality of life during the past week?', the response to which may be indicated on a seven-point scale with extremes labelled 'very poor' and 'excellent', whilst the SF-36[2] asks

'In general, would you say your health is "excellent", "very good", "good", "fair", "poor"?' These questions are intended to be assessments of overall QoL and health. Frequently, however, QoL questionnaires incorporate a number of questions that are intended to reflect each supposed latent variable. Thus the QLQ-C30 contains four questions related to 'emotional functioning', and the SF-36 has a similar set of five questions that are called 'mental health'. There are several reasons for using more than one question to measure latent variables such as emotional functioning and mental health. First, these are ill-defined concepts and it is often impractical to devise a single meaningful question which patients would understand. Second, a question of the form 'how good is your mental health' would, even if it is understood, be interpreted differently by different patients. Third, mental health and emotional functioning are compound concepts, embracing more specific aspects such as anxiety, irritability, nervousness, and depression; a patient with poor mental health would be expected to have high responses to all these items. Fourth, by asking a number of similar but distinct questions it is hoped that there will be improved reliability and consistency in the overall score for the latent variable. Therefore several individual items are commonly used in order to provide an indication of a latent variable. These items are assessed using separate questions, and are sometimes called manifest, or observed, variables.

In general, most QoL questionnaires are designed with the intention of tapping into a few general constructs or latent variables, such as physical functioning, emotional functioning, role functioning, cognitive functioning, and social functioning.[1] In order to achieve this, a number of questions (items) are used, these being the manifest variables. Now, if the questionnaire is well designed, each question should ideally be associated with a single latent variable.[3] For example, it is usually considered advisable that questions relating to, say, emotional functioning should not also relate to role functioning or other latent variables. It is also generally recommended that items should be selected such that a change in the underlying latent variable should be reflected by a corresponding change in the associated items; that is to say, for example, that if emotional functioning is to be assessed by four items, then low emotional functioning should tend to be manifested by low values for these four items.

Example – the HADS questionnaire

The Hospital Anxiety and Depression Scale (HADS)[4] is a general purpose instrument for assessing anxiety and depression which is widely used in many disease areas. As its name suggests, the HADS attempts to measure two constructs. There are 14 questions, each measured on a four-point scale; seven questions are intended to address anxiety, and the other seven depression. Half of the questions are deliberately worded positively, so that 'not at all' is the least favourable response, whilst the other half are worded negatively and 'not at all' is most favourable; this was done to introduce more balance into the questions posed to the patients.

The postulated structure of the HADS is relatively simple, with only two seven-item scales. It therefore provides a convenient example for examining the techniques associated with factor analysis.

Correlations

Suppose we have two variables called, say, x and y. Then x and y are described as (positively) correlated with each other if high values of x are associated with high values of y and low values of x are associated with low values of y. The level of association may be quantified by a statistical measure called a correlation coefficient, the most common of which is the Pearson product-moment correlation coefficient. If there is perfect correlation, such that if we know the value of x we can predict the value of y completely accurately, the correlation is 1. If there is no relationship between x and y, the correlation is 0. And if, on the other hand, high values of x are associated with low values of y and vice versa, there is an inverse relationship between x and y and thus a negative correlation; perfect negative correlation of -1 occurs if x is inversely related to y and it is possible to predict with complete accuracy the value of x (or y) for a given value of y (or x). Thus correlation coefficients vary between -1 and $+1$. Small values (close to 0) indicate weak correlation; a value of 0 indicates no correlation, or an absence of association between two items. Since a value of 1 is perfect correlation, such a value would imply that two items are measuring virtually the same thing since knowledge of either one would enable the other to be predicted with complete certainty; and a value of -1 would indicate a perfect inverse relationship, such that when one item is high the other is low and vice versa. It should be emphasized that the statement 'x is strongly correlated with y' carries no implication of causality or direction; it merely informs us that high x values are associated with high y values and, equivalently, high y values are associated with high x values.

Correlation coefficients play a major role in the validation of the structure of QoL instruments. A new instrument can be tested upon a sample of patients or other subjects, and from the data collected the correlations between all pairs of items can be calculated. In the example mentioned above, in which it was suggested that a low level of emotional functioning should be manifested by low levels of the all the corresponding questions used for its assessment, one would expect that the responses to these emotional functioning items would be correlated with each other; thus we would expect to find evidence of correlations between all pairs of these items.

When variables have a normal distribution the Pearson product-moment correlation coefficient, r, is generally used. For non-normal data other measures of correlation may be more suitable, such as Spearman's rho for non-normal continuous data or when variables have many discrete categories, and polychoric correlations for discrete data with fewer categories.

A closely related measure to correlation is 'covariance'. Most people find correlations easier to interpret since, unlike covariances, they are scaled from -1 to $+1$. However, many factor analysis programs use the equivalent covariances instead. This is because the underlying theory of factor analysis is more closely based upon covariances. One may draw an analogy with standard deviation (SD) versus variance; there is a direct relationship (square root) between SD and variance, but most people find SD is the easier measure to interpret. However, analysis of variance is invariably presented in terms of variances, since they are the more conveniently generalized measure. Therefore, in this chapter, we shall describe and illustrate the correlation structure of QoL data even though many factor analysis programs are, in fact, based upon analysis of covariances.

Worked example – the HADS questionnaire

The HADS questionnaire has been completed by patients in many of the UK Medical Research Council (MRC) randomized clinical trials of cancer therapy. The results from four recent MRC trials have been pooled, yielding a data set consisting of 1295 patients, and comprising advanced colorectal cancer patients (trial CR04), poor performance status patients with small cell lung cancer (LU12), good performance status patients with non-small cell cancer of the bronchus (CH01), and good performance status head and neck cancer patients (CH02).

The correlation matrix in Table 12.1 shows the correlations between all pairs of items. For simplicity, 'negative' items have been recoded so that in all cases a response of 0 is most favourable and 3 is least favourable. If this had not been done, some of the correlations would have been negative since negative items would tend to have low responses whenever related positive items have high responses. By introducing consistency of scoring it is easier to interpret the correlation matrix.

Table 12.1 only shows the 'lower triangle' of correlations; the correlation of x against y is the same as the correlation of y against x. Hence we only need to show Q1 against Q2 (0.36), as the correlation of Q2 against Q1 would be identical.

There are clearly many fairly highly correlated items, with correlations between 0.4 and 0.6. Although from prior knowledge we know that the odd numbered questions (Q1, Q3, Q5, ...) are the ones intended to reflect anxiety, it is difficult to see the pattern in this correlation matrix. However, rearranging the correlation

Table 12.1 Correlation matrix for HADS questionnaire, for 1295 patients in MRC trials CR04, LU12, CH01, CH02

	Q1	Q2	Q3	Q4	Q5	Q6	Q7	Q8	Q9	Q10	Q11	Q12	Q13	Q14
Q1	1.													
Q2	0.36	1.												
Q3	0.53	0.29	1.											
Q4	0.36	0.48	0.40	1.										
Q5	0.55	0.26	0.61	0.37	1.									
Q6	0.42	0.52	0.38	0.61	0.39	1.								
Q7	0.51	0.40	0.42	0.41	0.44	0.44	1.							
Q8	0.31	0.52	0.26	0.34	0.27	0.38	0.32	1.						
Q9	0.50	0.22	0.57	0.32	0.56	0.35	0.41	0.21	1.					
Q10	0.34	0.41	0.30	0.37	0.27	0.45	0.36	0.37	0.26	1.				
Q11	0.32	0.17	0.32	0.20	0.33	0.17	0.35	0.18	0.30	0.18	1.			
Q12	0.37	0.58	0.36	0.52	0.32	0.54	0.43	0.46	0.30	0.48	0.18	1.		
Q13	0.53	0.26	0.59	0.33	0.56	0.37	0.45	0.25	0.58	0.34	0.35	0.31	1.	
Q14	0.31	0.43	0.28	0.42	0.27	0.44	0.42	0.32	0.30	0.36	0.21	0.40	0.32	1.

Table 12.2   Correlations from Table 12.1 rearranged corresponding to the postulated subscales of anxiety (odd-numbered questions) and depression (even-numbered questions)

	Q1	Q3	Q5	Q7	Q9	Q11	Q13	Q2	Q4	Q6	Q8	Q10	Q12	Q14
Q1	1.													
Q3	0.53	1.												
Q5	0.55	0.61	1.											
Q7	0.51	0.42	0.44	1.										
Q9	0.50	0.57	0.56	0.41	1.									
Q11	0.32	0.32	0.33	0.35	0.30	1.								
Q13	0.53	0.59	0.56	0.45	0.58	0.35	1.							
Q2	0.36	0.29	0.26	0.40	0.22	0.17	0.29	1.						
Q4	0.36	0.40	0.37	0.41	0.32	0.20	0.33	0.48	1.					
Q6	0.42	0.38	0.39	0.44	0.35	0.17	0.36	0.52	0.61	1.				
Q8	0.31	0.26	0.27	0.32	0.21	0.18	0.25	0.52	0.34	0.38	1.			
Q10	0.34	0.30	0.27	0.36	0.26	0.18	0.34	0.41	0.37	0.45	0.37	1.		
Q12	0.37	0.36	0.32	0.43	0.30	0.18	0.31	0.58	0.52	0.54	0.46	0.48	1.	
Q14	0.30	0.28	0.27	0.42	0.30	0.21	0.32	0.43	0.42	0.44	0.32	0.36	0.40	1.

matrix (Table 12.2) makes the pattern very much clearer. Items in the two postulated scales are shown in two shaded triangles, anxiety being the upper area and depression the lower. It is now clear that there are fairly high (greater than 0.4, say) correlations between most items in each of the two scales, except Q11 is noticeably weaker. It is also reassuring to note that the unshaded area has lower correlations, which is consistent with the hypothesis that the anxiety items are only weakly correlated with the depression items.

Path diagrams

One way to represent the many inter-relationships between the items is by means of a path diagram. Adopting the usual conventions, we use circles to represent the latent variables or constructs, and boxes for the manifest variables or observable items. Lines link the items to their corresponding latent variable. Furthermore, if a construct is associated with particular items in the sense that a high value of the construct implies a high level for the item, then we add directional arrows to the lines. Thus we may regard the construct as implying a certain value of the item, or we might say the construct is manifested by the responses to the items, or, in extreme cases, that the latent variable causes an outcome value for the item. Figure 12.1 illustrates two latent variables, LV1 and LV2, with four questions associated with LV1 and three questions with LV2.

One implication of the arrows is that high (or low) values of LV1, for example, are expected to be associated with correspondingly high (or low) values of Q1 to Q4. Therefore we would expect Q1, Q2, Q3, and Q4 to be fairly strongly correlated.

Similarly, because there is no link between Q1 and Q5 (or Q6, Q7) we expect low correlations between Q1 and Q5 (and between Q1 and Q6, Q7); ideally, if there really is no relationship between Q1 and Q5, say, then the correlation ought

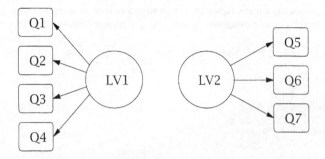

Fig. 12.1 Path diagram. Two latent variables, LV1 being represented by four items (Q1–Q4) on the questionnaire and LV2 by three items (Q5–Q7).

to be zero. In practice, particularly with QoL scales, there are nearly always relationships between most items and most latent variables. For example, anxiety is likely to have some effect upon social functioning, physical functioning, role functioning, and so on; thus an anxious athlete is unlikely to excel at his sport, and conversely poor physical functioning may make a person anxious. Hence it is more realistic to expect low correlations between items associated with different constructs, rather than zero correlations.

Example – the HADS questionnaire

The path diagram corresponding to the postulated structure of the HADS is shown in Fig. 12.2. This is similar in layout to Fig. 12.1 except that the two latent variables, anxiety and depression, are linked by a curved line with arrows at both ends; this indicates that the latent variables are expected to be correlated with each other, since persons with higher levels of anxiety are more likely also to have higher levels of depression, and vice versa.

This example is a very simple one, with only seven items and two postulated constructs. If we were analysing a more general QoL questionnaire there might be far more items and also more constructs.

Factor analysis

Factor analysis is a statistical technique that examines a correlation matrix and attempts to identify groups of variables such that there are strong correlations amongst all the variables within a group, but weak correlations between variables within the group and those outside the group. Thus if the model assumed in Fig. 12.1 is correct, we would expect each of the four items (Q1, Q2, Q3, Q4) to be correlated with each other, and that factor analysis would identify these as one 'factor'. If the items were highly correlated, as one might hope, the scale would be described as having strong internal structure. Similarly, Q5, Q6, Q7 are expected to be correlated and to form another factor. In principle one might be able to inspect a correlation matrix by eye, and verify whether this structure

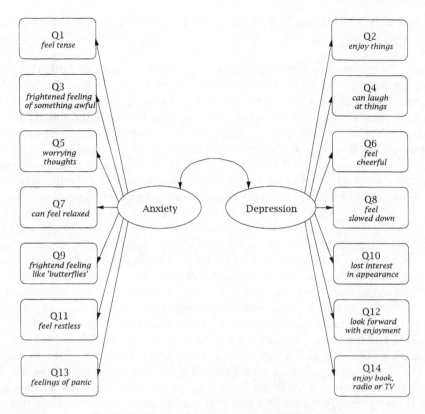

Fig. 12.2 Postulated structure of the HADS questionnaire.

pertains. In practice this is usually difficult to do for all but the simplest of models, and so we rely upon automatic techniques like factor analysis to explore the data.

Factor analysis as described here uses the correlation or covariance matrix as its starting point, and does not make use of any prior knowledge about the structure, or postulated structure, of the questionnaire. Therefore it is also termed 'exploratory factor analysis.'

Worked example – the HADS questionnaire

It is easiest to explain how factor analysis works by using an illustrative example. The correlation matrix presented in Table 12.1 showed the inter-relationships of the HADS items. Although pretreatment data were used for this example, we would expect to find very similar results if during- or post-treatment assessments were considered.

Let us now use a standard factor analysis program, to see how well the hypothesized structure is recovered. For the purpose of this exercise the statistical package SPSS[5] is used, and most of the SPSS default options are accepted. In general that might not be too wise; as will be discussed later, there are many choices to be made when carrying out factor analysis, and many of them can quite severely affect the analyses. However, to begin with we will ignore such complications.

An extract of the first part of the output from SPSS is shown in Table 12.3. The program starts by assuming there might be as many factors as there are variables (items). The reason for this is that we have not told the program that there are only two factors, and indeed perhaps the postulated model for the HADS is incorrect: how do we know that there are only two factors? Perhaps there are three or more. Thus the factor analysis program commences by calculating the import-ance of each of the possible factors – 14 in all. Why are there 14 possible factors? Because if each item proves to be completely independent of the other 13 items, we would have to regard each item as a separate construct or latent variable. If this is the case, it would be inappropriate to construct any scale scores and the data should be summarized by 14 factors that are the same as the original variables. Thus for each of the 14 potential factors there is a row in Table 12.3. The 'eigenvalues', or latent roots, in the table are obtained by matrix algebra; their precise mathematical meaning need not concern us, but a rough interpretation is that the eigenvalues are a measure of how much of the variation in the data is accounted for by each factor. Therefore the eigenvalues indicate the importance of each factor in explaining the variability and correlations in the observed sample of data. The first factor has an eigenvalue of nearly 6, and the second has an eigenvalue of 1.67. If all the eigenvalues are summed, the total will be found to be 14 – that is, eigenvalues are scaled such that the total variability of the data is equal to the number of variables. Therefore we can summarize the information contained by the eigenvalues in a way that is more easy to interpret if we express them as percentages – 5.967 is 42.6 per cent of 14. Examining Table 12.3, SPSS has calculated the percentage of variation that is explained by each factor and we see that the first two factors account for 55 per cent of the total variation.

Table 12.3 Eigenvalues and percentage of variance explained. The first two factors have eigenvalues greater than 1 and also account for 54.6 per cent of the total variance

Factor	Eigenvalue	Percentage of variance	Cumulative percentage
1	5.96709	42.6	42.6
2	1.67041	11.9	54.6
3	0.84458	6.0	60.6
4	0.75341	5.4	66.0
5	0.66332	4.7	70.7
6	0.63005	4.5	75.2
7	0.57912	4.1	79.3
8	0.48051	3.4	82.8
9	0.44994	3.2	86.0
10	0.43451	3.1	89.1
11	0.42338	3.0	92.1
12	0.38777	2.8	94.9
13	0.36427	2.6	97.5
14	0.35164	2.5	100.0

This information is used by the program to determine the number of factors that are present. The criterion used is the 'eigenvalues greater than 1' rule, which is discussed in more detail later. On this basis there are two factors, since only two eigenvalues exceed 1, as is noted in the table. This, of course, conveniently confirms our prior expectations that there are two latent constructs. The next stage is to examine whether the composition of these factors corresponds to the postulated constructs of anxiety and depression.

The output continues with Table 12.4, which gives the factor pattern matrix, or factor loadings, corresponding to the two-factor solution. These numbers indicate the importance of the 14 variables to each factor, and are equivalent to regression coefficients; unless an oblique rotation is used (as explained below), the loadings are also equal to the correlations between the factors and the items. At first sight Table 12.4 does not look too promising: the first factor has broadly similar loadings for all variables, and is thus little more than an average of all 14 items. Factor two is difficult to interpret, although it is noticeable that alternate items have positive and negative loadings.

The next stage in factor analysis is to 'rotate' the factors. It can be shown mathematically that the solution given in Table 12.4 is not unique. Other two-factor solutions are equally good at explaining 55 per cent of the variability, and in fact there are an infinite variety of alternative solutions. In general the initial factor solution will rarely show any interpretable patterns. Therefore it is usual to 'rotate' the factors until a solution with a simpler structure is found. One of the most commonly used methods is 'varimax', although many alternatives have been proposed; this and other methods are explained more fully later. Briefly, varimax attempts to minimize the number of variables that have high loadings on each factor, thereby simplifying the overall structure. Thus we hope to obtain a new set of loadings for factors 1 and 2, with fewer items having high values for each factor, but with 55 per cent of the total variance still explained by the two factors. If we proceed to use varimax rotation in SPSS, we obtain Table 12.5.

When reading Table 12.5 it is helpful to note which variables have loadings of at least 0.3 or 0.4. To simplify this, we have added shading to the SPSS output,

Table 12.4 Unrotated factor matrix. The initial, unrotated, solution for the factor loadings is shown (as printed by SPSS output; in practice, two decimal places should suffice)	Factor 1	Factor 2
Q1	0.68880	−0.19181
Q2	0.61452	0.43731
Q3	0.69948	−0.32483
Q4	0.64554	0.24986
Q5	0.68376	−0.34276
Q6	0.68442	0.27649
Q7	0.65949	0.00649
Q8	0.51257	0.29375
Q9	0.64239	−0.36330
Q10	0.54925	0.23137
Q11	0.40004	−0.18038
Q12	0.65710	0.37539
Q13	0.68305	−0.33262
Q14	0.54291	0.21062

Table 12.5 Rotated factor matrix – varimax rotation. Loadings greater than 0.4 have been shaded, showing the simplified factor structure after rotation

	Factor 1	Factor 2
Q1	0.33969	0.62916
Q2	0.74127	0.13922
Q3	0.25130	0.72913
Q4	0.62779	0.29161
Q5	0.22748	0.73026
Q6	0.67394	0.30113
Q7	0.46218	0.47048
Q8	0.56716	0.16538
Q9	0.18399	0.71470
Q10	0.54768	0.23508
Q11	0.14760	0.41326
Q12	0.72622	0.21284
Q13	0.23429	0.72271
Q14	0.52833	0.24491

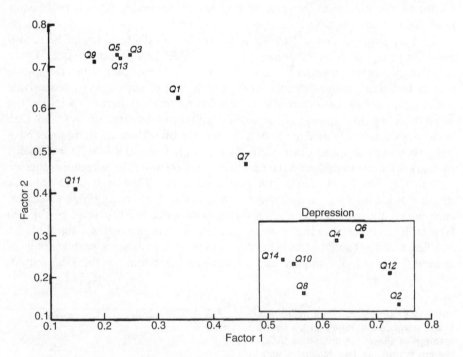

Fig. 12.3 Plot of factor 2 against factor 1. The depression items are clustered together, but Q11 is far from the other anxiety items and Q7 lies between depression and anxiety.

marking loadings above 0.4. In general, the expected relationships are apparent: the first factor relates to questions 2, 4, 6, (7), 8, 10, 12, and 14, whilst the second factor has questions 1, 3, 5, 7, 9, 11, and 13. Variable 11 in factor 2 is a bit weak (loading of 0.41), which corresponds to the low correlations that we noted in

Table 12.2. However, the only real surprise is variable 7 which is included in both factors. Inspecting Table 12.2 again, we see that Q7 (fourth column in Table 12.2) has correlations above 0.4 with several depression items (Q2, Q4, Q6, Q12, and Q14), which explains its appearance in the depression factor. Apart from that, the fit may be regarded as extremely good and provides adequate confirmation of the postulated structure of the HADS. It may be noted that other authors have applied factor analysis to the HADS questionnaire, with completely different data sets, and also found that item 7 was anomalous.[6] This question, 'I can sit at ease and feel relaxed', does not appear to perform very well and must be a candidate for revision in any future version of HADS.

Figure 12.3 shows the two orthogonal (varimax-rotated) factors diagrammatically. This simply plots the factor loadings of the 14 items, for factor 1 against factor 2. The even-numbered items cluster together, demonstrating that the depression scale is coherent and contains consistent items. Most items of the anxiety scale are also clustered together, with the exceptions of Q7 which is mid-way between the two scales, and Q11 which is rather an outlier. Plots like Fig. 12.3 can help by displaying graphically the factor space and the inter-relationship of the items. When there are more than two factors, pairwise plots can be made.

The uses of factor analysis

Historical perspective

A useful insight into the role of factor analysis may be obtained by considering its origins; this also provides a useful background for a discussion of the limitations of factor analysis when it is applied to QoL scales.

Factor analysis was initially developed by Spearman at the beginning of the twentieth century,[7] building upon earlier work by Karl Pearson. At that time Spearman was interested in modelling intelligence, with a view to testing whether intelligence could be regarded as having two components: a general ability, which was thought to be innate, and a specific ability which would vary according to subject (such as verbal skills, or mathematics) and which could be influenced by education. Therefore a student with high general intelligence would be expected to have high scores in most subjects, but specific intelligence would explain variations from subject to subject. Thus Spearman wished to show that the results from a battery of intelligence tests covering different school subjects would reveal one general factor, and that the remaining variability in the data could be explained by specific factors associated with each test. Although Spearman is commonly regarded as the father of factor analysis, over the years there has been much criticism of the way in which he used this technique;[8] there has been a long-standing discussion about the nature of intelligence. In particular, there has been recognition that unrotated factors almost invariably result in a model similar to that which Spearman was seeking, with one general factor; this is an artefact of the factor analysis as a method, and does not serve to verify the model. Furthermore, there is an awareness that rotation of factors is necessary yet also ill defined, since multiple solutions are possible. Therefore the modern view of factor analysis is that it is an exploratory technique, suitable for generating hypotheses about the structure of the data. In recognition of this, factor analysis is often given the name 'exploratory factor analysis' (EFA). Other, newer, techniques are available for testing whether a postulated model fits the data – in particular, confirmatory factor analysis (CFA).

Another characteristic of the original model is that intelligence tests, like most psychological tests, follow the basic pattern shown in Fig. 12.1 if the person being assessed has a high intelligence (or anxiety, depression in our example) we would expect this to be reflected in corresponding high scores for each of the individual items comprising the test. In fact, if any item in the test does *not* satisfy this requirement, under psychometric theory of tests it would be regarded as a poor test-item and would be a candidate for removal from the test instrument.[9] Psychological, psychometric, and educational tests are typically constructed with the intention of measuring a few, possibly as few as one or two, subscales and contain a number of items that are expected to be homogeneous within each subscale. The HADS instrument is thus fully representative of such a test. This is rather different from many QoL instruments, which may contain a few items for each of many subscales. For example, the EORTC QLQ C-30 contains five functional scales, three symptom scales, and a number of single items; further-more, only three of the scales comprise more than two items (physical functioning, five; emotional functioning, four; fatigue, three).

Scale validation

The main objective of applying factor analysis is scale validation. There are two situations: if the investigator has strong preconceptions concerning the structure of the scale, the investigator usually hopes that factor analysis will

(1) confirm that the postulated number of factors is present (two factors in the example of the HADS);

(2) confirm the grouping of the items.

However, if there is less certainty about the underlying model, the investigator would want to know

(1) how many factors (or scales or constructs) are present?

(2) how do the individual items relate to the factors?

(3) having identified the items that load on to each of the factors, does this lead to definition of the substantive content or a meaning for the factors?

Scale development

Another role for factor analysis lies in the checking of new scales. An illustration of this can be seen in the example of the HADS. The intention was that seven questions related to anxiety and seven to depression. The scoring of the HADS reflects this, since scores for each patient are formed by summing the items representing anxiety separately from those for depression (all items having been coded from 0 to 3, as described above, with 3 being the least favourable state);

therefore a high sum score represents anxiety or depression, respectively. However, item seven was seen to be related to both scales. Since this finding has been replicated by others,[6] it would suggest that perhaps the wording should be modified or a different and better targeted item substituted. The results from factor analysis imply that item seven is almost as strongly associated with depression as anxiety, and that either factor might influence the value of item seven.

Factor analysis can also draw attention to items which appear to contribute little to their intended scale. That, too, can be seen in the HADS example. Item 11 is a candidate for inspection, since it loads relatively weakly upon the anxiety scale. This suggests that item 11, 'I feel restless as if I have to be on the move', does not reflect anxiety very strongly, and that a better question should be devised.

Thus factor analysis can draw attention to items which load on to more than one scale, and also to items that do not load convincingly on to any scale. Another, related, use of factor analysis is that having identified clusters of items loading on to each construct, it is then easier to check whether there are excessively strong correlations between two or more items; to take an extreme case, if a correlation of 1.0 were observed between two of the items included in one factor, it would be sensible to drop an item since all information is already contained in the other item.

Scale scoring

When a scale or subscale is composed of several items, a scale score or summary statistic will be required; for example, individual patient scores for anxiety and depression are the natural summary from the HADS questionnaire. Quite often a simple summated score is used. Under the Likert summated scale method[9,10] the individual items are scored on a linear scale (for example, each item in the three-item fatigue scale of the EORTC QLQ is scored 1 = 'not at all', 2 = 'a little', 3 = 'quite a bit', 4 = 'very much'), and these items are then summed to provide the score for the attribute (in this example, the final score would therefore range from 3 to 12). Finally, since the range of values in each subscale will vary according to the number of items being summed, it is customary to standardize the scores using a linear transformation so that each will range from 0 to 100.

Of the assumptions built into the Likert approach, two are particularly important.

1. It is assumed that each item can be scored on a simple linear scale (for example, 1 to 4). It has frequently been found that complex weighting schemes offer little advantage over simple scoring methods.[11] This, together with the consideration that weights derived in any one context may be inappropriate for patients in another, has led to a general acceptance of simple scoring systems as being adequate for many situations.[12]

2. It is assumed that each item is measuring the same attribute, and therefore differential emphasis or 'weighting' should not affect the final result.[13] Empirical studies have tended to confirm this view[14] and have confirmed 'the robust beauty of improper linear models', leading many authors (for example, the influential

review by Cox *et al.*[15]) to advocate 'the use of simple weighting schemes within dimensions'. On the other hand, Olschewski and Schumaker[16] note that 'The simplicity of these single QoL indices is often subject to criticism. The main argument is the potential lack of differentiability. Low scores on some items may outweigh high scores on other items, yielding an intermediate overall score on average. It is argued therefore that simple addition should be restricted only to subscales of highly positively correlated items'.

However, Cox *et al.*[15] additionally note that any formal system for deriving weights is in no way guaranteed to be meaningful either clinically or to individual patients. Furthermore, since 'standard' weights derived for one study may be inappropriate for other investigations, there is the potential problem of study-specific weights which would destroy comparability between investigations.

Hence, despite the apparent *naïveté* of the assumptions of linearity and equal weighting, psychometricians often adopt the Likert method of summated scores because of its robust simplicity. Although the simple summated scale approach is frequently adopted, with the assumption of equal weighting being given to each item, various other methods are available for determining differential weights. In particular, the following methods may be adopted.

1. Clinicians' subjective opinions, based upon published knowledge and personal clinical experience.

2. Patient-derived weightings, based upon a variety of techniques for establishing preferences or utilities.

3. Data-derived weights, based upon the correlation structure of the instrument that is observed in a patient population.[16] Since factor analysis and related methods are commonly used to assess construct validity, a natural extension is to consider using the same techniques to ascribe weights to the items, based upon factor loadings. Applying the resultant weights to the observed item values results in 'factor scores' for each patient, with scores corresponding to each factor.

Psychometricians, however, rarely use factor scores as a method of deriving outcome scores; more commonly, factor analysis is used to identify those items that should be included in a particular factor or construct, and then either use equal weights or one of the other weighting methods described above. Reasons for exercising caution when using factor scores are that the scores are often neither very precise nor uniquely defined,[17] and any data-derived scores based upon one study may be inappropriate in the context of a different study drawn from another patient population. Thus, in general, we would advise against using scores as anything other than a numerical process for reducing dimensionality for subsequent analyses.

Applying factor analysis: choices and decisions

Unfortunately few factor analyses are as simple and as straightforward as in the above example. We were fortunate in that

(1) there were few variables (14) and, more importantly, few factors (2);

(2) the postulated model was well defined and the HADS scale had been carefully developed with items carefully chosen to load on to the two factors;

(3) the sample size was fairly large (1295 patients);

(4) the patients are likely to have a wide range of levels of anxiety and depression, making it easier discern the relationships.

Thus it was a relatively easy task to obtain a convincing confirmation of the HADS scale using our data. However, we shall now explore the problems of factor analysis in more detail, and discuss the range of decisions that must be made when carrying out analyses. As will be seen, some of the choices can be quite crucial to obtaining a satisfactory solution.

Sample size

Sample size influences factor analysis in a variety of ways. In factor analysis, where the factor structure is being explored, a small sample size will lead to large standard errors for the estimated parameters. Even more importantly, it may result in incorrect estimation of both the number of factors and the structure of the factors. As the sample size tends to infinity, even trivial factors will become statistically highly significant, and so there may be a tendency to extract too many factors when the sample size is large. Conversely, with a small sample size there will often be insufficient information to enable determination and extraction of more than one or two factors. Therefore caution must be exercised in interpreting the results from both large studies as well as small studies.

There is no general agreement about methods of estimating power and sample size. Sample size requirements will depend crucially upon the values in the between-item covariance matrix, and this is generally unknown before the study is carried out. Similarly, the power of the study will depend upon the distribution of responses to the questions, and this is likely to vary according to the population being studied and is rarely known in advance. Furthermore, many QoL items may be non-normal and strongly asymmetric, with high frequencies of subjects either reporting 'no difficulty' or 'very great difficulty' with individual items, thereby making simple approximations based upon normal distributions of little practical relevance.

When the distribution of the variables and their correlation (or covariance) matrix is either known or can be hypothesized it is possible to carry out simulation studies to evaluate the effect of different sample sizes. Although some such studies have been reported, these have generally been for simple situations such as models with two or three factors and normally distributed variables, and have assumed simple correlation structures. A few authors have suggested that 'saturation', the average correlation between the original variables and the factors, might be used as a broad indication of the likely level of correlations, and that sample size estimation can be based upon this. However, this, too, is usually difficult to estimate in advance of collecting the data.

Many authors have provided conflicting recommendations and rules of thumb, based upon combinations of simulations and experience. Recommendations for the number of subjects include 100,[18] 200,[19] 400,[20] 5 or 10 times the number of observed variables,[18,21] and various functions of the number of factors and observed variables.[22,23] In general there is no theoretical basis for any of these rules. In addition, Gorsuch[18] has pointed out that if the variables have low reliabilities or the phenomena are weak, then many more individuals will be needed, and Guadagnoli and Velicer[24] commented that 300 or more observations are required if a solution possesses many factor with only a few variables per factor and low factor loadings.

Although the issues we have described may make sample size estimation appear impractical, inadequate sample size has clearly been a problem in many studies even though this is often only appreciated with hindsight either upon completion of the study or when other investigators report conflicting factor analysis results. Thus sample size and power calculations cannot be simply dismissed. The best advice we can offer is to be conservative and aim for large sized studies. For QoL scales, which are often expected to have five or more factors, 30 or more items, possibly few items per factor, and with discrete and highly skewed scales for items, it seems likely that a minimum of several hundred patients is required and ideally there should be many hundreds.

Number of factors

The first step in factor analysis is to determine the number of factors that are to be extracted. This is one of the more important decisions to be made since a totally different and erroneous factor structure may be estimated if an incorrect number of factors is used.[18,25,26] If too many, or too few, factors are mistakenly entered into the model, the analyses often yield solutions that are extremely difficult to interpret. On the other hand, it is frequently possible to ascribe plausible meanings to many combinations of variables, and it can be very difficult to identify whether factors are meaningful and which models are likely to be correct. Therefore much research has been carried out into automatic or objective methods of deciding the number of factors that are present.

One of the oldest and most widely used approaches is Kaiser's 'eigenvalues greater than 1'[27] rule, as used in our example. Probably one (not very sound) reason for its near universal application in computer packages is the simplicity of the method. Various foundations have been proposed for this rule, such as noting that the average eigenvalue is 1.0 and so the rule excludes all eigenvalues below the average. On the other hand, if there are 10 variables this rule will include factors which explain at least 10 per cent of the variance; but if there are 50 variables, factors explaining as little as 2 per cent would be retained. In general, this rule tends to include too many factors.

Another widely used method is the 'scree plot', which is simply a plot of successive eigenvalues (Fig. 12.4). From factors 3 to 14, the eigenvalues lie more or less on a straight line. There is a clear elbow in the plot, with the first two factors lying above this line. This is taken to imply that a two-factor solution is

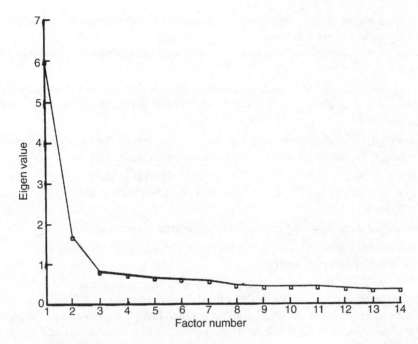

Fig. 12.4 'Scree' plot of eigenvalues from the HADS data in MRC patients. There is a clear 'elbow' to the plot, with eigenvalues corresponding to factors 1 and 2 being higher than expected on the basis of the other 'less significant' 12 factors.

appropriate. The scree plot is usually regarded as being fairly good at separating the important factors from the later 'factors' which are really little more than random noise; the scree is the random rubble at the foot of the cliff face. One slight disadvantage is that interpretation of scree plots suffer from subjectivity; fortunately, as in our example, a change in slope is often fairly evident.

Another widely used method is based upon the use of maximum likelihood (ML) estimation; unfortunately it has been shown that ML factor analysis is quite sensitive to residual variation and unless there are large sample sizes it can give unreliable estimates of the number of factors. In our example, ML estimation successfully identified the two-factor solution.

Many other methods exist, but are less widely used.[9,18]

Despite reservations, in practice both the eigenvalues >1 rule and the scree plot seem to have reasonable characteristics. When the same number of factors is suggested by all three methods, as in this example, the solution is quite convincing.

Method of estimation

A variety of methods is available for estimating the factors, all leading to different solutions. Most statistical packages offer several methods – for example, SPSS[5] and SAS[28] both offer seven methods for factor extraction, and these are not the same seven methods. The one thing in common with all estimation procedures is that they define some arbitrary measure of fit which is then maximized (or, if a measure of deviation from fit is used, minimized). Thus commonly used methods include

- maximum likelihood, which produces estimates that are most likely to have yielded the observed correlation matrix under assumptions of multivariate normality;

- unweighted least squares, which minimizes the sum of the squared differences between the observed and model-predicted correlation matrices;

- alpha factoring maximizes the Cronbach's alpha reliability of the factors, so that (for example) the first factor has the maximum reliability or internal consistency;

- principal axes factoring maximizes the variance accounted for;

- minimum residual factoring minimizes the off-diagonal residuals of the total variance–covariance matrix.

Similarly, various other methods exist, each with their proponents.

When the data possess a strongly defined factor structure it is likely that most methods of extraction will yield similar results. Both theoretical and empirical studies bear out this conclusion. However, in other situations there may be considerable divergence in the factor solutions, especially when there are small sample sizes, few explanatory variables, and a weak factor structure.

Statisticians generally prefer maximum likelihood (ML), because it is based upon sound mathematical theory which is widely applicable to many situations. ML estimation also provides foundations for hypothesis testing, including tests for the number of factors. Although estimation by ML is, computationally intensive, with modern computing power that is no longer a material disadvantage. Also, ML yields the same results whether a correlation matrix or a covariance matrix is factored, unlike other methods of estimation which most commonly assume that a covariance matrix is being used. Although it is commonly thought to be a disadvantage that ML estimation does explicitly assume that the sample is from a multivariate normal distribution, ML estimation of factor structure is fairly robust against departures from normality. However, the significance tests will be invalid; violation of the distributional assumptions reduces ML estimation to being more on a par with the other techniques. Thus, overall, we would recommend ML estimation as being the preferred estimation method.

The role of the factor estimation step is to find an initial solution, which can then be 'rotated' to provide a simpler structure that still suffices to explain the observed covariance matrix. Although the initial factor estimates may vary considerably according to the method used, it is often, but not necessarily, found that similar results are obtained after rotation, no matter which method of factor estimation was used.

Orthogonal rotation

There is in general no unique solution for a factor decomposition from a data set, and it is conventional to adopt an arbitrary procedure in which factors are rotated so that as many as possible of the items contribute to single factors. In other words, one of the aims of rotation is to simplify the initial factorization, to obtain a solution which keeps as many variables and factors distinct from one another. Frequently the initial solution is essentially uninterpretable, and rotation is an essential part of the factor analysis method. Of the many rotation procedures that are available, 'varimax', an orthogonal rotation (that is, which does not affect the between-factor correlation), is most widely used and generally appears to yield sensible solutions in practice.[18] In mathematical terms, varimax aims to maximize the variance of the squared loadings of variables in each factor; this has the effect of minimizing the number of high loadings associated with each factor. In practical terms, varimax results in a 'simple' factor decomposition, because each factor will include the smallest possible number of explanatory variables; if, according to widely held philosophy, a simple solution suffices, why should one choose a more complicated one? If there are preconceived ideas about the factor structure, it may be more appropriate to use goodness-of-fit tests to examine a specific hypothesis, but for exploratory analysis the apparent simplicity and the sensible results following varimax have led to its near universal implementation in all computer packages. However, other methods do exist, most notably quartimax, which attempts to simplify the factor loadings associated with each variable (instead of the variable loadings associated with each factor). Orthomax and equamax are yet two other methods, and combine properties of both quartimax and varimax. If you are not satisfied with the arbitrary choice of varimax, there are plenty of alternatives.

Oblique axes

One assumption built into the model so far is that the factors are orthogonal and are therefore uncorrelated with each other. In many cases that is an unrealistic assumption. For example, it is quite likely that there will be a tendency for seriously ill patients to suffer from both anxiety and depression, and it might be expected that these two factors would be correlated. In statistical terms, we wish to allow 'oblique axes' instead of insisting upon orthogonality. This leads to a whole set of other rotation methods, and Gorsuch lists a total of 19 orthogonal and oblique methods[18] out of the many that are available. Most statistics packages offer a variety of these methods. Unfortunately, different procedures will result in appreciably different solutions unless the underlying structure of the data happens to be particularly clear and simple. Promax, which is derived from varimax, is the most frequently recommended oblique rotation method. Starting from the varimax solution, promax attempts to make low variable loadings even lower by relaxing the assumption that factors should be uncorrelated with each other; therefore, promax results in an even simpler structure in terms of variables loading on to each factor. Promax is therefore simple in concept, results in identifying simple factor structures, and also happens to be easy to implement in programming terms. Thus it is widely used. Not surprisingly, given its nature, promax usually results in similar – but simpler – factors to those derived by varimax. The most widely used alternative is oblimin, which is a generalization of earlier procedures called quartimin, covarimin, and biquartimin; these attempt to minimize various covariance functions. As with so much of exploratory factor analysis it is difficult – and controversial – to make recommendations regarding the choice of method. One procedure of desperation that has been suggested is to apply several rotational procedures to each of two random halves of the total pool of individuals; if different rotational procedures result in the same factors, and if these same factors appear in both random halves, 'a factor would need to be taken very seriously indeed'.[18] In other words, rotation is a necessary part of the exploratory factor analysis procedure, but you should also be cautious and circumspect whenever using rotation methods.

Example of rotation – the HADS questionnaire

Table 12.5 showed the effect of a varimax rotation, which revealed the two factors postulated to underlie the HADS questionnaire. However, as shown in Fig. 12.2, it was also suggested that the anxiety and depression factors would be correlated. Therefore an oblique rotation is called for. Table 12.6 shows the effect of oblique rotation, using two different methods – direct oblimin and promax. Since SPSS version 6 does not provide promax, STATA[29] was used for this. As can be seen, the strong factor structure of the HADS prevailed, and both oblique rotations yielded similar solutions to the varimax rotation. The negative signs attached to factor 2 of the oblimin solution and factor 1 of the promax solution are

Table 12.6 Rotated factor matrix – oblique rotations. Direct Oblimin oblique rotation (SPSS) and Promax rotations (STATA) are compared. Loadings greater than 0.4 have been shaded, showing the simplified factor structure after rotation. The solutions are very similar (the negative signs to factors are arbitrary and can be ignored), and are also similar to the Varimax orthogonal rotation

	Direct Oblimin rotation		Promax rotation	
	Factor 1	Factor 2	Factor 1	Factor 2
Q1	0.15523	−0.61067	−0.17192	0.60396
Q2	0.82631	0.13189	−0.80916	−0.10682
Q3	0.01062	−0.76478	−0.03442	0.75132
Q4	0.63116	−0.09449	−0.62423	0.11012
Q5	−0.01815	−0.77566	−0.00645	0.76122
Q6	0.68227	−0.08730	−0.67431	0.10446
Q7	0.36357	−0.37321	−0.36955	0.37649
Q8	0.60895	0.03103	−0.59839	−0.01375
Q9	−0.06371	−0.77463	0.03843	0.75895
Q10	0.55825	−0.05951	−0.55134	0.07377
Q11	0.01216	−0.43139	−0.02549	0.42397
Q12	0.77931	0.03846	−0.76585	−0.01637
Q13	−0.00707	−0.76397	−0.01699	0.75004
Q14	0.53136	−0.07893	−0.52549	0.09210

immaterial, and reflect the arbitrary viewpoint from which the factors may be observed in geometrical space; the important features are the magnitudes of the loadings and the relative signs of the loadings within each factor. Perhaps the most noticeable difference from the varimax results in Table 12.5 is that the loadings of variable 7 have been diminished, yet again emphasizing that this variable does not perform satisfactorily.

Assumptions for factor analysis

As with any modelling technique, various assumptions are built into the factor analysis model and the estimation procedures associated with factor analysis. In many fields of research these assumptions may well be valid, but in the context of QoL scales there are a number of problems arising from violation of the inherent assumptions.

Distributional assumptions

The standard factor analysis model makes no special assumptions about data being continuous and normally distributed. However, as we have seen, the estimation procedures commonly used are based upon either ML or least squares, and assume continuous, normally distributed data. Furthermore, most methods of estimation of factors are based upon the Pearson product-moment correlation matrix (or, equivalently, the covariance matrix) with normally distributed error structure. In particular, if the distributional assumptions are violated then any test for goodness of fit may be compromised. This is central to maximum likelihood factor analysis, which requires goodness of fit measures in order to determine the number of factors to be retained, and as noted above this number is crucial to the subsequent extraction of the factor matrix.

Many investigators fail to specify the software that they have used. Unfortunately, even when published reports of QoL studies have indicated the software or model used, they invariably fail to discuss the distributional properties of their data. From the total lack of mention about the need for continuous normally distributed data one can only conclude that most authors are presumably unaware of the need for these assumptions.

The two main types of departure from the assumptions are that data may be discrete, possibly with only a few categories, or may be continuous but non-normal (for example, highly asymmetrical). Many forms of QoL data are both categorical and highly asymmetrical at the same time.

Categorical data

Although a few QoL instruments use linear analogue scales,[30] by far the majority are based upon items using questions with discrete ordinal responses. Usually these are either four-point (for example, QLQ and RSCL) or five-point scales. Various groups have been developing the mathematical theory for factor analysis of categorical data,[31-38] and software is beginning to become more widely available. However, this is largely an untested and unexplored area and it remains unclear as to how effectively these techniques will be able to estimate the underlying latent structure, and what sample sizes will be required in order to obtain stable and consistent estimation of factors. As Steiger[39] has commented, 'So far the amount of Monte Carlo evidence amassed concerning these questions would barely fill a thimble'.

Since most investigators use standard factor analysis even when they have four- or five-point scales, one should at least consider the effect of violation of the assumptions. How robust is factor analysis? Several reports, based upon experience or simulations, have claimed that scales with as few as five points yield stable factors.[40-43] However, it remains unclear whether factor analysis based upon Pearson's product-moment correlation coefficient is adequate provided the five-point scale can be regarded as arising from a normal distribution with cut-off points. Furthermore, the situation regarding four-point scales also remains uncertain although it has even been suggested that 'Correlations are fairly robust (that is, they can tolerate deviations from normality), so even ordinal scales with at least three points can be included.',[42] but this has not been supported by others[43] who recommend '5 response categories are a minimum'. However, using *reductio ad absurdum*, clearly a one-point scale would not permit factor estimation and so there must be some lower limit below which estimation becomes less reliable or impractical. It also seems likely that sample size may have to be increased to compensate for the loss of information in shorter scales.

Since the numerical solution of factor analysis uses the correlation (or sometimes the covariance) matrix, it is natural to consider techniques for estimating correlations based upon discrete ordinal data. Polychoric correlations are formed by assuming that the discrete categorical observed values are a manifestation of data with an underlying (normal) continuous distribution. The mathematical theory leads to relatively complex estimation procedures, but recently, numerical algorithms for their estimation have become available.[31,33,34] To date, few studies have made use of such methods and once again there are fears about the effect upon sample size: 'One should be *extremely* cautious in applying them to samples of less than several hundred',[9] and Potthast[44] recommends caution with less than 1000 observations. Rigdon[45] simulated five-point variables with underlying normal distribution, using a model of two factors, with each factor having four variables loading exclusively on to it, and wrote 'Can one use the polychoric correlation coefficient...? Depending upon what one is looking for, the answer is either 'yes' or 'not yet'!'.

Normality

Even less work has been done on the effect of non-normality upon factor analysis, and yet most QoL items are not only measured using discrete scales but are also highly skewed (see Fig. 12.5). We can see this effect clearly with the items in the HADS. Other general QoL scales will usually contain items that deviate markedly for normality. There are two reasons for anticipating problems contributing to the non-normality of the data. First, some of the items are likely to take extreme

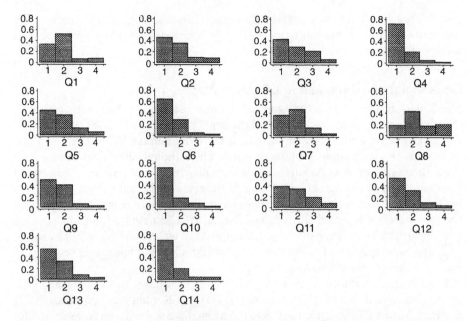

Fig. 12.5   Histograms of the 14 HADS items, using MRC data. The height of each bar represents the proportion of patients in each response category. The four responses were: 1, 'not at all'; 2, 'a little'; 3, 'quite a bit'; and 4, 'very much' (horizontal axis). Many items are markedly skewed, and all are four-point categories. They do not appear to follow normal distributions.

values depending upon the disease or the effects of its treatment. For example, patients receiving certain forms of chemotherapy will almost invariably experience considerable nausea, whilst this is unlikely to be a problem for patients undergoing surgery or patients receiving no active therapy. Hence, depending upon the therapy administered, items such as nausea may be expected to be highly skewed either towards 'not at all' or towards 'very much'. This is sometimes described as the 'floor' or 'ceiling' effect. In the case of the HADS, as is seen in Fig. 12.5, several items suffer from floor effects and tend to take minimum values for most patients, notably items Q4, Q6, Q10 and Q14, and all items except Q8 have very few patients with high responses. Second, there is no reason to assume that categories labelled 'not at all', 'a little', 'quite a bit', and 'very much' will yield equal-interval scales for patients' responses to any or all of the questions. Thus it is not surprising to find that the items follow highly skewed and non-normal distributions.

Although there have been attempts to develop asymptotically distribution-free (ADF) factor analysis,[31,35,36,46] this is still largely an exploratory area and early results suggest that huge sample sizes may be necessary for acceptable performance. For example, for ADF analysis on 15 variables and three 'strong' factors '...acceptable performance required samples of between 2500 and 5000 observations',[46] and when Muthén and Kaplan simulated five-point variables of various degrees of skewness for four models (2 to 4 factors, 6 to 15 variables), with 500 and 1000 observations they found 'Chi-squared tests and standard errors... are not as robust to non-normality as previously believed. ADF does not appear to work well'.[47]

Does violation of the assumptions matter?

Since most models for factor analysis assume continuous data with normally distributed error terms, whilst QoL data depart substantially from this both by being categorical and non-normal, what is the overall impact? The effect of these violations of assumptions is largely unknown, although empirical results and simulation studies suggest that the techniques may be relatively robust to reasonable degrees of departures. However, it seems likely that sample size, which in QoL studies is often small by any standards, should be increased to compensate for this. As already noted for ML estimation, it is commonly found in practice that departures from normality may have a marked effect upon hypothesis testing, such as for the number of factors or the goodness of fit, but has rather less impact upon the factor extraction.

The question remains: is there a simple rule of thumb to decide when ML estimation may be applied? Unfortunately, no. As Rigdon has commented (by Internet, SEMNET discussion list 1996) 'Any significant deviation from normality will be taken by critics as a weakness, while being dismissed by authors as inconsequential'.

Application of factor analysis in quality of life research

Given all the above attendant problems and difficulties it is perhaps surprising that factor analysis of QoL instruments so often results in apparently sensible factors! However, this may be simply a reflection of the strong and obvious correlation structure that underlies many 'constructs'; often the results, not surprisingly, confirm the expected QoL dimensions. Thus, provided there is adequate sample size, most studies do report finding factors that represent groupings of variables that could have been anticipated a priori to be correlated. Why, therefore, do so many authors report discrepancies in the factor structure when they repeat analyses with different data sets, as exemplified by the various analyses of the RSCL?

Contributory problems include the following.

1. Some variables have weak inter-correlations. This may occur because the underlying relationship really is weak, or because in a particular data set the observed correlations are weak.

2. Some studies may be under-sized. This will tend to result in unreliable estimation of the number of factors, and also in poor estimation of the factor structure.

3. Some studies may be too large: if care is not exercised, these may result in too many factors being identified, with even weak inter-correlations tending to pull variables together into a less meaningful factor.

4. Different patient data-sets may yield different factor structures. For example, in a cancer clinical trial involving both 'chemotherapy' and 'no-chemotherapy' arms, many chemotherapy patients might experience both nausea and hair loss, and the responses to such items on a questionnaire would probably show strong correlation; however, in a hormone therapy study these two items might appear uncorrelated or only weakly correlated. Thus there might be one side-effect related factor in the first study, but it would not appear (or appear only weakly) in the other study. Symptoms, side-effects and QoL issues are likely to vary in different subsets of patients, and for cancer patients may depend upon disease site (such as lung, prostate, stomach), stage of disease (advanced or early), treatment modality (such as chemotherapy, radiotherapy, or surgery), patients' sex, and patients' age.

5. Heterogeneous samples may yield strange factors. In a heterogeneous sample (different treatment modalities, for example) factor analyses may produce factors that are essentially group differences. These will be non-obvious, difficult-to-interpret factors that are not consistent with the investigator's expectations of the latent structure. A detailed analysis of this problem was presented by Meredith[48] who wrote 'The fourth factor is essentially uninterpretable unless one knows that it represents sex differences'. This problem is also discussed by Nunnally and Bernstein[9] who suggest that if one *knows* there are separate subgroups, one possibility is to use pooled within-group correlation matrices.

6. Some symptoms may be uncorrelated, yet contribute to the same scale. For example, it might be thought clinically logical to regard eating problems as part of a single scale. However, patients with head and neck cancer might have serious problems affecting their mouth, and hence preventing eating, whilst oesophageal patients might have problems swallowing. The correlation between oesophageal and oral-cavity problems might be low, yet for many quality of life purposes it might be convenient to regard them both as items in one scale, since a serious limitation with respect to either item reflects a major impact upon the patients' eating and quality of life.

Perhaps, after all, it is astonishing that exploratory factor analysis ever succeeds in confirming the postulated underlying latent structures.

Causal models

The models described so far have all been based upon the assumption that QoL scales can be represented as in Figs 12.1 and 12.2, with observed variables that reflect the value of the latent variable; presence of anxiety, for example, is expected to be manifested by high levels of Q1, Q3, Q5, Q7, Q9, Q11, and Q13 in Fig. 12.2. However, many QoL instruments include a large number of items covering diverse aspects of QoL. One such instrument is the Rotterdam symptom checklist (RSCL),[49] which includes 30 items relating to general QoL, symptoms, and side-effects; it also incorporates an activity scale and a global question about

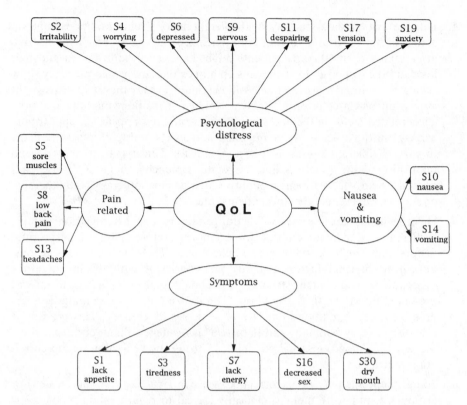

Fig. 12.6 Conventional factor analysis model for the Rotterdam symptom check list (RSCL), which is commonly postulated to consist of a psychological distress factor and other factors relating to symptoms and side-effects. Only 17 out of the 30 items on the main RSCL are shown.

overall QoL. For simplicity, we restrict consideration to 17 items. Adopting a conventional factor analysis model, a path diagram such as that of Fig. 12.6 might be considered. But is this a plausible model? It assumes that a latent variable 'psychological distress' tends to result in anxiety, depression, despair, irritability, and similar signs of distress, and that a poor QoL is likely to be manifested by psychological distress. This much does seem a plausible model. However, a patient with poor QoL does not necessarily have high levels of the treatment-related symptoms. That is to say, those patients receiving chemotherapy may well suffer from hair loss, nausea, vomiting, and other treatment related side-effects which cause deterioration in QoL, but other patients receiving non-chemotherapy treatments may be suffering from a completely different set of symptoms and side-effects which cause poor QoL for other reasons. Thus a poor QoL does not necessarily imply that, say, a patient is probably experiencing nausea; this is in contrast to the psychological distress indicators, all of which are expected to be affected if the patient experiences distress. On the other hand, if a patient *does* have severe nausea, that is likely to result in – or cause – a diminished QoL.

Therefore, a better model is to redraw Fig. 12.6 with symptoms and side-effects shown as 'causal indicators' and with the directional arrows pointing from the observed variables towards the 'symptoms and side-effects' factor, which in turn causes changes in QoL. This is shown in Fig. 12.7. The observed items reflecting psychological distress are commonly called effect indicators, to distinguish them from the causal indicators. The effect indicators provide a measure of the QoL likely to be experienced by patients, whilst the causal indicators affect or influence patients' QoL.

Exploratory factor analysis is ill equipped to deal with such situations. Instead, a more general approach has to be considered. This leads to models that can represent structures as shown in Fig. 12.7, and can estimate the coefficients and parameters that describe the various paths. This approach is known as structural equation modelling (SEM). At present, SEM requires the use of specialized software, and is not included as a standard part of statistical packages such as SAS, SPSS, and STATA. Programs that can handle SEM models include AMOS,[50] EQS,[51] or LISREL.[52]

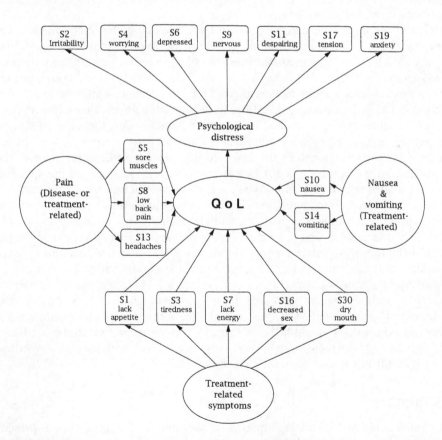

Fig. 12.7 Postulated causal structure for 17 items on the RSCL. Treatment- or disease-related symptoms and side-effects are more likely to be causal indicators than effect indicators.

One major difference between exploratory factor analysis and structural equation modelling is the emphasis that the latter places upon prior specification of the postulated structure. Thus many forms of SEM are also known as confirmatory factor analysis (CFA), since a factor-analytic structure is pre-specified and one major purpose of the modelling is to test – or confirm – how well the data fit this hypothesized structure. Thus the testing takes the form of 'goodness of fit' tests, with the model being accepted as adequate provided there is no strong counter-evidence against it. Although such techniques have been widely used in areas such as educational and personality testing, they are as yet little practised in the field of QoL. However, given the many disadvantages that we have described concerning exploratory factor analysis, it should be apparent that SEM is likely to be a far more appropriate approach. Despite this, it should still be emphasized that many of the problems we have raised remain unresolved for SEM just as much as for EFA; for example, categorical data are hard to handle, non-normality of data remains a major issue since normality underpins most of the goodness-of-fit measures, and sample size remains difficult to estimate in advance of carrying out the study.

One of the largest hurdles for SEM in QoL research is that many models will inevitably be complex. For example, feedback mechanisms may be present, and many variables may be a mixture of causal and effect indicators: difficulty sleeping may cause reduced QoL which may in turn cause anxiety which causes further sleeping problems and yet further affects QoL. In addition, it may be impossible to use data from ordinary QoL studies to distinguish between alternative models: when variables can be both effect and causal simultaneously, there are estimation problems and sometimes the solutions cannot be determined uniquely. Many alternative models may all fit the observed data equally well. In fact, one of the most important features of CFA is that it simply tests whether the pre-specified model is adequate to fit the observed data; this does not indicate that a model is correct, but merely that there is insufficient evidence against it. Thus a small study, with insufficient numbers of patients, will almost inevitably be unable to provide evidence of a poor fit unless a model is totally inappropriate; on the other hand, unless the model is perfect (by definition, a model is only a model and is never perfect) and if a study is large enough there will almost always be evidence of statistically significant departures from perfect fit. Therefore, statistical significance is only of minor relevance in CFA; small sized studies rarely have 'significant' goodness-of-fit indices, whilst very large studies almost always do. Instead, conclusions should be based largely upon the magnitude of the goodness-of-fit indices. Unfortunately there are many such indices, with varying properties, and it is difficult to choose between them.

Summary

Causal models, SEM, and CFA hold great potential for the future, but at present they have been little used in QoL research, and there remain many controversial issues to be resolved before they can be recommended for routine usage. On the other hand, EFA has many disadvantages, not the least of which is that it will frequently be an inappropriate model for QoL instruments because of the occurrence of causal indicators. Perhaps the main advantage of EFA is its relative ease of application. EFA is available through most of the larger statistical packages, and analysis using EFA can readily be carried out. SEM, on the other hand, requires specialized software. Also, SEM models are considerably more difficult to specify, even though most SEM packages are moving towards model specification using graphical path diagrams. The results of analyses as displayed by SEM packages are also more difficult to interpret.

One overall conclusion from this chapter should be that EFA, CFA, and SEM are not 'black box' procedures that can be applied blindly. Before embarking on any such analysis, the investigator must consider the possible path structures for the relationships between the explanatory variables and the latent structures. Usually there will be a number of alternative models that are thought plausible. The role of the approaches we have described is to examine whether any of these models appear reasonable, and if it does the investigator may feel satisfied. But this neither 'proves' that the model is correct, nor that the scale has been truly 'validated'; it only confirms that there is no evidence of bad fit.

Recommended reading

In addition to the references in the text, the book by Gorsuch[18] is recommended for a detailed description of factor analysis and related techniques – unlike many books on this topic, it covers factor analysis in depth whilst avoiding much of the heavier mathematics; for example, Gorsuch has a whole chapter about selecting the number of factors, and two chapters about rotation methods. However, the book by Nunnally and Bernstein[9] also contains extensive chapters about factor analysis and confirmatory factor analysis, and has the advantage of greater emphasis on psychometric scales. Structural equation and latent variable models are fully described by Bollen.[53]

References

1. Aaronson, N.K., Ahmedzai, S., Bergman, B., *et al*. The European Organization for Research and Treatment of Cancer QLQ-C30: A quality-of-life instrument for use in international clinical trials in oncology. *J. Natl Cancer Inst.*, 1993; **85**: 365–76.
2. Ware, J.E. and Sherbourne, C.D. The MOS 36-item short-form health survey (SF-36). 1. Conceptual-framework and item selection. *Med. Care*, 1992; **30**: 473–83.
3. DeVellis, R.F. *Scale development: theory and application*. Newbury Park, California: Sage, 1991.
4. Zigmond, A.S. and Snaith, R.P. The Hospital Anxiety and Depression Scale. *Acta Psychiatr. Scand.*, 1983; **67**: 361–70.
5. SPSS Inc. *SPSS Professional Statistics 6.1*. Chicago: SPSS Inc., 1995.
6. Moorey, S., Greer, S., Watson, M., *et al*. The factor structure and factor stability of the Hospital Anxiety and Depression Scale in patients with cancer [see comments]. *Br. J. Psychiatry*, 1991; **158**: 255–9.

7. Spearman, C. General intelligence objectively determined and measured. *Am. J. Psychol.*, 1904; **15**: 201–93.

8. Burt, C. The two factor theory. *Br. J. Psychol: Statist. Section*, 1949; **2**: 151–79.

9. Nunnally, J.C. and Bernstein, I.H. *Psychometric theory*. New York: McGraw-Hill, 1994.

10. Likert, R.A. A technique for the development of attitude scales. *Educ. Psychol. Meas.*, 1952; **12**: 313–15.

11. Jenkinson, C., Ziebland, S., Fitzpatrick, R., and Mowat, A. Sensitivity to change of weighted and unweighted versions of two health measures. *Int. J. Health Sci.*, 1991; **2**: 189–94.

12. Fletcher, A., Gore, S., Jones, D., Fitzpatrick, R., Spiegelhalter, D.J., and Cox, D. Quality of life measures in health care. II: Design, analysis, and interpretation. *Br. Med. J.*, 1992; **305**: 1145–8.

13. Wright, J.G. and Feinstein, A.R. A comparative contrast of clinimetric and psychometric methods for constructing indexes and rating-scales. *J. Clin. Epidemiol.*, 1992; **45**: 1201–18.

14. Dawes, R.M. The robust beauty of improper linear models. *American Psychologist*, 1979; **34**: 571–82.

15. Cox, D.R., Fitzpatrick, R., Fletcher, A.E., *et al*. Quality-of-life assessment: can we keep it simple? *J. Roy. Statist. Soc.*, 1992; **155**: 353–93.

16. Olschewski, M. and Schumacher, M. Statistical analysis of quality of life data in cancer clinical trials. *Stat. Med.*, 1990; **9**: 749–63.

17. Krzanowski, W.J. *Principles of multivariate analysis*. Oxford: Clarendon Press, 1988.

18. Gorsuch, R.L. *Factor analysis*, (2nd edn). New Jersey: Lawrence Erlbaum, 1983.

19. Boomsma, A. The robustness of LISREL against small sample sizes in factor analysis models. In: *Systems under indirect observation*, (Joreskog, K.G., Wolf, H., eds). Amsterdam: North Holland, 1982.

20. Aleamoni, L.M. Effects of sample size on eigenvalues, observed communalities and factor loadings. *J. Appl. Psychol.*, 1973; **58**: 266–9.

21. Nunnally, J.C. *Psychometric theory*, (2nd edn). New York: McGraw-Hill, 1978.

22. Cattell, R.B. *The scientific use of factor analysis*. New York: Plenum Press, 1978.

23. Baggaley, A.R. Deciding on the ratio of number of subjects to number of variables in factor-analysis. *Multivariate Experimental Clinical Research*, 1983; **6**: 81–5.

24. Guadagnoli, E. and Velicer, W.F. Relation of sample size to the stability of component patterns. *Psychol. Bull.*, 1988; **103**: 265–75.

25. Zwick, W.R. and Velicer, W.F. Factors influencing 4 rules for determining the number of components to retain. *Multivar. Behav. Res.*, 1982; **17**: 253–69.

26. Zwick, W.R. and Velicer, W.F. Comparison of 5 rules for determining the number of components to retain. *Psychol. Bull.*, 1986; **99**: 432–42.

27. Kaiser, H.F. The application of electronic computers to factor analysis. *Educ. Psychol. Meas.*, 1960; **20**: 141–51.

28. SAS Inst. Inc. *SAS/STAT User's guide, version 6, Vols 1 and 2*. Cary, North Carolina: SAS Inst. Inc., 1996.

29. Stata Corp. *Stata reference manual: release 4.0*. College Station, TX, USA: Stata Corporation, 1995.

30. Selby, P.J., Chapman, J.A., Etazadi-Amoli, J., *et al*. The development of a method for assessing the quality of life in cancer patients. *Br. J. Cancer*, 1984; **50**: 13–22.
31. Lee, S.Y., Poon, W.Y., and Bentler, P.M. Structural equation models with continuous and polytomous variables. *Psychometr.*, 1992; **57**: 89–105.
32. Lee, S.Y., Poon, W.Y., and Bentler, P.M. A 3-stage estimation procedure for structural equation models with polytomous variables. *Psychometr.*, 1990; **55**: 45–51.
33. Lee, S.-Y. and Poon. W.-Y. Maximum likelihood estimation of polyserial correlations. *Psychometr.*, 1986; **51**: 113–21.
34. Lee, S.Y., Poon, W.Y., and Bentler, P.M. A 2-stage estimation of structural equation models with continuous and polytomous variables. *Br. J. Math. Stat. Psychol.*, 1995; **48**: 339–58.
35. Bartholomew, D.J. *Latent variable models and factor analysis*. London: Charles Griffin, 1987.
36. Bartholomew, D.J. Factor analysis for categorical data. *J. Roy. Statist. Soc.*, 1980; **42**: 293–321.
37. Jöreskog, K.G. Latent variable modelling with ordinal variables. In *Statistical modelling and latent variables*, (Haagen, K., Bartholemew, D.J., Deistler, M., eds). London: Elsevier, 1993.
38. Jöreskog, K.G. and Sörbom, D. *LISREL VII. A guide to the program and applications*. Chicago: SPSS Inc., 1988.
39. Steiger, J.H. Factor analysis in the 1980s and the 1990s: some old debates and some new developments. In *Trends and perspectives in empirical social research*, (Borg, I., Mohler, P.P., eds). Berlin: Walter de Gruyter, 1994.
40. Bollen, K.A. and Barb, K.H. Pearson's *r* and coarsely categorized measures. *Amer. Soc. Rev.*, 1981; **46**: 232–9.
41. Babakus, E., Ferguson, C.E., and Jöreskog, K.G. The sensitivity of confirmatory maximum-likelihood factor-analysis to violations of measurement scale and distributional assumptions. *Journal of Marketing Research*, 1987; **24**: 222–8.
42. Streiner, D.L. Figuring out factors: the use and misuse of factor analysis. *Can. J. Psychiatry*, 1994; **39**: 135–40.
43. Dolan, C.V. Factor-analysis of variables with 2-response, 3-response, 5-response and 7-response response categories – a comparison of categorical variable estimators using simulated data. *Br. J. Math. Stat. Psychol.*, 1994; **47**: 309–26.
44. Potthast, M.J. Confirmatory factor-analysis of ordered categorical variables with large models. *Br. J. Math. Stat. Psychol.*, 1993; **46**: 273–86.
45. Rigdon, E.E. and Ferguson, C.E. The performance of the polychoric correlation-coefficient and selected fitting functions in confirmatory factor-analysis with ordinal data. *Journal of Marketing Research*, 1991; **28**: 491–7.
46. Hu, L.T., Bentler, P.M., and Kano, Y. Can test statistics in covariance structure-analysis be trusted? *Psychol. Bull.*, 1992; **112**: 351–62.
47. Muthén, B.O. and Kaplan, D. A comparison of some methodologies for the factor-analysis of non-normal Likert variables – a note on the size of the model. *Br. J. Math. Stat. Psychol.*, 1992; **45**: 19–30.
48. Meredith, W. Measurement invariance, factor-analysis and factorial invariance. *Psychometr.*, 1993; **58**: 525–43.

49. de Haes, J.C.J.M., Olschewski, M., Fayers, P.M., *et al*. *The Rotterdam symptom checklist (RSCL): a manual*. Groningen: Northern Centre for Healthcare Research, 1996.
50. Arbuckle, J.L. *Amos users' guide version 3.6*. Chicago: SmallWaters Corporation, 1997.
51. Bentler, P.M. *EQS structural equations program manual*. Encino, California: Multivariate Sofware, Inc., 1995.
52. Jöreskog, K.G. and Sörbom, D. *LISREL 8: user's reference guide*. Chicago: Scientific Software International, 1996.
53. Bollen, K.A. *Structural equations with latent variables*. New York: Wiley, 1989.

Appendix: Statistical background

Factor analysis can be expressed in mathematical terms as follows. Let us assume that there are v observed variables, called x_i, where $i = 1 \ldots v$, and that the model will contain k factors. Then factor analysis consists of fitting a model of the form

$$x = \Lambda f + \varepsilon \qquad (12.1)$$

where Λ is the $v \times k$ common factor pattern matrix (or factor loadings), f is called the 'common factor' vector, and ε consists of the residual terms including random error terms.

Superficially, eqn 12.1 is very similar to the equation for multiple regression, which may be written either as $Y = \alpha + X\beta + \varepsilon$ or, in an equivalent but more general format in which α is included with the β terms, by

$$Y = X\beta + \varepsilon.$$

However, for multiple regression both Y and X are known, and the object is to estimate β; this is fundamentally different from the situation in which the objective is to obtain a solution for Λ, and where the aim is to find such a solution with as few columns k as are necessary for a clinically meaningful fit.

To solve eqn 12.1, we first assume that the common factors f are uncorrelated with each other, that they are uncorrelated with the residual terms ε, and that they have mean of zero with unit variance. Writing the $v \times v$ population covariance matrix as Σ, it can be shown that

$$\Sigma = \Lambda\Lambda' + \psi$$

where ψ is the $v \times v$ diagonal matrix of variances of the residuals, ε.

The covariance matrix Σ is estimated by the sample covariance matrix S, which is calculated from the observed responses of the patients; in fact, the mean levels of the patient responses to the QoL questions are not used, and estimation of the factor structure is based solely upon the covariance matrix S. Thus the importance of increasing n, the sample size or number of patients, is to ensure that the estimate of S is sufficiently precise.

For maximum likelihood estimation, it is assumed that multivariate normality applies to the patients' observations, leading to S having a Wishart distribution with a known likelihood function. This then enables the equations to be solved, yielding numerical estimates of the Λ factor loadings.

However, as has been well recognized by statisticians and psychometricians, there are a multiplicity of solutions to the basic equation, all of which fit equally well. In particular, if Λ is a solution to eqn 12.1, then $\Lambda M'$ is another equally good solution whenever $M'M = I$; M' is then called an 'orthogonal rotation matrix', and it can be shown that an infinite variety of solutions for M' exists.

This has had two consequences. First, mathematical constraints are generally placed upon the equations, to ensure that a unique solution may be obtained for Λ. Two conventions, out of the many available, are to start by assuming that the factors are orthogonal and therefore uncorrelated with each other, and that each successive factor makes the maximum contribution to explaining the total variance so that, as can be shown mathematically, $\Lambda'\psi\Lambda$ is diagonal. Second, after finding an initial solution, a 'rotation' is used. Most commonly, a 'Varimax' rotation is often used on the factor matrix Λ so that the new loadings are either relatively large or relatively small; this is done by seeking a rotation that maximizes the variance of the squared factor loadings. The effect of these constraints is to lead to a simple structure for the model and the relationships between the variables and the factors. Thus the Varimax rotation tends to result in each item loading upon one and only one factor, while the orthogonality results in factors that are uncorrelated with each other. Although, fortuitously, this frequently leads to models that appear to be sensible, it is difficult to believe that these constraints correspond to reality. Also, and perhaps more importantly, there is nowadays an acceptance that when factor analysis is applied in this manner it is largely exploratory and model-forming – and hence often called exploratory factor analysis (EFA). Further studies are usually required to validate or confirm the results.

V

Data analysis

13 *Methods of analysis for longitudinal studies of health-related quality of life*

Diane L. Fairclough

Most studies of health-related QoL consider measurement from one of two perspectives. In the first, the end-points are expressed in the metric of the QoL scales, whereas in the second group the outcome is expressed in the metric of time. The latter group includes outcomes such as QALYs and Q-TWiST that are discussed in other chapters of this book (Chapters 7 and 15) and will not be included here. In studies where the end-points are expressed in the metric of the QoL scales, QoL assessment is generally incorporated into the study by administering questionnaires at multiple time points before, during, and sometimes after an intervention, with the goal of characterizing the patient's QoL in a longitudinal fashion. The number of planned assessments may be as few as three[1] or as many as nine.[2,3]

There are three basic approaches to the analysis of these longitudinal studies which should primarily depend on the research questions of interest. The first is to conceptualize the study as a repeated measures design, with assessments planned during particular phases of the patient's treatment and/or disease progression. An example is a study by the Eastern Cooperative Oncology Group of two adjuvant therapy regimens for patients with hormone-receptor negative, node-positive breast cancer.[1] In this study there were three planned assessments: one prior to therapy, another during therapy, and a final assessment four months following therapy, representing three phases of the patient's treatment. The second approach is to focus on the change in QoL over time using a growth curve model. This approach is appropriate in settings where duration of treatment may not be determined *a priori* but depends on disease status and continues as long as therapy appears to be effective, as often occurs in patients with chronic or advanced disease. The third approach is to reduce the longitudinal information to a single summary measure (or global statistic). These summary measures include the average rate of change (slope) and area under the QoL v. time curves (area under curve, AUC).

The choice of the appropriate methods of analysis is also influenced by two other issues: missing data (see Chapter 14) and multiple end-points and comparisons.[4] Missing data is a concern because of the potential for biased estimates of QoL when the reasons for missing data are related to factors that affect the patient's QoL. The presence of multiple end-points presents two potential problems: that of controlling type I errors (see below) for multiple comparisons and finding strategies for presenting QoL results in a way that is clinically meaningful and easily interpretable. These two issues are central to the discussion of alternative methods of analysis presented in this chapter.

Repeated measures analysis of variance

Multiple univariate analyses

The most commonly used method of analysis consists of univariate analyses at each time point using test procedures such as t-tests, ANOVA, or Wilcoxon rank sum test. While simple to implement, this approach has several disadvantages.[5-7] First, the large number of comparisons often fails to answer the clinical question but rather presents a confusing picture. The potential for a large number of comparisons is illustrated by an international breast cancer study group trial with four schedules of adjuvant therapy with five measures of QoL and nine scheduled assessments[2] where there is the *potential* for up to 135 $[(4-1) \times 5 \times 9]$ separate tests. Further, the results of multiple univariate analyses may not be statistically valid as the significance tests are not independent. Specifically, the probability of concluding that there are significant differences in QoL when none exist (the type I error) increases as the number of comparisons increases. In some cases, these univariate methods can be difficult to implement if measurements are mistimed due to delays in therapy or other factors.

One strategy for handling the multiple testing is to specify a limited number of comparisons (no more than three) in the design of the trial.[8] While this is a valid approach, in practice investigators are reluctant to ignore the remaining data. There is also an ethical question about collection of data that are not intended to be used in the analysis. An alternative method to address this problem is to utilize a multiple-comparisons procedure, such as the Bonferroni, or Scheffe corrections. For example, the Bonferroni procedure is to accept as statistically significant only those tests with p values that are less than α/n, where α is the overall type I error and n is the number of tests (or comparisons) performed. In the above example, if the type I error rate was set to be 5 per cent, then comparisons would be statistically significant if the p values where less than $0.05/135 = 0.00037$. While addressing the type I error problem, this approach significantly reduces the 'power' to detect real differences in QoL. This example is somewhat extreme because of the four treatments, but it is typical to have studies of two treatments with 3-9 repeated measures and 4-6 measures of QoL, and thus 12-54 potential multiple comparisons.

Multivariate analysis

A second analytic approach for repeated measures is to perform multivariate analyses. These procedures include multivariate analysis of variance (MANOVA), when the proportion of subjects with missing assessments is very small and the data are missing completely at random (MCAR), or likelihood-based multivariate methods such as mixed effects or repeated measures models[9,10] when the data are missing at random (MAR). (See Chapter 14 and below for more detailed discussion of missing data.) Multivariate tests such as Hotelling's T and likelihood ratio tests can be used to control the type I error of the multiple comparisons. These statistics, however, test a hypothesis of 'no treatment' differences against a general alternative. Specifically, they ask the general question, 'Are there differences in QoL at *any* point in time?' and are not sensitive to persistent differences over time. These tests may sometimes be hard to interpret when the results are counterintuitive.[5] For example, the test may be 'statistically' significant when QoL is better in one treatment arm at one time point and the other treatment at another time point, and not significant when one treatment appears to have consistently better QoL over time.[11]

Growth curve models

Growth curve models are most useful for clinical trials with missing and mistimed observations, time-varying covariates, and a large number of potential repeated measures. In most cases, these models include polynomial functions of the actual time of assessment relative to some reference point. An example is a prospective longitudinal study of QoL in 68 terminal cancer patients in which patients were assessed every three to six weeks until death;[12] the research focus was on the patterns of change in QoL over time prior to death. A second example is a proposed phase III study by the Eastern Cooperative Oncology Group of HIV patients with Karposi sarcoma. In this study, the primary research question is 'Is QoL better or worse because of disease changes or toxicity', which will be assessed by including time-varying covariates, including changes in disease status and the occurrence of treatment-related toxicity, in a growth curve model.

Latent variable models

Health-related QoL is generally considered to be a multidimensional construct, with physical, function, emotional, social, and spiritual components. As such, the multiple measures of the different aspects of QoL can be considered to be measurements of an unobservable latent variable. Latent variable models for longitudinal studies have been used by Zwinderman[13] for dichotomous outcomes and by Busch *et al.*[14] for continuous, normally distributed outcomes. In both applications, the issue of missing assessments was addressed with the subsequent analyses based on the assumption of MAR (see Chapter 14).

Summary measures

An alternative approach to either multiple univariate analyses or multivariate analyses is the use of summary measures[5,6,15] or global statistics.[16] Examples of summary measures include post-treatment mean,[5,7,17] mean change relative to baseline,[17] last value minus baseline,[17] average rate of change over time (or slope),[7] maximum value,[5-7] area under the curve,[7,15] and time to reach a peak or a pre-specified value.[6,7] There are several reasons for the use of summary measures in the analysis of a longitudinal study of QoL.[11] The primary advantage of these summary measures is that they are often easier to interpret than the multivariate methods described previously. Not only are the number of comparisons reduced, but measures such as the rate of change and the area under the curve are familiar concepts in clinical medicine. In addition, depending on the summary measure selected, they often have greater power to detect clinically relevant differences in QoL that persist over time.

Patterns of change across time

The choice of which summary measure should be selected as the end-point in a clinical trial depends on the objective of the investigation, expected pattern of change across time, and patterns of missing data. Consider several possible patterns of change in QoL across time (Fig. 13.1). One pattern might be a steady rate of change over time reflecting either a constant improvement in QoL over

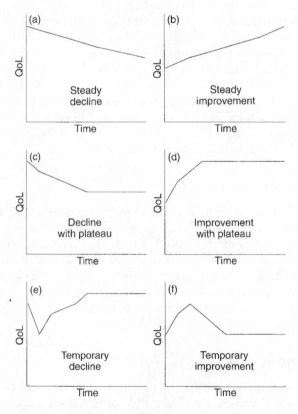

Fig. 13.1 Examples of patterns of change in QoL over time.

time or a constant decline over time. This pattern of change suggests that the rate of change or slope would be a good choice of a summary measure for this population. In contrast, other measures, such as the change from baseline to the last measure, might not be desirable if patients who fail earlier and thus drop out from the study earlier have smaller changes than those patients with longer follow-up.

An alternative profile might be a rapid change initially with a subsequent plateau after the maximum therapeutic benefit is realized. Examples include two clinical trails of adjuvant therapy for breast cancer.[2,18] This profile illustrates the importance of identifying the clinically relevant question *a priori*. If the objective is to identify the therapy that produces the most rapid improvement in QoL, the time to reach a peak or pre-specified value would be good choice. If, in contrast, the ultimate level of benefit is more important than the time to achieve the benefit, then a measure such as the post-treatment mean or mean change relative to baseline might be desirable.

A third pattern of change might occur with a therapy that has transient benefits or toxicity. For example, individuals may experience transient benefits and then return to their baseline levels after the effect of the therapy has ceased. Alternatively, a toxic therapy for cancer may significantly reduce QoL during therapy but ultimately result in a better QoL following therapy than the patient was experiencing at the time of diagnosis.[18] For these more complex patterns of change over time, a measure such as the area under the curve might be considered as a summary of both early and continued effects of the therapy.

Constructing summary measures

There are two fundamental approaches to constructing summary measures, which differ primarily by the manner in which one handles missing data.[11] In the first approach, one first summarizes the data within an individual subject by constructing a single value for each individual and then performs a univariate test. In the second approach, data are initially summarized within each treatment group and summary measures are constructed from these population estimates.

For example, in the first approach, the rate of change experienced by each individual could be estimated using ordinary least squares (for individuals with at least two measurements) and a two-sample t-test could be used to compare the estimates in two treatment groups. In the second approach, the mean rate of change (or slope) for each treatment group would be estimated using a mixed effects model and the differences in the slopes between the two treatment group tested. If there are no missing data, then the two approaches are virtually identical. However, when there are missing data, missing assessments are handled on an individual basis in the first approach and on a population basis in the second approach.

Within individuals

First, consider the construction of summary measures that reduce the set of n (or $n_{ik} < n$) measurements (Y_{ijk}) on the ith individual in the kth group to a single value (S_{ik}) by computing a weighted sum of the measurements (Y_{ijk}) or a function of the measurements ($f(Y_{ijk})$):

$$S_{ik} = \sum_{j=1}^{n_{ik}} w_j \, f(Y_{ijk}).$$

O'Brien[19] proposed several methods for complete data. In the first, the measurements on all subjects are ranked at each time point and then the average of the ranks across the n time points is computed for each individual. If the reasons for missing data were known and one could make reasonable assumptions about the ranking of QoL in patients at each time point, one could possibly adapt this approach to a study with missing data. For example, it would not be unreasonable to assume that the QoL of patients who died or left the study due to excessive toxicity was worse than the QoL of those patients who remained on therapy. They would then be assigned the lowest possible rank for measurements scheduled after death or during the time of excessive toxicity.

In the second approach proposed by O'Brien,[19] the measurements at each time point are converted to z scores by subtracting the overall mean ($\bar{Y}_j$) and dividing by the standard deviation of the pooled sample: $z_{ijk} = (Y_{ijk} - \bar{Y}_j)/\mathrm{SD}(Y_{ijk})$. The measurements are then averaged by using either equal weights ($w_j = 1/n$) or weights derived by summing the columns of the inverse correlation (R^{-1}) of the n repeated measures. This later approach down-weights the more highly correlated measurements. Based on studies of the power and size of the test, O'Brien[19] recommended the average of the ranks for general use and the second approach with the weights derived from the inverse correlation, for normally distributed data with moderate or large sample sizes.

Matthews[7] and Cox et al.[15] suggest an approach that provides a measure of QoL over time. The summary statistic is the area under the curve (AUC) of the QoL scores (Y_{ijk}) plotted against time (t). The AUC for the ikth individual can be estimated using a trapezoidal approximation:

$$S_{ik} = \mathrm{AUC}_{ik} = \sum_{j=1}^{n} (t_j - t_{j-1}) \frac{Y_{ijk} + Y_{i(j-1)k}}{2}, \qquad j = 0, \ldots, n.$$

When the data are complete, this computation is straightforward. However, with this approach strategies for handling missing data need to be developed. For example, if intermediate observations are missing, one could interpolate between observations. If a patient dies during the study, the minimum QoL score could be assigned at that time point. For a patient who dropped out, the last measurement could be inferred either by carrying the last value forward or extrapolating from the last two observations. Each of these approaches makes assumptions that may or may not be reasonable in specific settings and it would be advisable to examine the sensitivity of the conclusions to the various assumptions.

An alternative strategy for handling censoring due to drop-out or administrative censoring is proposed by Korn.[20] Initially, it would appear that one could present the AUC values calculated to the time of censoring as one would present survival data. This approach would appear to have the advantages of displaying more information about the distribution of the AUC values and accommodating administrative censoring. Unfortunately, administrative censoring is informative on the AUC scale[21,22] and the usual Kaplan–Meier estimates will be biased. Specifically, if the censoring mechanism is due to staggered entry and incomplete follow-up is identical for two groups, the group with poorer QoL will have lower values of the AUC and will be censored earlier on the AUC scale. Korn suggests a procedure to reduce the bias of the estimator by assuming that the probability of censoring in short intervals is independent of the QoL measures prior to that time. While this assumption is probably not true, if the QoL is measured frequently and the relationship between QoL and censoring is weak, the violation may be small enough that the bias in the estimator will also be small.

Across individuals

The second approach to constructing summary measures is to obtain parameter estimates for each treatment group ($\hat{\beta}_{kj}$) and then reduce the set of estimates to a single summary measure for each treatment group:

$$\hat{S}_k = \sum_{j=1}^{n} w_j\, g(\hat{\beta}_{kj}).$$

In general, $g(\hat{\beta}_{jk})$ are the estimates of the mean ($\hat{\mu}_{kj}$) of the jth measurement of QoL in the kth treatment group adjusted for important covariates.[11] Alternatively, $g(\hat{\beta}_{jk})$ may be a direct estimate of the summary measure such as the slope. If the data are complete, one can use multivariate analysis of variance or growth curve models to estimate β_{kj}. When data are missing, one can use the appropriate methods discussed later in this chapter for obtaining unbiased estimates depending on whether the data are missing at random[9,10] or non-ignorable.[23–27] In practice, the second strategy may be preferable because it may be much easier to develop a model-based method for handling missing data than to develop strategies on an individual basis.

A simple example of this second class of summary measures is the average of the r post-baseline means. This approach of constructing summary measures can also be used to estimate the area under the curve (AUC) for the kth treatment group. The AUC can be estimated by using a weighted function of the means (trapezoidal approximation),

$$\hat{S}_k = \sum_{j=1}^{n} (t_j - t_{j-1})\frac{\hat{\mu}_{jk} + \hat{\mu}_{(j-1)k}}{2}.$$

Alternatively, if a polynomial model is used to estimate the change over time then the AUC can be estimated by integration

$$\hat{S}_k = \int_{t=0}^{t_n} \sum_{j=0}^{n} \hat{\beta}_{kj} t^j = \sum_{j=0}^{n} \hat{\beta}_{kj} t^{j+1} \Big/ (j+1).$$

Pocock *et al.*[28] suggest an extension of O'Brien's weighted average z scores to the combination of any asymptotically normal test statistics, illustrating the concept with the log-rank statistics and a binary end-point. Fairclough[11] describes an application to repeated assessment of QoL and survival where the logarithmic transformation of the survival times is assumed to be normally distributed.

Since $\hat{S}_k$ is a linear combination of asymptotically normal parameter estimates, the asymptotic variance of the summary measure is $\text{Var}(\hat{S}_k)=W'\text{Cov}[g(\hat{\beta}_{jk})]W$ where $W=(w_1,\ldots,w_n)$. For two treatment groups, we can test the hypothesis $S_1=S_2$ using a t-statistic, $t=(\hat{S}_1-\hat{S}_2)/\text{Var}(\hat{S}_1-\hat{S}_2)^{1/2}$ with $df=N-4$ for small samples.[28] More generally, for large samples, we can test the hypothesis $S_1=S_2=\cdots=S_K$ using a Wald chi-square statistic: $\chi^2_{K-1}=\hat{\phi}'[\text{Cov}(\hat{\phi})]^{-1}\hat{\phi}$, where $\hat{\phi}=(\hat{S}_2-\hat{S}_1,\ldots,\hat{S}_n-\hat{S}_1)$.

Missing data

Missing data are inevitable in any longitudinal study; over an extended period of time patients will potentially experience morbidity or mortality due to disease or its treatment. As described in Chapter 14, missing data may result from administrative problems, such as staff forgetting to give the forms to the patient during a very busy time. Other reasons are directly related to the patient's quality of life, such as the patient being unable to complete the questionnaire because of severe toxicity or death.

There are three classes of missing data that determine which methods of analysis are appropriate for longitudinal studies.[29] Briefly, if the reasons for missing assessments are completely unrelated to the patient's QoL, then we consider the data to be missing completely at random (MCAR). Common sense and historical evidence suggest that this assumption will not be true in most clinical trials. If the probability of a missing assessment only depends on the observed measures of QoL and other explanatory factors, we consider the data to be missing at random (MAR). Finally, missing data are considered to be not missing at random (NMAR) or non-ignorable if the probability that an observation is missing depends on the value of the missing observation. Formal definitions and further discussion of these three types of missing assessments are presented in Chapter 14. Various formal approaches to testing the assumption of MCAR include those described by Little,[30] Diggle,[31] Engleman,[32] Ridout,[33] and Park and Davis.[34]

Missing data present difficulties in the design and analysis of longitudinal QoL studies for several reasons. First is the loss of power to detect change over time or differences between groups as a result of a reduced number of observations. However, in many large (phase III) trials the sample size has been based on other clinical end-points and the power to detect meaningful differences in QoL measures is generally adequate. If not, increasing the sample size of the trial may be feasible depending on patient and economic resources. Second is the potential for bias of the estimates as a result of non-randomly missing data (see Chapter 14). For example, patients who are experiencing a negative impact of the disease or therapy on their lives may be less likely to complete the QoL assessments. In other settings, patients who have had an excellent response to therapy may feel that they no longer need to continue their participation in the treatment study. In either case, as will be illustrated below, a clear understanding of the reasons for missing assessments is a critical factor in the selection of the appropriate method of analysis for these longitudinal studies.

Analysis of complete cases (MCAR)

The most often used methods of analysis for longitudinal data are methods such as multivariate analysis of variance (MANOVA) or growth curve models that include data from patients who have completed *all* of the scheduled assessments (complete cases). These methods are popular because they are taught in most intermediate statistical courses and are available in almost every statistical analysis package. If the proportion of subjects with any missing assessments is very small (<5 per cent of the cases), these methods may be reasonable. However, in many studies with extended follow-up and patients who may be experiencing morbidity and/or mortality, these methods could easily exclude more than half of the subjects from the analysis. More critically, these approaches are based on the very strong assumption of MCAR; if that assumption is violated then the estimates may be seriously biased. The assumption is that the probability than an observation is missing does not depend on the QoL of the patient at the time of any of the planned assessments. To illustrate this concept, consider a longitudinal study conducted by the International Breast Cancer Study Group (IBCSG)[2] of 1475 premenopausal breast cancer patients. Figure 13.2 presents the available scores from the perceived adaptation to chronic illness scales (PACIS)[3] for patients who did not experience disease progression during the first 18 months of follow-up. The relationship of missing assessments to the QoL measured during the non-missing assessments is demonstrated by the higher scores reported by the 344 patients who completed all seven assessments, with the scores dropping for the 403 patients who missed one or two assessments, and the lowest scores for the 224 patients who completed only one to four assessments. Thus, even after excluding patients with missing assessments due to disease progression, the probability that an observation is missing does depend on the QoL that the patient is experiencing. Thus, an analysis of the complete cases (the 344 patients with all seven assessments) would be biased and not representative of the entire group of patients.

Analysis of all available data (MAR)

The assumption that data are MCAR, required in the analysis of complete cases, can be relaxed to the assumption that data are missing at random (MAR)[29] or ignorable.[35] In this situation, the probability that an observation is missing may depend on observed data and covariates, but still must be independent of the value of the missing observation(s) after adjustment for the observed data and covariates. Likelihood based methods,[9,10] which use all the available data, result in unbiased estimates when the data are MAR. These methods are also accessible in many of the major statistical software packages.[36,37]

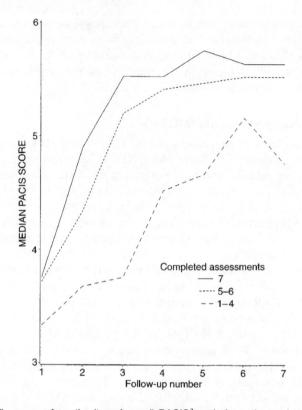

Fig. 13.2 Median scores from the (transformed) PACIS[3] scale for patients who completed 1–4 (N=224), 5–6 (N=403), or all seven (N=344) of the scheduled assessments. Patients who experienced disease progression are excluded. Higher scores indicate better QoL.

One approach to understanding the assumption of MAR is to consider a study where the assumption is incorrect. In this observational study,[12] 68 patients with metastatic or progressive disease completed an assessment of QoL every 3–6 weeks. When the data are analysed using a model that assumes the data are MAR, there is only a small insignificant decrease in the estimates of QoL over time (Fig. 13.3(a)). However, when stratified by the duration of follow-up (or survival), patients who died earlier experienced a rapid rate of decline in QoL over time (Fig. 13.3(b)). The counterintuitive results displayed in Fig. 13.3(a) are the consequence of the MAR assumption. In this setting, the estimates obtained from the MAR models describe the average QoL of the surviving patients rather than the entire population.

Methods for non-ignorable missing data (NMAR)

Non-ignorable missing data are probably the most likely type of missing data in QoL studies in clinical trials where there is drop-out due to toxicity, disease

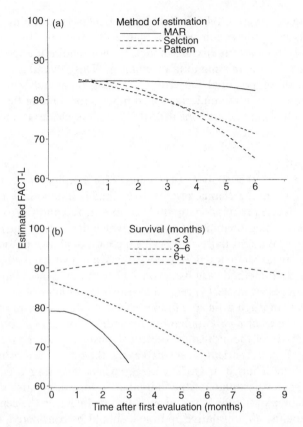

Fig. 13.3 Functional Assessment of Cancer Therapy-General (FACT-G) assessments in terminal cancer patients. (a) Estimated FACT-G scores from three different methods of analyses. 'MAR': mixed-effects model assuming data are missing at random; 'Selection': selection model for non-ignorable dropout; and 'Pattern': pattern mixture model for non-ignorable dropout. (b) Estimated FACT-G scores by length of survival (mixed-effects model).

progression, or even therapeutic effectiveness. Studies with this type of missing data are also the most difficult to analyse. The primary reason is that there are numerous potential models and it is impossible to verify statistically the 'correctness' of any model because the data required to distinguish between models are missing. A secondary reason is that software for these methods of analysis is not available in statistical analysis packages.

Little[23] describes two general classes of models, selection and pattern mixture. The choice between the two classes depends partially on whether the missing data mechanism is viewed to be solely a 'nuisance' or not. In the class of selection models, a statistical model is specified for the missing data mechanism. In addition to adjusting the estimates for the missing data, these models allow the investigator to make inferences about the relationship of QoL and other explanatory factors causing missing observations. This might be particularly interesting, for example, if death or disease progression was the cause of drop-out. In contrast to the selection models, the pattern mixture models do not require the specification of a particular model for the missing data mechanism. This advantage is balanced by the large number of potential patterns of missing data and the difficulties of estimating parameters in the underidentified models for some of the missing data patterns. The following two sections describe these two classes of models in more detail.

Selection models

Selection models for the analysis of studies with non-ignorable missing data include models where the change in QoL over time is functionally related to the time of death, disease progression, or study drop-out. Wu and Carroll[24] proposed a probit model for the probability of drop-out which depends on the linear change in QoL over time. Wu and Bailey[25] describe a conditional linear model where the rate of change in an individual is modelled as a polynomial function of the drop-out time. Both methods are based on a growth curve model approach with the individual slope parameter(s) related to censoring of later observations (right censoring) either through a linear random effects model with a probit model for the censoring process or a conditional linear model. Mori et al.[26] propose empirical Bayes estimates of the individual subject slopes which adjust for informative right censoring. When a patient is censored early, the time of censoring dominates the estimate of the change in QoL, whereas when censoring occurs later, the ordinary least squares estimate of the individual's slope dominates the estimate.

When the change over time is not expected to be linear or the censoring times vary across patients, an alternative approach should be considered. Schluchter[27] and DeGruttola and Tu[38] have proposed extensions of the random effects or two-stage mixed effects model. The time of censoring (or death) is incorporated into the second-stage model of the population parameters by allowing the time of censoring to be correlated with the random effects of the longitudinal model for QoL. The conditional expectation of the random effects is a function of the censoring time.

Returning to the previous example of the study of 68 terminal cancer patients, the results displayed in Fig. 13.3(b) suggest that it might be reasonable to assume that the rate of decline in the Functional Assessment of Cancer Therapy-General (FACT-G) over time, β_{1i} (and possibly the baseline values β_{0i}) are correlated with the time of death in these patients. Using the models proposed by Schluchter[27] and DeGruttola and Tu,[38] the estimated correlation of the random intercept and slope terms with the log of the survival times was 0.38 and 0.89 respectively. Thus, patients who died earlier had both lower initial values of the FACT-G and a more rapid rate of decline in their FACT-G scores. Further, there was a significant and clinically relevant decline in the estimated mean FACT-G score for the entire study population over a six month period (labeled 'Selection' in Fig. 13.3(a)).

In addition to these monotone patterns of missing data due to drop-out or censoring, non-monotone patterns may exist. Robins et al.[39] describe a weighted generalized estimating equations (GEE) approach for non-monotone patterns that are missing at random. Troxel and Harrington[40] describe a likelihood method with Markovian correlation structure in which the 'missingness' follows a logistic model.

Pattern mixture models

The basic concept behind the pattern mixture models described by Little[23] is that the distribution of the measures of QoL, Y_i, may differ across the k different missing data patterns, having different means, μ^k and variance, Σ^k. For example, patients who die earlier (with missing data due to death) may have lower QoL scores (different means) and also may have more or less variability in their scores (different variance) than patients who survive longer. The true distribution of the measures of QoL for the entire group of patients will be a mixture of the distributions of each of the k groups of patients. The general method of analysis is to stratify the patients by the missing data patterns. Then the mean and variance parameters $\hat{\mu}^k$, $\hat{\Sigma}^k$ are estimated within each strata. Weights are determined by the number of subjects within each of the k missing data patterns ($w_k = n_k/N$). The population estimates are the weighted average of the estimates from the K missing data patterns, ($\hat{\mu} = \Sigma w_k \hat{\mu}^k$). The advantage of these models is that one doesn't have to define a model for the missing data mechanism. One of the difficulties of this approach is the large number of missing data patterns that occur in actual studies where there may only be a few subjects with some patterns. But more critically, for all but the one pattern where there are no missing observations, the model may be underidentified. Specifically, there may not be enough data in certain patterns to estimate all the parameters of the model without making additional assumptions. The most obvious example of an underidentified model occurs for the pattern where all the observations are missing. The assumptions that allow for estimation of the model parameters are often difficult to communicate and can not be validated because they depend on the values of the missing data.

An application of a pattern mixture model for random-effects-dependent drop-out[23] is illustrated using the previously described study of terminal cancer patients. In this study, each patient had a unique pattern of observations and the number of patterns is almost equal to the number of patients. So, to simplify the problem, the patients are stratified into three groups based on their duration of survival or follow-up: less than three months ($n_1 = 24$), 3–6 months ($n_2 = 19$), and greater than six months ($n_3 = 25$). A mixed-effects model was used to estimate the parameters in each of the three strata (Fig. 13.3(b)). The assumption in this application is that the quadratic model used to estimate the changes in the FACT-G over the first three months for the first group can be extrapolated to estimate the unobserved QoL during the second three months. Using this method, the estimated decline in QoL over a six-month period, labeled 'Pattern' in Fig. 13.3(a), is similar to that estimated using the selection model described above with overlapping confidence intervals (not shown).

In practice, current application of methods (selection models and pattern mixture models) for non-ignorable missing data is limited by several factors. The first is the large number of subjects that will be required to distinguish between alternative models. The second is the restriction of some assumptions such as linear changes over time and the inability of any one technique to deal with both the monotone and non-monotone patterns. In addition, the sophisticated programming required for these methods and the lack of generally available software are barriers to implementation. However, the most significant barrier may be how to present these complicated models in a manner that is readily interpretable in the clinical literature.

Imputation: model fitting by estimating missing data

An alternative method of analysis uses the strategy of imputation to estimate the missing data.[41-44] (See Chapter 14.) The motivations for this approach are that complete data methods such as MANOVA can be used to analyse the imputed data sets and information about the reasons for missing data can be incorporated into the imputation scheme. These methods include both single and multiple imputation using both model-based and sampling methods for imputation. Detailed discussion of several methods of imputation is presented in Chapter 14.

The choice of the method for imputation should consider the missing data mechanism. For example, methods such as normal regression models or hot-deck imputation assume that the data are MAR. A popular approach is to use the last observation (or value) carried forward (LOCF or LVCF), where the patient's last available assessment is substituted for each of the missing assessments. This approach has limited utility[45] and should be employed with great caution. For example, in a study where QoL is decreasing over time, a treatment with early drop-out could possibly look better than a treatment where tolerance to the therapy was better.

Lavori et al.[44] propose a strategy for multiple imputation based on a 'propensity score' for the probability of drop-out. The idea is to find a univariate score that summarizes the multiple variables defining the history of each patient, stratify patients using the quintiles of the score, and then use an approximate Bayesian bootstrap[42] to impute the missing values within each of the strata. A multistep process is used to compute the score for each of the planned observation times. One of the advantages of this approach is that a single set of propensity scores is computed, which can be used for multiple QoL outcomes. This approach assumes that, conditional on the propensity score, the data are MAR. As the number of assessments increases with multiple causes for missing data, these strategies can quickly become very complex. Rubin and Schenker[42] suggest that sensible rather than 'pristine' methods are generally adequate and balance the effort expended with the extent of the missing data problem.

Single and multiple imputation

Single imputation methods include 'mean imputation' and 'regression imputation'. In 'mean imputation', the average value of the measure of QoL is substituted for the missing observations. In 'regression imputation', the predicted value of the measure of QoL estimated using a regression model is substituted for the missing assessments. The criticism of the single imputation methods is that most methods of analysis treat imputed values just like observed values in the analysis and underestimate the uncertainty by ignoring the measurement error, among-subject variability, and the incomplete knowledge of the reason for non-response.

Multiple imputation[41,42] retains many of the advantages of single imputation, but rectifies this problem. The basic strategy of multiple imputation is to impute three[42] to 10[44] sets of values for the missing data which incorporate both sampling variability and the uncertainty about the reasons for non-response. Methods of sampling can include explicit models such as a fully normal regression model, or implicit models such as approximate Bayesian bootstrap.[42] Each set of data is then analysed using complete data methods and the analyses are combined in a way that reflects the extra variability due to missing data.[42,43]

Non-parametric analysis using ranked data

Gould[46] describes a practical method for the analysis of clinical trials with withdrawal. If there is adequate documentation concerning the reasons for missing assessments, it may be possible to determine a reasonable ordering (or ranking) of QoL among the subjects. For example, it would be reasonable to assign patients who withdraw because of disease progression, excessive toxicity, or death a rank that is lower than that observed for patients remaining on the study. The advantage of this approach is that we do not have to impute the specific value. Heyting[45] identifies some limitations, including multiple reasons for drop-out, that are not clearly ordered. Methods for non-parametric analysis of repeated measures are proposed by Wei and Johnson.[47]

Sensitivity analyses

Given the numerous potential methods of analysis, how do we choose between different strategies? In some cases, we will have information such as the reason for missing assessments or a clearly defined objective that will determine the 'best' approach. But in general, while certain approaches may be eliminated from consideration, we will be left with several possibilities. A sensitivity analysis in which the effect of the different methods of analysis is examined may be informative. There are two likely outcomes of the sensitivity analysis. The first is that the conclusions are consistent regardless of the approach. An example of this is a sensitivity analysis of four methods of handling missing data in a clinical trial of two adjuvant therapies for breast cancer.[1] The patients were randomized to either standard cyclophosphamide, doxorubicin and 5-flurouricil (CAF) or a experimental 14 week multidrug regimen. In both arms, 9 per cent of the patients were missing the assessment that occurred during therapy. The end-point was the change in QoL (during-before therapy) as measured by the Breast Chemotherapy Questionnaire BCQ.[18] In a non-parametric, two-sample comparison (Wilcoxon rank sum test), the four strategies considered included:

(1) analysis of available data,

(2) assigning the lowest rank when missing data occurred in patients discontinuing treatment because of toxicity or relapse,

(3) simple imputation of the missing data using regression, and

(4) assigning the lowest rank when missing data occurred regardless of the reason.

The median, interquartile ranges, and p values associated with the treatment comparisons are displayed in Fig. 13.4.[48] Regardless of the approach taken, medians and interquartile ranges were similar and the treatment differences were statistically significant.

The alternative outcome of a sensitivity analysis is that the conclusions are dependent on the method of analysis or the summary measure selected. When this occurs, the methods should be examined to ascertain the reason for the discrepancy. For example, in an Eastern Cooperative Oncology Group trial of three regimens of chemotherapy for patients with advanced non-small lung cancer

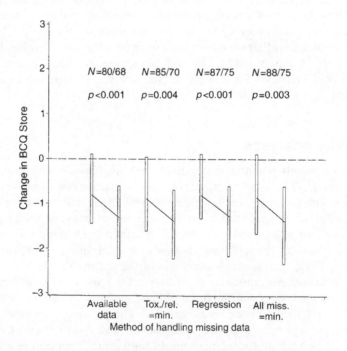

Fig. 13.4 Comparison of four methods of analysis (see text for detailed description). Scores represent the difference between BCQ scores measured prior to and during therapy. The first bar of each pair represents change in scores for patients on the standard CAF therapy and the second bar represents patients on the experimental multidrug therapy. The vertical bars show the interquartile ranges (25–75 percentiles) of the distribution of scores and the horizontal lines connect the median scores for the two treatment groups. p values correspond to the Wilcoxon rank sum test for the treatment comparisons.

Table 13.1   Sensitivity analysis of Non-small cell lung cancer (NSCLC) trial

Treatment arm[2]		VP16		Taxol		Taxol+G-CSF		p-value[1]
Assumptions/Analysis		Estimate	SE	Estimate	SE	Estimate	SE	
		Summary Statistic: Change over 6 months						
1: MCAR	Complete case	−1.8	2.7	−5.2	2.1	−5.0	2.2	NS
2: MAR	Available data	−8.0	2.3	−6.7	2.1	−6.0	2.0	NS
3: NMAR	Selection model[3]	−14.5	1.6	−11.7	1.4	−12.3	1.4	NS
		Summary Statistic: Area under the curve						
MCAR	Complete case	53.8	1.1	56.8	0.9	53.2	0.8	0.01
MAR	Available data	50.3	0.7	52.8	0.7	51.1	0.7	0.03
NMAR	Selection model[3]	49.1	0.5	51.3	0.5	49.4	0.5	<0.01

[1] H_0: Likelihood ratio test of equality of three treatment groups.
[2] Patients received either cisplatin and etoposide (VP-16), cisplatin and paclitaxel (Taxol),
or cisplatin, paclitaxel and filgrastim (Taxol+G-CSF)
[3] Joint model of FACT-L and log time until death.

(NSCLC), two summary statistics were considered. The first was the change in QoL (measured by the Functional Assessment of Cancer Therapy-Lung (FACT-L))[50] over a six month period and the second was the AUC under the QoL vs. time curve for the same period. In the sensitivity analysis, three different analysis models were considered,[49] including an analysis of complete cases (MCAR), all available data (MAR), and a selection model (NMAR).[27] The results, summarized in Table 1, demonstrate both the sensitivity of the estimates to the method of analysis and the choice of the summary measure. Specifically, analyses that assume the missing data are ignorable (either MCAR or MAR) underestimate the six month change in QoL and overestimate the AUC in all three treatment arms relative to the analyses that assume the missing data are not random (NMAR). This result was expected in this trial of patients with advanced disease and is consistent with other information obtained from this trial concerning the reasons that QoL assessments were missing. The most striking result was that tests of treatment differences were sensitive to the summary measure selected. Specifically, the tests were non-significant for the change over time, but generally significant for the AUC (Table 13.1). Further examination indicated that baseline and follow-up scores were consistently higher in one of the treatment groups (Taxol only). As a result, the average AUC for that treatment group was higher despite similar rates of change for all three groups. In this trial, the explanation for the discrepant results was clear, and the results were reported using the selection model for the analysis of the change in QoL over 6 months.

Summary and implications for design and conduct

With the incorporation of QoL into an increasing number of clinical trials, there is an urgent need to develop practical methods for the analysis of these longitudinal studies.[48] Methods of analysis for trials where the data can safely be assumed to be MAR are well established with easily accessible software. However, in most trials some of the missing data associated with QoL assessment is likely to be non-ignorable. The question then becomes, when is it critical to use more sophisticated methods? For example, will it make a difference in the treatment comparisons if only 5 per cent of the subjects have missing data? What about 10 per cent or 20 per cent? Can we say that if the proportion of missing data is the same in two treatment arms, treatment comparisons will be valid even if the estimates are biased? Clearly, there are many questions that need to be addressed in the context of actual clinical trials. The challenge will be to adapt theoretical methods to settings where there are multiple reasons for missing data.

The issues of missing data and multiple comparisons have strong implications for the design and conduct of these studies.[8,48] The first step is to specify a well defined objective. Vague aims such as 'to compare the quality of life patients on the two treatment arms' do not help the investigators to specify a limited number of end-points or to develop a strategy to minimize multiple comparisons. Clearly, strategies to minimize missing data will also be important (see Chapter 14). For example, linking the timing of the QoL assessments with another assessment may reduce the number of assessments that are omitted. Careful consideration of whether to continue QoL assessment when a patient discontinues treatment early will affect what hypotheses can be tested and the ability to generalize the results. Careful prospective documentation of the reasons for missing assessments will give the analyst a basis for choosing a particular analysis strategy.

Acknowledgements

This work was supported by grants CA23318 awarded by the National Cancer Institute, DHHS, and PBR-53 from the American Cancer Society and a faculty research grant to the Department of Biostatistics, Harvard School of Public Health, by the Schering-Plough Corporation. We thank the following for allowing us to use the data appearing in the figures: Fig. 13.2, International Breast Cancer Study Group; Fig. 13.3, Victor Chang, MD and Shirley Wang, RN; and Fig. 13.4, the Eastern Cooperative Oncology Group.

References

1. Fairclough, D.L., Fetting, J., Cella, D., *et al*. Quality of life on a breast cancer adjuvant trial comparing CAR with a 16-week regimen. *Proc. Am. Soc. Clinical Oncology*, 1995; **114**: Abstract 890.
2. Hurny, C., Bernhard, J., Coates, A.S., *et al*. for the IBCSG. Counting the cost of adjuvant therapy: impact of treatment on quality of life in node-positive patients with operable breast cancer. *Lancet*, 1996; **347**: 1279–84.
3. Hurny, C., Bernhard, J., Gelber, R.D., *et al*. Quality of life measures for patients receiving adjuvant therapy for breast cancer: an international trial. *Eur. J. Cancer*, 1992; **28**: 118–24.
4. Korn, E.L. and O'Fallon, J. Statistical considerations, statistics working group. *Quality of life assessment in cancer clinical trials*, Report on Workshop on Quality of Life

Research in Cancer Clinical Trials, Division of Cancer Prevention and Control. National Cancer Institute, 1990.

5. DeKlerk, N.H. Repeated warnings re repeated measures. *Aust. NZ J. Med.*, 1986; **16**: 637–8.
6. Pocock, S.J., Hughes, M.D., and Lee, R.J. Statistical problems in the reporting of clinical trials: a survey of three medical journals. *New Engl. J. Med.*, 1987; **317**: 426–532.
7. Matthews, J.N.S., Altman, D.G., Campbell, M.J., and Royston, P. Analysis of serial measurements in medical research. *British Medical Journal*, 1990; **300**: 230–5.
8. Gotay, C.C., Korn, E.L., McCabe, M.S., Moore, T.D., and Cheson, B.D. Building quality of life assessment into cancer treatment studies. *Oncology*, 1992; **6**: 25–8.
9. Dempster, A.P., Laird, N.M., and Rubin, D.B. Maximum likelihood from incomplete data via the EM algorithm (with discussion). *J. Roy. Statist. Soc. B*, 1972; **39**: 1–38.
10. Jennrich, R. and Schluchter, M. Unbalanced repeated-measures models with structured covariance matrices. *Biometrics*, 1986; **42**: 805–20.
11. Fairclough, D.L. Summary measures and statistics for comparisons of quality of life in a clinical trial of cancer therapy. *Stat. Med.* 1997; **16**: 1197–1209.
12. Hwang, S.S., Chang, V.T., Fairclough, D.F., Koch, K., Latorre, M., and Corpion, C. Longitudinal measurement for quality of life and symptoms in terminal cancer patients. *Proceedings of the American Society for Clinical Oncology*, Abstract 1737, 1996.
13. Zwinderman, A.H. The measurement of change of quality of life in clinical trials. *Statistics in Medicine*, 1990; **9**: 931–42.
14. Busch, P., Schwenderner, P., Leu, R.E., *et al.* Life quality assessment of breast cancer patients receiving adjuvant therapy using incomplete data. *Health Economics*, 1994; **3**: 213–20.
15. Cox, D.R., Fitzpatrick, R., Fletcher, A.I., Gore, S.M., Spiegelhalter, D.J., and Jones, D.R. Quality-of-life assessment: can we keep it simple? (with discussion). *J. Roy. Statist. Soc. A*, 1992; **155**: 353–93.
16. Tandon, P.K. Application of global statistics in analyzing quality of life data. *Stat. Med.*, 1990; **9**: 819–27.
17. Frison, L. and Pocock, S.J. Repeated measures in clinical trials: analysis using mean summary statistics and its implications for design. *Stat. Med.*, 1992; **11**: 1685–1704.
18. Levine, M., Guyatt, G., Gent, M., *et al.* Quality of life in stage II breast cancer: an instrument for clinical trials. *J. Clin. Oncol.*, 1988; **6**: 1798–1810.
19. O'Brien, P.C. Procedures for comparing samples with multiple endpoints. *Biometrics*, 1984; **40**: 1079–87.
20. Korn, E.L. On estimating the distribution function for quality of life in cancer clinical trials. *Biometrika*, 1990; **30**: 535–42.
21. Gelber, R.D., Gelman, R.S., and Goldhirsh, A. A quality of life oriented endpoint for comparing therapies. *Biometrics*, 1989; **45**: 781–95.
22. Glasziou, P.P., Simes, R.J., and Gelber, R.D. Quality adjusted survival analysis. *Stat. Med.*, 1990; **9**: 1259–76.
23. Little, R.J.A. Modeling the drop-out mechanism in repeated-measures studies. *J. Am. Stat. Assoc.*, 1995; **90**: 1112–21.
24. Wu, M.C. and Carroll, R.J. Estimation and comparison of changes in the presence of informative right censoring my modeling the censoring process. *Biometrics*, 1988; **44**: 175–88.

25. Wu, M.C. and Bailey, K.R. Estimation and comparison of changes in the presence of informative right censoring: conditional linear model. *Biometrics*, 1989; **45**: 939–55.

26. Mori, M., Woodworth, G.G., and Woolson, R.F. Application of empirical Bayes inference to estimation of rate of change in the presence of informative right censoring. *Stat. Med.*, 1992; **11**: 621–31.

27. Schluchter, M.D. Methods for the analysis of informatively censored longitudinal data. *Stat. Med.*, 1992; **11**: 1861–70.

28. Pocock, S.J., Geller, N.L., and Tsiatis, A.A. The analysis of multiple endpoints in clinical trials. *Biometrics*, 1987; **43**: 487–98.

29. Little, R.J. and Rubin, D.B. *Statistical analysis with missing data*. New York: John Wiley, 1987.

30. Little, R.J.A. A test of missing completely at random for multivariate data with missing values. *J. Am. Stat. Assoc.*, 1988; **83**: 1198–1202.

31. Diggle, P.J. Testing for random dropouts in repeated measurement data. *Biometrics*, 1989; **45**: 1255–8.

32. Engelman, L. BMDP 8D: correlations with missing data. In *BMDP statistical software*, Dixon, W.J. (ed.). Berkeley: University of California Press, 1990.

33. Ridout, M.S. Testing for random dropouts in repeated measurement data. *Biometrics*, 1991; **47**: 1617–21.

34. Park, T. and Davis, C.S. A test of the missing data mechanism for repeated categorical data. *Biometrics*, 1993; **49**: 631–8.

35. Laird, N.M. Missing data in longitudinal studies. *Stat. Med.*, 1988; **7**: 305–15.

36. Schluchter, M.D. BMDP 5V: unbalanced repeated measures models with structured covariance matrices. In *BMDP statistical software*, Dixon, W.J. (ed.). Berkeley: University of California Press, 1990.

37. The MIXED procedure. Chapter 16 in SAS technical report P-229, SAS/STAT software: changes and enhancements. SAS Institute Inc. Cary, NC, 1992; pp. 289–366.

38. DeGruttola, V. and Tu, X.M. Modeling progression of CD4-lymphocyte count and its relationship to survival time. *Biometrics*, 1994; **50**: 1003–14.

39. Robins, J.M., Rotnizky, A., and Zhao, L.P. Analysis of semiparametric regression models for repeated outcomes in the presence of missing data. *J. Am. Stat. Assoc.*, 1995; **90**: 106–20.

40. Troxel, A.B. and Harrington, D.P. Longitudinal responses with nonignorable non-monotone missing data. International Biometric Society ENAR Spring Meetings 1995. Program and Abstracts, p. 89.

41. Rubin, D.B. *Multiple imputation for nonresponse in surveys*. Wiley, New York, 1987.

42. Rubin, D.B. and Schenker, N. Multiple imputation in health-care data bases: an overview and some applications. *Stat. Med.*, 1991; **10**: 585–98.

43. Crawford, S.L., Tennstedt, S.L., and McKinlay, J.B. A comparison of analytic methods for non-random missingness of outcome data. *J. Clin. Epidemiol.*, 1995; **48**: 209–19.

44. Lavori, P.W., Dawson, R., and Shera, D. A Multiple imputation strategy for clinical trials with truncation of patient data. *Stat. Med.*, 1995; **14**: 1913–25.

45. Heyting, A., Tolboom, J.T.B.M., and Essers, J.G.A. Statistical handling of drop-outs in longitudinal clinical trials. *Stat. Med.*, 1992; **11**: 2043–61.

46. Gould, A.L. A new approach to the analysis of clinical drug trials with withdrawals. *Biometrics*, 1980; **36**: 721–7.

47. Wei, L.J. and Johnson, W.E. Combining dependent tests with incomplete repeated measurements. *Biometrika*, 1985; **72**: 359–64.

48. Fairclough, D.L. Quality of life in cancer clinical trials: now that we have the data, what do we do? *J. Appl. Stat. Sci.* 1996; **4**: 253–269.

49. Fairclough, D.L., Peterson, H., Cella, D., and Bonomi, P. Comparison of model based methods dependent on the missing data mechanism in two clinical trials of cancer therapy. *Stat. Med.* (In press.)

50. Cella, DF., Bonomi, A.E., Llyod, S.R., *et al*. Reliability and validity of the functional assessment of cancer therapy-lung (FACT-L) quality of life instrument. *Lung Cancer*, 1995; **12**: 199–220.

14 Analysis of incomplete quality of life data in clinical trials

Desmond Curran, Peter M. Fayers, Geert Molenberghs, and David Machin

Introduction

Assessment of quality of life (QoL) is rapidly becoming an integral part of randomized clinical trials, especially in diseases involving unpleasant symptoms or side-effects of treatment. However, difficulties with data collection and compliance appear to be the most important barriers to the successful implementation of QoL assessments in clinical research settings. Poor compliance also poses problems with QoL analyses, due to the bias that may be introduced, either by patients dropping out of the trial completely or by not participating comprehensively in the QoL assessment.[1] Olschewski et al.[1] provided the following extreme hypothetical situation: an ineffective treatment not preventing disease, and leading to a deterioration of patients' well-being, which the patients are no longer capable of documenting on a QoL form. Owing to their non-compliance these patients would no longer contribute to the analysis of QoL. This is compared with a treatment that is effective but induces side-effects that reduce the well-being, but not so severely that the patient refuses QoL assessment. An analysis based on the available QoL forms may falsely lead to declaring the worst treatment superior. In addition, if deteriorating health or advancing disease prevents patients from participating in the QoL assessment, consideration of only patients who complete the questionnaire might lead to too optimistic a view of the treatment under study with respect to the QoL of patients.

A search of the QoL literature reveals very few methodological papers handling the problem of missing data. Also, very few published clinical trial results indicate clearly the extent of missing forms or how they are handled. Hopwood et al.[2] discussed this issue and illustrated methods for presenting the proportion of missing forms. Zwinderman[3] proposed a number of solutions to the problem of missing forms and provided some computer programming code in BMDP® and SAS® for modelling the data using repeated measures analysis of variance, assuming that missing data are missing at random. Zee and Pater[4] suggest that one method of analysing incomplete quality of life data is to use a growth curve model, in conjunction with the EM (expectation–maximization) algorithm.[5]

A vast amount of work on missing data has been carried out in other research fields such as agriculture,[6] clinical trials,[7,8] and survey sampling.[9-11]

QoL data are usually collected using a self-assessment questionnaire, such as the EORTC QLQ C-30.[12] QoL data tend to be multidimensional since a questionnaire usually consists of a series of questions which are subsequently collapsed into a number of scales or domains, such as physical, role, emotional, cognitive. In addition, QoL data tend to be longitudinal with the questionnaire administered at regular intervals during treatment and subsequent follow-up of patients in the trial. QoL data differ from clinical data for various reasons. In particular, clinical data may often be collected retrospectively, for example from the patient's medical charts. However, once a patient has missed a QoL assessment the retrospective collection of the data is hampered by the recall abilities of the patient.

In QoL research there are two main types of missing data,

(1) *item non-response* for missing data in a questionnaire where a response has not been provided for at least one question;

(2) *unit non-response* when the whole questionnaire is missing for a patient. We distinguish several types:

   (a) intermittent missing forms,

   (b) drop-out from the study,

   (c) late entry into the study.

To explain the different types of unit non-response we provide an example as follows. Consider a study where QoL is assessed every month. Suppose a patient completed assessments at months 0, 2, 3, 5, and 6. There are intermittent missing questionnaires at months 1 and 4. At month 7 the patient dropped out of the study and therefore no additional assessments were received. Suppose a second patient was registered into the trial in September 1996 and the analysis was performed in the beginning of December 1996. The patient completed questionnaires at months 0, 1, and 2. However, one would not expect additional questionnaires for this patient as he was only recently registered in the study, that is, late entry into the study.

In cancer clinical trials, especially in advanced disease, it is evident that not all patients will complete the same number of assessments due to attrition caused by death and other medical reasons. In addition, QoL assessments are frequently limited to the period during which a patient remains on protocol treatment. Thus, patients who remain on protocol treatment for a longer period may complete more QoL questionnaires. Figure 14.1 presents a Kaplan–Meier plot of time on protocol treatment and a table of QoL assessment compliance. In this phase III trial of breast cancer, patients with newly diagnosed bone metastases were requested to complete a QoL questionnaire at baseline (pre-treatment), each month for the first seven months, and every three months thereafter until progression, at which time patients stopped receiving protocol treatment. The median time on treatment was 6.4 months. As may be seen in the figure, the attrition of patients is

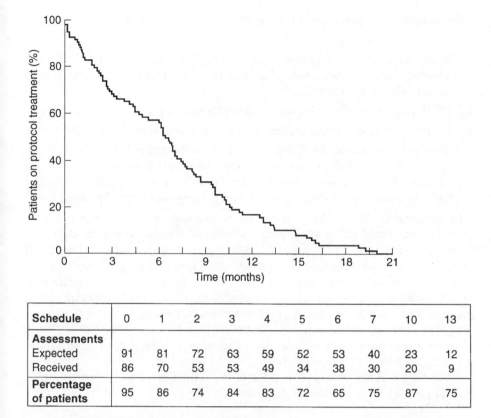

Fig. 14.1   Kaplon–Meier estimates of time on protocol treatment and a table of compliance for breast cancer patients with newly diagnosed bone metastases.

Schedule	0	1	2	3	4	5	6	7	10	13
Assessments Expected	91	81	72	63	59	52	53	40	23	12
Received	86	70	53	53	49	34	38	30	20	9
Percentage of patients	95	86	74	84	83	72	65	75	87	75

substantial, for example less than 20 per cent of patients were still on protocol treatment at 12 months.

Why do missing data matter?

The main cause for concern is that missing data may result in bias, and that the results of a trial will therefore be uninterpretable. Essentially, a key question is 'Are the characteristics of patients with missing data different from those for whom complete data are available?' For example, it might be that more ill patients, or patients with more problems, are less willing or less able to complete the questionnaires satisfactorily. Alternatively, perhaps patients with no problems are less convinced about the need to return comprehensive information. Thus, any analyses which ignore the presence of missing data may result in biased conclusions about the changing patterns, or between-treatment differences, in the QoL of patients, and will be open to criticism.

Considerations of potential bias raise the following questions.

1. Is the missing data random or non-random?

2. What is the impact of ignoring the missing data? If, in a clinical trial, the patterns of missing data are similar in all treatment groups, will the treatment comparisons remain unbiased?

3. What proportion of missing data is acceptable in a trial?

4. How can one best estimate or allow for the missing data when analysing the trial?

5. Some methods of analysis, and some computer software implementations, allow incomplete data in the sense that patients with partial information are also included. However, this is usually tantamount to assuming that the missing data are missing at random. How do these assumptions affect the conclusions?

In addition to the problems of treatment (between group) comparisons, it should also be noted that another potential effect of bias due to missing data may be underestimation of the impact of treatment and disease on QoL. This could arise if patients with the worst QoL fail to return information. One might expect that the patients who are generally in a poor condition drop out of the trial early. Of course this is speculation and the converse might equally apply, especially when patients have received potentially curative treatment. Perhaps the most ill patients are more aware of the need to complete the questionnaires. This speculation is removed if the reasons why patients do not participate in the QoL assessment are routinely documented.

Proceeding with the example provided in Fig. 14.1, Fig. 14.2 presents the physical functioning score by time of drop-out. This figure is useful for investigating

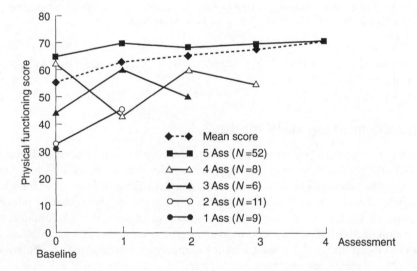

Fig. 14.2 Physical functioning score by time of drop-out for breast cancer patients with newly diagnosed bone metastases.

whether or not the drop-out of patients was completely random or not. Note that scale scores were calculated by averaging items within scales (Fig. 14.4 presents the single items, later) and transforming average scores linearly to a 0 to 100 scale, with higher scores representing a higher level of functioning (for more detail see 'Methods of handling missing items', which gives the formula for constructing scales).

As may be seen from Fig. 14.2 patients with a low physical functioning score tended to drop out earlier than patients with a high physical functioning score. We can therefore conclude that the drop-out is not completely at random. Therefore, there is a selection bias in the inclusion of patients into the QoL analysis at later time points. Care should therefore be taken in the interpretation of any graphs which include mean scores as they may be misleading. For example, if we study the overall mean physical functioning scores at the first five assessment points, one might conclude incorrectly that the physical functioning score improves substantially with time, i.e. from 55.4 at baseline to 70.8 at the last assessment. As mentioned earlier, this deception occurs because of the patients with lower physical functioning scores dropping out earlier.

One of the simpler and more obvious forms of non-compliance is for some patients to refuse to continue completing QoL questionnaires. Clearly the reduced number of patients available for analysis means that the effective sample size is reduced, and thus there will be a loss of statistical power. If this were the only effect of non-compliance, a naïve solution would be to recruit additional patients to the trial, to compensate for the losses. However, the bias caused by missing data is not removed simply by increasing the sample size, as discussed later in the chapter. In practice, however, missing data may also occur both as intermittent missing forms during the follow-up period, and as missing items within a form. Thus it can often arise that many patients will have at least one missing form or at least a few missing items during the course of the trial. Much statistical analysis software assumes that complete, balanced data matrices are available, that is, all patients return the same number of QoL assessments at fixed, scheduled time points. Hence it may be necessary to exclude a whole form or even a whole patient from an analysis. If for example, we wish to perform a repeated measures analysis of the data presented in Fig. 14.2 over the first five assessments, using some standard software only the 52 patients for whom all five assessments are available may be included in the analysis.

Even when there is only a small proportion of missing values for each item, the result may be a substantial proportion of patients having at least one or more missing items during their follow-up period. Analyses which are based solely upon those patients for whom complete data are available may find that the cumulative exclusion of patients results in far too few patients remaining in the final analyses and hence a severe loss of power. In addition, there is a process of selection of patients into the analysis (i.e. patients with complete data), and subsequently the subset of patients who have complete data may not be representative of all the patients in the trial.

Improving compliance

Administration of QoL

For QoL to be incorporated successfully into clinical trial methodology, very practical steps have to be taken to ensure good standards of data collection. Fortunately, as cancer research activity has increased, oncology nurses in various settings are more involved in the conduct of clinical trials. As pivotal members of the research team, nurses and data managers need a clear view of their specific tasks to improve efficiency and quality data. Research nurses play a major role in the education of patients and therefore may be influential in generating interest in the QoL part of the study. Due to excessive workload many clinicians are unable to give the necessary attention to data collection in a QoL study. Suitably trained personnel should be employed to lift some of the burden from the clinician and ensure better compliance of QoL data, for example, to ensure standardization and continuity of working procedures.

Hurny et al.[13] reported that in their trial larger institutions had higher rates of compliance. Smaller institutions may be at a disadvantage as they usually do not have the resources to dedicate a full-time staff member to data management and quality assurance. However, he added that with an organized effort at the local institutional level, high quality data collection can be achieved. Hurny et al.[13] suggested that to achieve good quality QoL data, there is a need for systematic training and commitment of staff at all institutions. Studies should be designed and carried out to investigate what problems with data collection are encountered in institutions, and to find solutions to these problems. Perhaps, in order to enhance the use of existing instruments (QoL questionnaires), more effort needs to be spent on making the administration simpler.

Recommendations for conducting QoL assessment

1. During the design stage of a study sufficient financial resources should be available to provide an adequate infrastructure to manage the study (e.g. appropriate personnel and materials) and to integrate the QoL assessment into the normal daily practises of a clinic.

2. Objectives of the study should be presented clearly in the protocol, such as the rationale for including QoL, the main QoL end-point.

3. It is preferred that QoL is not an optional evaluation.

4. Based on the objectives of the study an appropriate valid instrument should be selected and, if necessary, additional treatment-specific questions should be developed, tested and added if appropriate. However, for feasibility reasons the number of items should be kept to a minimum.

5. The QoL questionnaire should be available in the appropriate languages in relation to potential participants in the clinical trial. If additional translations are required, they should be developed using tried and tested translation procedures.

6. The schedule of assessments should not be too much of a burden for the patient, while at the same time it should be frequent enough and at appropriate time points to provide a relevant picture of the patients' QoL over the study period. For practical reasons, the schedule of QoL assessments should coincide with the routine clinical follow-up visits for the trial.

7. Statistical considerations in the protocol (e.g. effect size, sample size, and analysis plan) should be clear and precise.

8. Protocols should include guidelines on data collection procedures for research nurses and data managers.

9. A cover form should be attached to the questionnaire: this form should be completed if the patient did not complete the questionnaire, providing reasons for non-completion.

The Southwest Oncology Group suggests that in the cooperative group setting, recommendations for conducting QoL assessment should include[14]

(1) building support for QoL assessment among the group leadership;

(2) involving physicians and nurses in the study design;

(3) identifying a QoL liaison person at each participating institution; and

(4) aggressive monitoring of the quality and timeliness of data collection.

Education

Osoba discussed barriers to measuring QoL and how these barriers are perceived by individuals such as researchers, clinicians, and policy makers.[15] He distinguished between (1) attitudinal, (2) conceptual and methodological, and (3) practical barriers. He suggested that to overcome the attitudinal barriers we need to educate key individuals on the scientific validity of QoL data by dissemination and diffusion of clinically meaningful information coming from psychometrically reliable measures.[16] QoL researchers should try to reach people at all levels of involvement: QoL assessors, policy makers, planners of clinical trials, developers of clinical practice guidelines, and those at the level of patient clinical decision making.[16] The various individuals involved should be convinced that QoL is a serious end-point of a trial and not just a fashionable add-on.[1] Till et al.,[16] in a workshop report, suggest the introduction of QoL perspectives into education and health service programmes, especially for health professionals. The authors also advised that initially, emphasis should be placed on QoL assessments in areas of potentially high impact on the burden of disease, and where major differences in the outcome of such assessments are anticipated. They also commented on the large amount of data (especially from clinical trials) that is beginning to accumulate, and the need for the data to be analysed and published, preferably in clinical journals.

Many clinicians believe that the most important information regarding a patient's physical well-being (e.g. performance status, pain, nausea and vomiting, etc.) can be judged accurately by an experienced clinician.[17,18] They feel that the additional effort required to collect QoL data does not yield further information than that reported on the case report forms (CRFs).[18] However, during recent years these beliefs have been questioned by several authors.[19,20] In addition, QoL assessment measures emotional and social domains. However, Osoba suggests that clinicians may not wish to know about functional impairments in these domains as they may not know how to deal with this information.[15]

Da Silva *et al.*[18] have reported that the low level of recruitment they found in their QoL substudy did not reflect a lack of willingness on the part of the patient to complete the requisite questionnaires. Many patients have a positive attitude to being questioned about their well-being and it may even improve the doctor–patient relationship.[1]

Missing items

The problem

MRC and EORTC experience in a variety of trials suggests that for most items, between 0.5 per cent and 2.0 per cent of values will be missing from returned EORTC QLQ C-30 forms, and similar figures apply to most of the items on the Rotterdam symptom check list (RSCL). Thus, overall, the problem of missing items might be regarded as unimportant. However, there are two important considerations.

First, since each questionnaire contains about 30 questions, a 1 per cent missing rate would, if it occurred at random, imply that about a quarter of patients could have a missing item on their initial QoL assessments whilst even a 0.5 per cent rate could result in 14 per cent of patients with missing data. Furthermore, at each subsequent assessment there will be additional missing data and thus many patients are likely to have some degree of missing data. Any method of analysis which excludes patients who have missing values may result in a seriously reduced data set. However, analysis of the patterns of missing data reveals that it does not occur at random; patients who omit answers to one question are more likely to omit answers to other questions. If the process were purely random, one would expect a binomial distribution with hardly any patients returning forms with three or more missing items; in practice, there were some patients, albeit only 3 per cent of the total, omitting responses to anything from 3 to 25 questions. Also, missing items within forms often take the form of a run of adjacent questions, even though successive questions are usually unrelated to each other. Therefore far fewer forms contained missing values than would be expected by chance. Review of 7000 forms in six MRC trials indicates that 92 per cent of forms contained complete information regarding 29 out of the 30 questions in the first section of the RSCL, although one question (as explained below) presented particular problems. The proportion of forms with missing data varied considerably from study to study, from 4 per cent to 14 per cent. Unfortunately even 9 per cent of forms with missing data is a sufficiently high proportion to cause considerable concern, and means that perhaps a third of patients will have some missing data at some stage during their follow-up.

Second, some items may present particular problems. In particular, the question about decreased sexual interest on the RSCL produces far more serious problems with patient compliance and for that reason was excluded when estimating the overall missing item rate of 1 per cent. For example, in a wide range of MRC trials including lung, bronchus, bladder, renal, and head and neck cancers, approximately 19 per cent of patients left the question about sexual interest blank when completing the RSCL (the percentages varied between 9 and 25 per cent across the trials). This and similar questions addressing sexuality issues on the EORTC QLQ C-30 supplementary modules frequently present high rates of missing values.

Some questions manifested age or gender differences with respect to the completion of certain items, with older patients being more likely to leave questions unanswered.[21] These associations with gender and age suggest that 'missing' data may be informative, with patients experiencing problems being less likely to admit to them.

Methods of handling missing items

When individual items are missing there are problems in calculating values for the summated scales. For a scale which is based upon a number of items, of which one or more is missing, there are in general three main methods that may be adopted.

Treat the score for the scale as missing

If any of the constituent items are missing, the scale score for that patient is excluded or treated as missing for all statistical analyses. When data are missing completely at random, this reduced data set represents a randomly drawn sub-sample of the full data set. Hence inferences about the values of the sample parameters can be considered reasonable.

This method is the simplest and most naïve approach to the analysis, but results in overall loss of data since the scores based upon several items are excluded whenever even a single item is missing. Far more importantly, however, it may lead to serious bias when there is informative censoring. For example, the RSCL includes an item with a question '(to what extent you have been bothered by) decreased sexual interest'; this question, as discussed earlier, is frequently unanswered. One plausible assumption is that patients experiencing problems are likely to be more reticent concerning this question, and that therefore missing items occur more frequently when there are sexual problems. Thus 'missing' might frequently imply 'very much problem'. This is also supported by the analyses of the data: there was a marked gender difference, with a greater proportion of female patients omitting to answer this question, together with a comparable reduction in the number of female patients reporting decreased sexual interest. Simply excluding the scores for these patients might result in misleading and biased conclusions about the prevalence and severity of problems.

Simple mean imputation

The scale score can be estimated from the mean of those items that are available. This is a widely adopted approach which is very simple to implement.[22] There are two ways of describing this method, both of which are mathematically equivalent. Suppose two items are missing from a five-item scale. The mean of the three known results may be calculated, and this mean is then used to replace the two missing values. The scale score can then be estimated. However, this is also equivalent to calculating the scale score using only those three items for which we do have known values. Thus, irrespective of which formulation is used, this method effectively assumes that any missing item would have had a value equal to the average of the non-missing items within the same scale. In its most common form, application of this rule is usually restricted to cases where the respondent has completed at least half of the items in the scale.

The EORTC QLQ C-30 scoring manual describes how to implement simple mean imputation.[22] For example, the emotional functioning scale of the QLQ C-30 is formed by summing four items (see Fig. 14.3). Since the above rule states that at least half the items should have been answered, we can estimate a scale score provided only one or two items are missing. The responses to the answered questions are then averaged, to give a 'raw score'. This is then transformed to the standardised score as shown below. In the EORTC QLQ C-30, emotional functioning (EF) is assessed by four items corresponding to questions 21 to 24, each on a four-point scale. Let us call the n questions contributing to a scale Q_i, where in this example the $n = 4$ questions which are Q_{21}, Q_{22}, Q_{23}, Q_{24}.

If no items are missing, the 'raw score' is calculated as the average of the items:

$$\text{Raw score} = \sum_i Q_i / n$$
$$= (Q_{21} + Q_{22} + Q_{23} + Q_{24})/4.$$

Since different scales include items with different ranges of values, they will have various minimum and maximum values; these items are on four-point scales and thus the raw score lies between 1 and 4. Therefore, a linear transformation is applied, to standardize the score to 0 to 100; also, this scale is reversed so that high scores indicate a high or healthy level of functioning. The range is the difference between the maximum and minimum values (here, range = $4 - 1 = 3$).

$$\text{Standardized score} = [1 - (\text{Raw score} - 1)/\text{Range}] \times 100$$
$$= [1 - (\text{Raw score} - 1)/3] \times 100. \tag{14.1}$$

	Not at all	A little	Quite a bit	Very much
21. Did you feel tense?	1	2	3	4
22. Did you worry?	1	2	3	4
23. Did you feel irritable?	1	2	3	4
24. Did you feel depressed?	1	2	3	4

Fig. 14.3   EORTC QLQ C-30 emotional functioning scale (©1992).

Suppose Q_{22} were missing. The raw score becomes

$$\text{Raw score} = \sum_i Q_i / n$$
$$= (Q_{21} + Q_{23} + Q_{24})/3.$$

The equation (eqn 14.1) for transforming the raw score to the final score remains unchanged.

The beauty of this method is its simplicity, and for many homogeneous scales it may be an entirely satisfactory way of estimating the scale scores. However, there are a number of situations in which it may be found to result in misleading scores, as described below.

Hierarchical scales

Some scales are 'hierarchical', and have an implicit ordering of responses. An example of this is the EORTC QLQ C-30 (version 1.0 and version 2.0) scale for physical functioning, which is based upon questions 1 to 5 (Fig. 14.4). If a patient replies 'Yes' to question 3, about difficulties with a short walk, it would not be sensible to base a missing value for question 2 on the average of the answered items; clearly those who have difficulty with short walks would have even greater problems with a long walk. In this case the structure of the questionnaire may imply that the replies to some questions will restrict the range of plausible answers to other questions.

If we consider the 'long walk' and 'short walk' questions, two simple cases are straightforward: (a) assume the answer to 'long walk' is missing. If the patient has difficulty with short walks, then it would seem reasonable to assume that long walks would cause difficulty too. (b) Assume 'short walk' is missing. If the patient has no difficulty with long walks, we may assume there is unlikely to be difficulty with short walks. However, simple mean imputation may be more appropriate for the other two possible situations (no difficulty with short walks, but long walk missing; difficulty with long walks, and short walk missing). In the EORTC QLQ C-30 the proportion of missing questions in the physical functioning scale

	No	Yes
1. Do you have any trouble doing strenuous activities, like carrying a heavy shopping bag or suitcase?	1	2
2. Do you have any trouble taking a <u>long</u> walk?	1	2
3. Do you have any trouble taking a <u>short</u> walk outside of the house?	1	2
4. Do you have to stay in a bed or a chair for most of the day?	1	2
5. Do you need help with eating, dressing, washing yourself or using a toilet?	1	2

Fig. 14.4   EORTC QLQ C-30 physical functioning scale (©1992).

is minimal and the majority of missing questions are thought to be missing completely at random. Therefore this method has been advocated for this scale.

Score depends upon external variables

The value of an item may be more strongly associated with variables external to the scale (e.g. clinical or demographic variables) than with other items within the scale. We demonstrate this situation with an extreme hypothetical example, using the RSCL gastrointestinal scale which contains vomiting as one of its five items. In a clinical trial comparing 'chemotherapy' with 'no-chemotherapy', suppose the chemotherapy regimen causes all patients to vomit; for some cancer chemotherapies this might be a reasonable assumption. Equally, many no-chemotherapy treatments would be unlikely to induce vomiting. However, the other four items in the scale might be less strongly associated with the two treatment arms in the trial. When the vomiting question is unanswered, any estimated score that fails to allow for the strong association with treatment would be biased.

Informative censoring

Informative censoring may apply if 'decreased sexual interest' is missing. If missing implied problems with decreased sexual interest it would be inappropriate to assume that the average value of the other items should be used to calculate the score. If missing tends to imply that the patient has problems, the estimated score should in some way reflect this.

Item 'not applicable'

It is questionable how to estimate scale scores when some constituent items are missing through not being applicable. For example, patients may not reply to Question 1 (see Fig. 14.4) in the EORTC QLQ C-30 physical functioning scale because they never try to perform such activities. It is debatable as to how best to allow for non-applicable items, and the decision will partly depend upon the scientific question being posed. However, in the example cited, it might be argued that 'not applicable' represents problems in terms of physical functioning and will thus be reflected by the other items in the scale.

General imputation methods

In other research fields, particularly survey sampling, statistical methods have been developed to estimate or 'impute' the most likely values for the missing data. The objective of imputation is to replace the missing data with estimated values which preserve the relationships between items, and which reflect as far as possible the most likely true value. If properly carried out, imputation should reduce the bias that can arise by ignoring non-response. By filling in the gaps in the data, it also restores balance to the data and permits simpler analyses. Hence imputation is an attractive procedure – provided one can be sure that the conditions are appropriate and that unintended bias is not being introduced.

A variety of techniques has been proposed, some of which are mathematically quite difficult to apply.[11,23-25] Perhaps as a consequence, general imputation methods do not appear to have been widely used with QoL instruments. However, in survey sampling a large literature has developed on imputing missing items.[10-12]

One straightforward imputation technique is that of 'last value carried forward', which takes the previously completed value for that patient. However, this method assumes that the patient score remains constant over time. An improvement to this method might be produced by adjusting this value for any shift in the general population over time. Suppose at the previous assessment the previous mean (μ_1) and standard deviation (σ_1) for a single item are 2.0 and 1.5 respectively and at the current assessment the corresponding values are $\mu_2 = 2.4$ and $\sigma_2 = 1.6$ respectively. Suppose a patient responded with a 1 (x_1) at the previous assessment. Then the standardized last value is given by

$$z = (x_1 - \mu_1)/\sigma_1$$
$$= (1.0 - 2.0)/1.5 = -0.67.$$

Assuming that there is a missing value at the current assessment, we take forward the previous standardized value and estimate the missing value x_2 as follows:

$$z = (x_2 - \mu_2)/\sigma_2.$$

Thus

$$-0.67 = (x_2 - 2.4)/1.6$$

and hence

$$x_2 = (-0.67 \times 1.6) + 2.4 = 1.3.$$

Of course, this method assumes that the scores for the item form approximately a normal distribution. This may not be true for all items. However, this method is very simple to implement, takes into account the previous score and also allows for a shift in the population scores.

Other adjustments to the above method could be performed, that is, instead of adjusting for the mean and standard deviations of the current and previous scores one could adjust for the mean and standard deviation of the current item and the mean and standard deviation of the current scale (excluding the missing item from the scale). Other methods of imputation are described in detail later in this chapter.

Missing forms

The problem

This tends to be a far more serious problem. Phase III cancer trials normally require several hundreds of patients to be recruited, and thus such trials are frequently organized on a multicentre basis. Whereas a single-centre trial may be able to assemble an enthusiastic team that is committed to assessing QoL, there may be severe problems in motivating some participants of larger multicentre trials. This can lead to major problems in compliance, especially if collaborating clinicians only receive nominal or relatively small amounts of money in return for their participation – as happens with many MRC and EORTC clinical trials. In common with the experience of many other groups, patient compliance has been a problem in many studies assessing QoL. In common with other groups,[26,27] we have also found that it is most difficult to collect QoL data from patients with a poor health status and progressing disease. In general, multicentre trials are the most demanding environment for conducting QoL assessments.

Thus Ganz et al.,[26] using the FLIC scale, reported that 87 per cent of patients returned a baseline questionnaire, but overall only 58 per cent of expected forms were completed. Finkelstein et al.,[27] on behalf of the ECOG group using the FLIC assessment, achieved 76 per cent compliance during second and later cycles of therapy. Hurny et al.[13] reported a compliance rate of about 50 per cent when using the EORTC QLQ C-30 together with a linear analogue scale (LASA) and a mood-adjective checklist (BF-S), and noted that the institution, not the patients, appeared to be the major variable contributing to high or low compliance rates. They suggested that pre-treatment QoL assessment should be performed as a prerequisite for randomization, and recommended that there should be a policy of systematic training and commitment of staff at participating institutions.

The MRC experience has been similar. Bleehen et al.,[28] for the MRC lung group, found that only 47 per cent of the expected patient 'diary cards' were returned, with a third of the patients providing no data at all; however, they noted that there were major differences in compliance rates according to the centre responsible for the patient, providing strong support for the belief that much of the problem is institution compliance rather than patient compliance. Earl et al.,[29] in a UK Cancer Research Campaign trial, obtained better compliance using a similar form of assessment, but acknowledged that this was probably due to the study being in a single centre with a research nurse assigned solely for this purpose. Geddes et al.,[30] on behalf of the same group, reported 68 per cent compliance, and opined that patients find it difficult to continue completing the assessment when they become ill with progressive disease, 'and this poses a methodological problem for investigators who wish to assess effects throughout an entire treatment programme.' MRC studies using the RSCL have reported 75 per cent of patients completing the RSCL and hospital anxiety and depression scale (HADS) questionnaires at baseline, with 53 per cent overall compliance.[2]

Statistical analyses with missing forms

Introduction

However good the design of the study, administrative procedures, and effort made, a residual non-response problem will remain.[31] Therefore statistical techniques need to be developed which reduce the potential bias caused by non-compliance.

Due to the nature of the problem certain assumptions need to be made. One assumption which is frequently made in other research fields is that the respondents are not dissimilar from the non-respondents, given additional characteristics (e.g. age, income, and so on). However, in QoL research this may not be the case, especially if the main reason for non-response is that patients stop filling out QoL questionnaires after disease progression.

As will be shown, missing data can be handled either by imputing (filling in) the missing values and then performing the analysis as with complete data, or by directly estimating the parameters from the incomplete data. Also, different methods are required depending on whether the data are cross-sectional or longitudinal in nature.

The sample size, proportion of missing data, and the mechanism creating the missing data determine the degree to which missing data are a problem.[32] In addition, the type of analysis and number of variables used determine the degree of problem. A low rate of 'missingness' may be tolerable in a cross-sectional analysis but may be problematic in a longitudinal analysis. Even in the situation where data is missing completely at random and 5 per cent is missing at each assessment, then as many as 20 per cent of patients may be omitted from a complete case analysis based on five assessments.

Bias

The main concern when analysing incomplete QoL data is that of bias. Consider the case of a randomized clinical trial where we wish to estimate the overall QoL score of patients at one time point on treatment A. Suppose that there is a proportion of patients who respond (return a completed questionnaire) in each treatment arm P^A and P^B, so the proportions who do not respond are $1 - P^A$ and $1 - P^B$, respectively. We assume that the responders (R) and the non-responders (NR) may have different means, which in turn may differ between treatment groups. Let μ_r^A be the mean score of respondents in treatment A, and μ_{nr}^A be the mean score of non-respondents in treatment A if they had responded.[31] In Appendix 1, we show that the bias is proportional to difference in mean QoL of score between respondents and non-respondents $(\mu_{nr}^A - \mu_r^A)$ and to the proportion of non-responders $(1 - P^A)$. It should be noticed that this bias is not reduced simply by increasing the sample size.

In a clinical trial, usually the objective is to investigate the difference in QoL in both treatment arms. In Appendix 1, we illustrate that the bias in a treatment comparison is equal to difference in bias observed in each treatment arm. A treatment comparison is therefore considered unbiased if the bias is the same in both treatment arms. One may calculate the proportion of respondents in both treatment arms, but it is not possible to calculate the difference in mean QoL score between respondents and non-respondents in both treatment arms. If the reason for non-response is known, then this information may be useful in determining whether the analysis is biased or not. Additionally, if the probability of response is associated with some patient characteristics measured at entry into the trial (e.g. age, performance status, clinical stage of disease), then it may be possible to reduce the bias by adjusting for these factors when performing a treatment comparison.

Current methods of analysis

To date, most publications on the analysis of QoL data have used only a proportion of the data collected. For example, some authors have preferred to use analyses where the complete data set is available for a subgroup of patients, other authors have studied the effect of treatment at individual time points, neglecting to take the repeated structure of the data into account. Additionally, some authors have chosen summary measures and graphical procedures to describe the most important features of the data. In this section we will describe these more commonly used methods of analyses and later we will describe new and future developments in the analyses of incomplete QoL data.

Describing compliance

The first step in any analysis of QoL data should involve the description of compliance (which individuals have missing data at which assessments) and the reasons for missing data. Compliance is defined as the number of forms actually completed at each time point as a proportion of those expected (e.g. as defined in the clinical trial protocol). One advantage of studying QoL as an integral part of a clinical trial is that additional clinical information is collected at each visit of the patient. In the majority of cancer clinical trials information related to the patients' survival status, disease status, symptoms, and toxicity are collected. This information may be useful in determining why further QoL data had not been attained. Additionally, some cancer cooperative groups include a cover sheet with the QoL questionnaire. If the questionnaire has not been completed then the reason for not completing the questionnaire is filled out on the cover sheet. An example of the questions included is presented in Fig. 14.5. At the time of the analysis this information may be summarized in a table (see Appendix 2).

Has the patient filled in the current quality of life questionnaires, 0 = no, 1 = yes

If no, please state the main reason
    1 = patient felt too ill
    2 = clinician or nurse felt the patient was too ill
    3 = patient felt it was inconvenient, takes too much time
    4 = patient felt it was a violation of privacy
    5 = patient didn't understand the actual language / illiterate
    6 = administrative failure to distribute the questionnaire to the patient
    7 = other, please specify

Fig. 14.5   Assessment of missing QoL questionnaires.

Complete case analysis

The most simple, but least desirable approach to a missing data situation is to remove the patients with incomplete data from the analysis.[23] In QoL studies, especially for patients with advanced disease, this generally means deleting an unacceptable amount of information. It does, however, mean that standard complete data methods of analysis can be used (e.g. repeated measures analysis of variance). When data are missing completely at random (MCAR), the reduced data represent a randomly drawn subsample of the original data set and thus inferences about the values of the population parameters can be considered reasonable. However, in QoL research in cancer clinical trials patients who are in a generally good condition would be expected to have more complete follow-up. Consequently, the QoL of patients may be overestimated at later time points. Therefore this method has two distinct disadvantages: (1) it reduces the sample size and (2) it may produce biased results if data are not MCAR. In the breast cancer example, if we consider cases for whom up to five assessments are available, we may incorrectly assume that the overall mean was 64.6 at baseline and that by the assessment at four months the mean score was 70.8. As one may see from Fig. 14.2, this method of analyses considerably over estimates the mean score at all assessment time points.

Available case analysis

Complete case analysis appears to be wasteful for analysis such as estimation of means and frequency distributions. An alternative procedure is to use all available cases on a certain variable. For example, in a clinical trial we may wish to compare two treatments with respect to QoL at individual time points (e.g. using a t-test or a Wilcoxon test). Recall, earlier, we discussed the issue of bias in a cross-sectional treatment comparison and we concluded that it may be possible to reduce any bias by adjusting for factors which are measured before treatment, such as age, clinical stage of disease, performance status. Although the sample size may vary at each time point, this method makes use of all available data. The main disadvantage of this method is that different sets of patients contribute at different time points depending on the pattern of missing data. Thus, this method yields problems of comparability across time points if the data are not MCAR. Additionally, most statisticians would agree that overall tests of significance are preferable to simple comparisons per time point. Overall tests allow general statements about effects, are statistically more powerful, and provide a safeguard against multiple comparisons. Naturally, overall tests can be followed by comparisons per time point when a significant treatment by time effect is present in order to provide an indication for the cause of the significant interaction.

Summary measures

A widely used method for analysis of data collected serially over time is to reduce the data on each patient to a single summary that reflects some important aspect of the response. For example, in clinical trials, data on toxicity is usually sumarized by taking the worst value recorded during the treatment period. The summaries for all patients are then analysed using an appropriate univariate test. In QoL analyses, summary measures may be useful for simplifying the repeated structure of the data. Summary measures which could be considered in QoL data are the mean, median, minimum, and maximum recorded for each individual patient. In some circumstances, the summary measure could be expressed as a change score (e.g. minimum, maximum) from baseline.

In palliative trials, where a treatment is provided with the intent of alleviating a certain symptom, a useful summary statistic could be the worst score for that symptom. Another possibility is to define a certain change score from baseline to be clinically or subjectively important. The time taken to reach this change score may then be analysed using a time-to-event analysis.[33]

Tannock *et al.*[34] used two summary measures in analysing their data. Each of the patient's scores for each domain of QoL was summarized by the median and the best score. These were subsequently converted to median and best change scores by subtracting the patient's baseline score. Differences in the summary scores between the two treatment groups were assessed with the Wilcoxon rank-sum test.

The area under the response curve (sometimes referred to as relative operating characteristic or ROC, curves) is another possible summary statistic if the primary question of interest is the comparison of the overall value of the QoL scores in different groups. The area under the curve may be interpreted as a type of weighted average of the scores at each assessment time point. Appendix 3 provides a method for calculating the area under the curve.

As mentioned earlier the advantages of summary measures is that they are quite easy to calculate and once the appropriate summary measure has been obtained for each patient the values can be used in a simple treatment comparison (e.g. using a *t*-test or Wilcoxon test). Of course, the summary measure should have some clear clinical or subjective relevance and ideally should be reported in the protocol with some rationale for its selection.

When using summary statistics, as with any type of statistical analysis, care has to be taken that bias is not being introduced into the analysis. For example, in the palliative setting, where the worst score for a symptom is taken as a summary statistic, the results may be biased if patients with a high level of a symptom are unable to complete a self-assessment questionnaire and thus are not able to report their worst level of symptoms. Bias may also be introduced if the follow-up periods and the rates of completing questionnaires are not equivalent in both treatment arms.

Graphical representations

Graphs are an effective way to display data and illustrate results. Fig. 14.1 presented a Kaplan–Meier plot of time on protocol treatment and a table of QoL assessment compliance. This figure is useful in determining what type of analyses are feasible. For example, it is clear that in any complete case analysis the number of patients with complete cases will only be a small proportion of the total number of patients accrued into the trial. Similarly, available case analyses will be restricted by the small number of patients at later stages.

Graphical representations may also be useful in describing how QoL scores change over time. The most informative graph shows separate curves of the individual patients' profiles over time. However, in a large scale clinical trial it is clearly not practical to include all the individual patient profiles in the plot. Therefore, it may be more appropriate to present summary statistics, over time. However, care must be taken to ensure that plots presenting summary statistics are not misleading. For example, in Fig. 14.2, if the overall mean physical functioning score was plotted on its own one might incorrectly conclude that the physical functioning score improves substantially with time. This deception would be caused by different patients contributing to the plot at different time points. At minimum, the number of patients contributing at each time point should be reported to alert potential readers of possible misinterpretation. In addition, lines connecting points representing means of different subgroups should be broken to indicate that there is no direct relationship.

If summary statistics are used in analyses then it may be useful to display these statistics graphically to gain some insight and a better understanding of the data. For example, if the summary statistic of interest is the maximum (or minimum) score it may be useful to plot the value for each patient against the time that the maximum (or minimum) occurred.

Imputation-based approaches to the analysis of missing data

The main problems associated with the analysis of QoL data are its multidimensional and longitudinal nature, and attrition caused by the reduction of patient numbers through death and missing data. An ideal method of analysis is one which could take all of these adequately into account. Imputation techniques may be useful in partly filling the void. In survey sampling a large literature has developed on imputing (filling in) missing items.[9-11] A major advantage of imputation is that, once the values have been filled in, standard complete data methods of analysis can be used. Methods of imputation include mean imputation, last value carried forward (LVCF), hot deck imputation, cold deck imputation, and regression imputation.[11,23]

Last value carried forward

'Last value carried forward' refers to filling in the previously observed value for the missing value. This method and adjustment of this method were described earlier. To illustrate this and some further methods of imputation we will use a practical example from a clinical trial: a phase III trial comparing orchidectomy alone or orchidectomy with mitomycin C treatment in patients with poor prognosis metastatic prostate cancer. According to the protocol, QoL should have been assessed at baseline (pre-treatment), every six weeks during the first year, every three months thereafter until progression of disease, and at the time of progression. A modified version of the EORTC QLQ C-30 was used to assess QoL.[12] The questionnaire included two of the QLQ C-30 functional scales (physical, role); the three symptom scales (fatigue, pain, and nausea/vomiting);

the global health/QoL scale; and five of the single-item scales (dyspnoea, insomnia, appetite loss, constipation, and diarrhoea). Five additional questions assessing urinating functioning were also included. In this example we concentrate on the physical functioning (PF) scale (see Fig. 14.4). For simplicity, we developed a model consisting of four states: good PF score (PF score ≥ 60), poor PF score (PF score < 60), progression, death. A typical patient might therefore have a sequence of scores as shown below, i.e. the patient is initially in a good state of physical functioning, drops temporarily to a poor state but improves, there are then two missing assessments, thereafter the patient is in a poor physical functioning state, has a progression of disease, and eventually dies. Note that once a patient enters state 3 (progression) or state 4 (death) the patient cannot return to one of the previous states.

$$1 \quad 1 \quad 2 \quad 1 \quad - \quad - \quad 2 \quad 2 \quad 3 \quad 3 \quad 4.$$

Using the 'last value observed carried forward' rule, the missing value would be replaced by a 1. The complete sequence is therefore

$$1 \quad 1 \quad 2 \quad 1 \quad 1 \quad 1 \quad 2 \quad 2 \quad 3 \quad 3 \quad 4.$$

Imputation using a Markov chain

The Markov chain is an important concept in probability theory. Applications of Markov chains occur in many fields; in particular, they appear in agriculture, biology, economics, engineering, and medicine. A complete treatment of the subject may be found in the book by Bailey.[35] Let i denote the ith assessment. Using the observed data we produce a table (transition matrix) of transitions between states as shown in Table 14.1, that is, of the patients who were in a good PF state at assessment i, at assessment $i+1$, 76.0 per cent were still in that state, 11.4 per cent had moved to the bad PF state, and 12.6 per cent had moved to a state of disease progression. In total, six transition matrices were generated to represent the trial period. Separate transition matrices were produced for each treatment arm as the transition percentages differed between the two treatment groups. Additionally, the transition percentages changed over time, therefore one transition matrix was produced to represent the first three transitions (assessment time points), a second represented the subsequent three assessments, and the third transition matrix represented the final transitions. The transition matrix displayed in Table 14.1 presents the transitions matrix in treatment arm 1 for the second time period (i.e. transitions 4 to 6).

Table 14.1 Transition matrix of transitions between states

State	Good PF	Bad PF	Progression	Death
Good PF	76.0	11.4	12.6	0.0
Bad PF	11.1	75.0	13.9	0.0
Progression			91.4	8.6
Death				100.0

In the incomplete patient sequence given above the last value observed before the first missing value was a one. Taking into account the fact that the patient was in state 2 at the next observed value we know that the missing values must be replaced by a 1 or a 2, since a patient can not return to state 2 from a state of progression or death. Thus possible transitions are $1 \rightarrow 1$ (76.0 per cent), or $1 \rightarrow 2$ (11.4 per cent), which gives a total of 87.4 per cent. We therefore adjust the percentages to ensure that they add up to 100 per cent (i.e. 76.0/87.4 = 87.0 per cent and 11.4/87.4 = 13.0 per cent). Similarly, the restricted transition percentages for $2 \rightarrow 1$ and $2 \rightarrow 2$ are 11.1/86.1 = 12.9 per cent and 75.0/86.1 = 87.1 per cent, respectively (see Table 14.2).

Using a random number generator, we may then select a number randomly from a uniform distribution from 0 to 100. If the number selected is less than 87.0 we impute a value of 1, otherwise we impute a value of 2. Thus, if the process of selecting numbers is repeated infinitely, 87 per cent of times the number will be less than 87.0 and a 1 will be imputed, and 13 per cent of times the number will be greater than or equal to 87.0 and a 2 will be imputed.

Using a random number generator in SAS® the first value generated was 10.083165 and thus the value imputed was a 1. The second number generated was 68.462263 and therefore the second value imputed was also a 1. The complete sequence is therefore

$$1 \quad 1 \quad 2 \quad 1 \quad 1 \quad 1 \quad 2 \quad 2 \quad 3 \quad 3 \quad 4.$$

In the previous method we used the fact that the missing values could not have been a 3 (progression) or a 4 (death) and thus we restricted our transition matrix accordingly as shown in Table 14.2. We can therefore improve the imputation process by taking into account the specific value of the next observation after the missing values. In the incomplete patient sequence given above the last value before the missing values was a 1 and the first value after the missing sequence was a 2. All possible intermittent sequences are given in Table 14.3 with the associated transition probabilities in brackets underneath each value. The probability of each sequence occurring is then calculated by multiplying the probabilities of each individual transition; for example, for sequence $1: 0.87 \times 0.87 \times 0.13 = 0.098$. The probabilities are then adjusted to ensure that the sum of the probabilities is 1.0. Thus the adjusted probability for sequence 1 is $0.098/(0.098 + 0.099 + 0.002 + 0.099) = 0.329$. The cumulative probability is then calculated by adding the probabilities of the individual sequences.

Using a random number generator, we may then select a number randomly from a uniform distribution from 0.0 to 1.0. We then compare the number generated with the cumulative probabilities, that is, if the number selected is less than 0.329

Table 14.2   Restricted transition matrix of transitions between states

State	Good PF	Bad PF
Good PF	87.0	13.0
Bad PF	12.9	87.1

Table 14.3 Potential imputation sequences and their associated probabilities

					Probability	Adjusted probability	Cumulative probability
Original sequence	1	–	–	2	–	–	–
Sequence 1	1	1	1	2	0.098	0.329	0.329
		(0.870)	(0.870)	(0.130)			
Sequence 2	1	1	2	2	0.099	0.332	0.661
		(0.870)	(0.130)	(0.871)			
Sequence 3	1	2	1	2	0.002	0.007	0.668
		(0.130)	(0.129)	(0.130)			
Sequence 4	1	2	2	2	0.099	0.332	1.000
		(0.130)	(0.871)	(0.871)			

sequence 1 is taken, if the random number falls between 0.329 and 0.661 sequence 2 is taken, and so on. Using the random number generator the first number randomly generated was 0.82740854. Thus, sequence 4 was taken. The complete sequence for the patient is therefore

$$1 \quad 1 \quad 2 \quad 1 \quad 2 \quad 2 \quad 2 \quad 2 \quad 3 \quad 3 \quad 4.$$

Hot deck imputation

Hot deck imputation refers to selecting at random a score from patients with observed data and substituting it for the missing value. The hot deck literally refers to the deck of responses of patients with observed data from which we may select a score. Hot deck imputation may involve very elaborate schemes for selecting responses for substitution. For example, one might only select a response from patients with matching patient covariates (e.g. treatment, sex, age group, performance status, previous QoL scores). In the prostate cancer example provided above, suppose we wish to impute values at each assessment time point taking into account matching covariates. To identify which covariates were associated with a good or bad PF score we used the logistic regression model.[36] A two-sided test was used at the 5 per cent significance level to test the value of each variable. The importance of a factor was expressed by the percentage of poor PF score observed in the patients presenting a specific value of the variable, odds ratio (OR: the odds of a bad PF score versus a good PF score in patients with that specific value as compared to the odds in the reference category), its 95 per cent confidence interval (95 per cent CI) and the P value of the chi-squared statistic.

Starting at the baseline assessment, the factors that were thought to have an effect on the QoL score were WHO performance status (0, 1, 2), age (≤ 63, 64–70, ≥ 71 years), pain (no pain, mild, moderate, severe, intractable), and transurethral resection (no, yes). In a backward selection model, the only significant factor remaining in the model was WHO performance status. In Table 14.4, 73.3 per cent of patients with WHO performance status 0 at baseline were in the good PF state and the remaining 26.7 were in the bad PF state. Thus, using the hot deck imputation procedure, if a patient with a missing value at baseline has WHO performance status 0 at baseline, using a random number generator as described

Table 14.4   Hot deck imputation taking into account the baseline performance status

WHO performance status	Good PF	Bad PF
0	73.3	26.7
1	47.6	52.4
2	20.0	80.0

Table 14.5   'Nearest neighbour' hot deck imputation taking into account several factors

Patient no	Treatment	WHO performance status	Pain	Distance score	State
50	1	1	2	3.110	1
51	0	2	1	3.405	2
52	0	2	1	3.405	–
52	1	2	0	3.540	2

above a 1 (good PF state) would be substituted for the missing value with probability 0.733 and a 2 (bad PF state) would be substituted with probability 0.267.

A follow-up clinical case record form should have been completed for each patient according to the same schedule as for the QoL assessment. Quite frequently the clinical form was available when the QoL questionnaire had not been completed. The WHO performance status, pain score, and information on whether a transuretheral resection had been performed or not were recorded on the follow-up form. Taking these variables into account, the treatment group (0 = orchidectomy, 1 = orchidectomy + mytomycin C), assessment time point (1, 2, 3), and age group, we fitted the logistic regression model to identify what factors were associated with the three states (good PF, bad PF, and progression). The final logistic regression model retained the three variables: WHO performance status ($P < 0.001$), pain score ($P = 0.001$), and treatment group ($P = 0.006$). For each patient, a 'distance' score was calculated using the parameter estimates:

$$\text{Distance score} = 1.448 \text{ (WHO performance status)} + 0.644 \text{ (treatment group)} + 0.509 \text{ (pain)}.$$

Thus, a patient with WHO performance status 2, in the 'orchidectomy alone' treatment group, and having mild pain (i.e. = 1), would have a distance score of $(1.448 \times 2) + (0.644 \times 0) + (0.509 \times 1) = 3.405$. Similarly, a distance score is calculated for each patient (see Table 14.5). If a patient has a missing QoL value, the response from the 'nearest' patient to the patient with the missing value is taken. For example, patient 52 has a distance score of 3.405 and has a missing QoL score. Patient 51 also has a distance score of 3.405 and is in state 2. Therefore, we substitute a 2 for the missing value of patient 52.

Cold deck imputation

Cold deck imputation refers to replacing a missing value of an item by a constant value from an external source, such as a value from a previous study.

Mean imputation

Simple mean imputation generally refers to substitution of the mean scores of a group of patients with observed data for the score of patients with unobserved data. A result of mean imputation is that the estimate of the variance and standard deviation will be artificially reduced. An improvement to simple mean imputation is produced by taking the mean score of a subset of patients with similar characteristics to the patient with missing data. One might also consider the option of substituting the mean of the patient's previous score for the missing value. This method of imputation is sometimes referred to as horizontal mean imputation. If there is a constant decline in a patient's QoL score over time then it may be unwise to use this method.

Regression imputation

Regression imputation replaces missing values by predicted values from a regression of the missing item with both previously observed scores for that patient and associated variables. Mean imputation can be regarded as a special case of regression imputation. More generally, regression imputation is basically a modelling technique.

As with complete case analysis, a major advantage of imputation is that, once the values have been filled in, standard complete data methods of analysis can be used. In contrast, some mathematical statistical approaches to non-response require new and specialized computer programs in order to handle the problem of missing data. Of great importance also is that acceptance and understanding of statistical conclusions may be lost if sophisticated mathematical techniques are used for analysis. The choice and the design of an imputation technique also allows the user's prior knowledge and experience to be incorporated into the imputation process. Consequently, theoretically sound methods of imputation may be advantageous as the imputation method may be applied on only one occasion and may yield easily comprehensible conclusions.

Some problems do exist using single imputation, for example, when complete data methods are used, an imputed value is treated as if it were an observed value. This can cause problems, as summary statistics such as percentiles, variances, and confidence intervals may have incorrect estimates and hence any inferences which are drawn may be misleading. This is especially true for mean and regression imputation. 'Last value carried forward' assumes a continuous process. However, one might expect that QoL scores do not remain constant over time and subsequently this method of imputation may be inappropriate. Of the imputation techniques mentioned above the Markov chain and hot deck imputation methods seem the most efficient, as they take additional patient information into account in the imputation process.

Multiple imputation

The idea of multiple imputation is that several values, say m, are imputed instead of just one.[11,23] As a result, m data sets are created. In current imputation practice, m is often small (e.g. $m \leq 5$).[37] Conducting a multiple imputation analysis requires repeating the same standard complete analysis several times, such as calculating the summary statistic and variance for each of the m imputed data sets. The m separate analyses may then be combined into one inference using the rules given by Rubin.[11] With the rapid development of computer technology this has become relatively straightforward. Thus, multiple imputation retains the advantage of allowing complete data analysis as in single imputation whilst at the same time reflecting the uncertainty of the imputed value. Multiple imputation also has the advantage that when imputations are randomly drawn in an attempt to represent the distribution of data, the efficiency of the estimator is improved. It also allows the researcher to perform various types of sensitivity analysis.

Likelihood-based approaches to the analysis of missing data

Let us assume that there is a mechanism or process which causes the missing data. Rubin[11] and Little and Rubin[23] made distinctions between three different missing value processes (completely random, random, or not missing at random). The mathematical formulae describing these missing data mechanisms are given in Appendix 4.

Missing completely at random (MCAR)

A QoL questionnaire is MCAR if the probability of having a missing questionnaire is independent of scores on previous observed questionnaires and independent of the current and future scores, had they been observed. Thus, a QoL questionnaire may be MCAR if the reason for missingness is that the nurse/data manager forgot to ask the patient to complete the questionnaire, that is, the reason for missingness is independent of the patients QoL. MCAR also includes cases where the missing data depends on the values of fixed covariates. For example, rates of missing data may vary across age groups or treatment groups.

Missing at random (MAR)

For MAR data, the probability of having a missing questionnaire may depend on previous scores but must be independent of the current and future scores. In Fig. 14.2, we illustrated that patients with a lower physical functioning tended to drop out of the study earlier than patients with a higher physical functioning score. Therefore, the probability of having a missing QoL questionnaire depended on the previous physical functioning score and hence the missing QoL assessments were not MCAR but may have been MAR. Since both MCAR and MAR data are independent of unobserved scores, an unbiased repeated measures analysis may be performed using only the available data. For example, 'Proc Mixed' in SAS may be used to perform a repeated measures analysis with incomplete data.

Not missing at random (NMAR)

If the missing data depend on the unobserved scores then the missing data mechanism cannot be ignored. For example, the reason why patients stop filling out QoL forms may be due to increased toxicity or disease progression. In QoL studies it is likely that there are a number of mechanisms responsible for missing data. If sufficient data are collected relating to why QoL questionnaires have not been completed, then one may be able to distinguish the missing data mechanisms. In some cases it may be possible to determine the QoL scores of a random sample of patients by using alternative modes of administration such as telephone interview or by obtaining proxy scores from members of the patient's family.

When the missing values arise through a known censoring mechanism, the EM algorithm[38] provides a possible theoretical framework for dealing with informative, intermittent missing values. The EM algorithm is a very general iterative algorithm for ML estimation in incomplete data problems. The basic procedure of the EM algorithm is

(1) to replace missing values by estimated values,

(2) estimate model parameters,

(3) re-estimate the missing values assuming the new model parameters are correct,

(4) re-estimate parameters

and so on, iterating until convergence. A more detailed account of this topic may be found in the book by Little and Rubin.[23]

Zwinderman investigated the problem of missing forms.[3] He discussed the situation where a specific mechanism may produce missing data, that is, patients with a high mobility impairment may have a higher likelihood of dropping out of the study or dying. He assumed that all patients within the same treatment group, independent of their mobility impairment, are expected to have the same change pattern over time. The assumption that a patient's mobility score depends only on the previously observed mobility scores and not on the current or unobserved future is a strong one, which may be violated in QoL studies where many patients may drop out of the QoL study due to progression or toxicity. Zwinderman suggests that in this type of situation, that is when drop-out is associated with a breakdown or threshold mechanism, then the process is not observed and hence the data do not depend on the past but on the unobserved future, so that MAR is invalid.

To determine which methods of analysis are appropriate one should initially distinguish the pattern of missing data and identify the mechanism which generates the missing data. Curran et al.[39] demonstrated that in the setting of a cancer clinical trial, drop-out was often not completely at random. Thus complete case analyses may be biased. In addition, graphical presentations of summary statistics (e.g. means or proportions) of available cases over time may be misleading, as scores at later time periods may be seriously biased. The authors also illustrated in one example that the change score between the two previous assessments was predictive of drop-out, indicating that patients with a decreasing score were more likely to drop out. Thus, in this example, imputation methods such as 'last value carried forward' are not suitable.

Distinguishing between MCAR and MAR is often not a primary concern. Recall that if either MCAR and MAR hold then the analysis may be performed solely on the basis of the observed data. The main issue is distinguishing between

MAR and NMAR. In the paper by Curran et al.,[39] the authors demonstrate that testing the assumptions of MAR, or alternatively NMAR, is not trivial. The authors suggest that testing will almost always depend on strong assumptions that are often untestable.

When fitting a non-ignorable model certain assumptions are made in the specification of the model, that is, assumptions about the relationship of the missing data process and the unobserved data are made. These assumptions are fundamentally untestable. Molenberghs et al.[40] demonstrated examples where models provided almost similar fits to the observed data, but yielded completely different predictions for the unobserved data.

Sensitivity

Sensitivity to model specification may be a serious problem. For non-imputation based approaches it is prudent to calculate estimates on a variety of models, rather than rely exclusively on one model, especially when the 'amount of missingness' is considerable. It may also be sensible to test the sensitivity of the model to the assumption of the distribution of the missing data mechanism. As discussed earlier, problems encountered with the use of single imputation is that there remains some uncertainty with the single imputed value. Sensitivity analysis for the method of imputation may also be performed.

There is always a reason why the QoL questionnaire has not been completed. If this reason can be associated with any measured variable or characteristic then that characteristic may be used to make an estimate of the missing values. Additional follow-up information on a random sample of non-respondents may also help in performing an adjustment of differences between respondents and non-respondents.

Conclusion

Sufficient care and attention should be taken at the design stage of a study to ensure an adequate infrastructure, including appropriate personnel and material to carry out the study. No matter how well the analysis is thought out and how accurate assumptions are about missing data mechanisms, inferences in the presence of incomplete data are not as convincing as inferences based on a complete data set.

For QoL analysis in the presence of incomplete data, neither complete nor available case analysis seem appropriate if data are not expected to be MCAR. Summary measures may also be biased since they ignore the problem of missing forms. Single imputation methods may be useful if data are expected to be MCAR or MAR. Hot deck imputation sounds the most promising of the single imputation techniques as it allows for a large variety of schemes, and depending on the scheme chosen it generally provides a more accurate estimate of the true variance than mean or regression imputation. Multiple imputation appears quite promising in the context of QoL analyses, as do model-based approaches which take into account the non-ignorable missing data mechanisms in repeated measures assessments. It may be wise to investigate the sensitivity of the results of analysis to the method of handling missing forms, especially if the number of missing forms is substantial.

The methods presented here are relatively new to the field of QoL research. We hope that these ideas and methods will inspire and encourage researchers to investigate the potential of these techniques in quality of life analyses.

References

1. Olschewski, M., Schulgen, G., Schumacher, M., and Altman, D.G. Quality of life assessment in clinical cancer research. *Br. J. Cancer*, 1994; **70**: 1–5.
2. Hopwood, P., Stephens, R.J., and Machin, D. Approaches to the analysis of quality of life data: experiences gained from a Medical Research Council Lung Cancer Working Party. *Qual. Life Res.*, 1994; **3**: 339–52.
3. Zwinderman, A.H. Statistical analysis of longitudinal quality of life data with missing measurements. *Qual. Life Res.*, 1992; **1**: 219–24.
4. Zee, B. and Pater, J. Statistical analysis of trials assessing quality of life. In *Effects of cancer on quality of life*, (ed. D. Osoba). Florida: CRC Press, 1991.
5. Dempster, A.P., Laird, N.M., and Rubin, D.B. Maximum likelihood from incomplete data via the EM algorithm. *J.R. Statist. Soc. B*, 1977; **39**: 1–38.
6. Diggle, P.J., Liang, K.Y., and Zeger, S.L. *Analysis of longitudinal data*. Oxford: Clarendon Press, 1994.
7. Molenberghs, G. and Lesaffre, E. Marginal modelling of correlated ordinal data using a multivariate Plackett distribution. *J. Am. Stat. Assoc.*, 1994; **89**: 633–44.
8. Lesaffre, E., Molenberghs, G., and Dewulf, L. Effect of dropouts in a longitudinal study: an application of a repeted ordinal model. *Stats. Med.*, 1996; **15**: 1123–41.
9. Madow, W.G., Nisselson, H., and Olkin, I. *Incomplete data in sample surveys: report and case studies*. New York: Academic press, 1983.
10. Pregibon, D. Typical survey data: estimation and imputation. *Survey Methodol.*, 1977; **2**: 70–102.
11. Rubin, D.B. *Multiple imputation for nonresponse in surveys*. New York: John Wiley, 1987.
12. Aaronson, N.K., Ahmedzai, S., Bergman, B., *et al.* The European Organization for Research and Treatment of Cancer QLQ-C30: A quality-of-life instrument for use in international clinical trials in oncology. *J. Natl. Cancer Inst.*, 1993; **85**: 365–76.
13. Hurny, C., Bernhard, J., Joss, R., *et al.* Feasibility of quality of life in a randomized phase III trial of small cell lung cancer—a lesson for the real world. *Ann. Oncol.*, 1992; **3**: 825–31.
14. Hayden, K.A., Moinpour, C.M., Metch, B., *et al.* Pitfalls in quality-of-life assessment: lessons from a Southwest Oncology Group breast cancer clinical trial. *Oncol. Nurs. Forum*, 1993; **20**: 1415–19.
15. Osoba, D. Measuring the effect of cancer on quality of life. In *Effects of cancer on quality of life*, (ed. D. Osoba). Florida: CRC Press, 1991.

16. Till, J.E., Osoba, D., Pater, J.L., and Young, J.R. Research on health-related quality of life: dissemination into practical applications. *Qual. Life Res.* 1994; **3**: 279–83.

17. Fossa, S.D., Aaronson, N.K., Newling, D., *et al*. Quality of life and treatment of hormone resistant metastatic prostatic cancer. *Eur. J. Cancer*, 1990; **26**: 1133–6.

18. Da Silva, C.F., Fossa, S., Aaronson, N., *et al*. The quality of life of patients with newly diagnosed M1 prostate cancer. Experience with EORTC trial 30853. *Eur. J. Cancer*, 1996; **32**: 72–7.

19. Slevin, M.L., Plant, H., Lynch, D., Drinkwater, J., and Gregory, W.M. Who should measure quality of life, the doctor or the patient? *Br. J. Cancer*, 1988; **57**: 109–12.

20. Weeks, J. Quality-of-life assessment: performance status upstaged? *J. Clin. Oncology*, 1992; **10**: 1827–9.

21. Fayers, P., Curran, D., and Machin, D. Aspects of incomplete quality of life data in randomized trials: missing items. *Stat. Med.*, 1997.

22. Fayers, P.M., Aaronson, N.K., Bjordal, K., and Sullivan, M. *EORTC QLQ-C30 scoring manual*. Brussels: EORTC, 1995.

23. Little, R.J.A. and Rubin, D.B. *Statistical analysis with missing data*. New York: John Wiley, 1987.

24. Laird, N.M. Missing data in longitudinal studies. *Stat. Med.*, 1988; **7**: 305–15.

25. Kenward, M.G., Lesaffre, E., and Molenberghs, G. An application of maximum likelihood and generalized estimating equations to the analysis of ordinal data from a longitudinal study with cases missing at random. *Biometrics*, 1994; **50**: 945–53.

26. Ganz, P.A., Haskell, C.M., Figlin, R.A., La-Soto, N., and Siau, J. Estimating the quality of life in a clinical trial of patients with metastatic lung cancer using the Karnofsky performance status and the functional living index–cancer. *Cancer*, 1988; **61**: 849–56.

27. Finkelstein, D.M., Cassileth, B.R., Bonomi, P.D., *et al*. A pilot study of the functional living index–cancer (FLIC) scale for the assessment of quality of life for metastatic lung cancer patients: an Eastern Cooperative Oncology Group study. *Am. J. Clin. Oncol.*, 1988; **11**: 630–3.

28. Bleehen, N.M., Girling, D.J., Fayers, P.M., Aber, V.R., and Stephens, R.J. Inoperable non-small-cell lung cancer (NSCLC): a Medical Research Council randomized trial of palliative radiotherapy with two fractions or ten fractions. Report to the Medical Research Working Party. *Br. J. Cancer*, 1991; **63**: 265–70.

29. Earl, H.M., Rudd, R.M., and Spiro, S.G. A randomized trial of planned versus as required chemotherapy in small cell lung cancer: a Cancer Research Campaign trial. *Br. J. Cancer*, 1991; **64**: 566–72.

30. Geddes, D.M., Dones. L., Hill, E., *et al*. Quality of life during chemotherapy for small cell lung cancer: assessment and use of a daily diary card in a randomized trial. *Eur. J. Cancer*, 1990; **26**: 484–92.

31. Holt, D. Missing data and nonresponse. In *Eductional research, methodology, and measurement: an international handbook*. (ed. J.P. Keeves). Oxford: Pergamon Press, 1988.

32. Kim, J.O. and Curry, J. The treatment of missing data in multivariate analysis. *Sociological methods and research*, 1977; **6**: 215–40.

33. Buyse, M.E., Staquet, M.J., and Sylvester, R.J. *Cancer clinical trials*. Oxford: Oxford University Press, 1983.

34. Tannock, I.F., Osoba, D., Stockler, M.R., *et al.* Chemotherapy with mitoxantrone plus prednisone or prednisone alone for symptomatic hormone-resistant prostate cancer: a Canadian randomized trial With palliative end points. *J. Clin. Oncol.*, 1996; **14**: 1756–64.
35. Bailey, N.J. *Elements of stochastic processes.* New York: John Wiley, 1964.
36. Cox, D.R. *Analysis of binary data.* London: Chapman and Hall, 1970.
37. Meng, X.L. Multiple-imputation inference with uncongenial sources of input. *Stat. Sci.*, 1994; **9**: 538–73.
38. Dempster, A.P., Laird, N.M., and Rubin, D.B. Maximum likelihood from incomplete data via the EM algorithm. *J. R. Statist. Soc. B.*, 1977; **39**: 1–38.
39. Curran, D., Bacchi, M., Hsu-Schmitz, S.F., Molenberghs, G., and Sylvester, R.J. Identifying the types of missingness in quality of life data from clinical trials. *Stat. Med.*, 1997.
40. Molenberghs, G., Goetghebeur, E.J.T., and Lipsitz, S.R. Non-random missingness in categorical data: limitations. *American Statistician*, 1997.

Appendix 1: Estimation of bias caused by QoL non-response in clinical trials

The mean QoL score for all patients in treatment A would be $\mu^A = P^A \mu_r^A + (1 - P^A)\mu_{nr}^A$. However, as our sample only contains information on respondents, the observed mean score estimate is μ_r^A. The bias in treatment arm A by using only the respondents is

$$\begin{aligned} \text{Bias}_A &= \mu^A - \mu_r^A \\ &= P_r^A \mu_r^A + (1 - P^A)\mu_{nr}^A - \mu_r^A \\ &= (1 - P^A)(\mu_{nr}^A - \mu_r^A). \end{aligned}$$

In a clinical trial, usually the objective is to investigate the difference in QoL in both treatment arms, i.e. $\delta = \mu^A - \mu^B$. However, the observed difference is $\delta_r = \mu_r^A - \mu_r^B$. Thus, the bias in the treatment difference is

$$\begin{aligned} \text{Bias}_T = \delta - \delta_r &= (\mu^A - \mu^B) - (\mu_r^A - \mu_r^B) \\ &= (\mu^A - \mu_r^A) - (\mu^B - \mu_r^B) \\ &= \text{Bias}_A - \text{Bias}_B. \end{aligned}$$

Appendix 2: Compliance of quality of life questionnaires

Assessment	0	1	2	3	4
Expected (alive)					
Received					
Not received					
Patient felt too ill					
Patient felt it was a violation of privacy					
Administrative failure to distribute the form					
Patient progression/moved to another hospital					

Appendix 3: Calculation of the area under the curve

The area under the curve is calculated by adding areas under the graph between each pair of consecutive observations. Using the trapezium rule, the area under the curve is calculated from the equation

$$\text{AUC} = \frac{1}{2} \sum_{i=0}^{n-1} (t_{i+1} - t_i)(y_i + y_{i+1})$$

where y_i is the scale score at time t_i. In the example provided in Fig. 14.6, measurements are available at one-monthly intervals, thus $(t_{i+1} - t_i) = 1$ for all i measurements. Thus

$$
\begin{aligned}
\text{AUC} &= \frac{1}{2} \sum_{i=0}^{6} (y_i + y_{i+1}) \\
&= \frac{1}{2} ((80+60) + (60+80) + (80+100) + (100+60) \\
&\quad + (60+40) + (40+60) + (60+60)) \\
&= 470.
\end{aligned}
$$

Appendix 4:

Suppose in a clinical trial we intend to assess quality of life at several time points $(t_1, \ldots, t_j)$. Y_{ij} represents the QoL score for patient $i(i = 1, \ldots, N)$ at assessment time j $(j = 1, \ldots, J)$. Let Y_{ij}^o denote the observed values of Y_{ij} and Y_{ij}^m denote the missing values of Y_{ij} for those not observed because of missing forms.

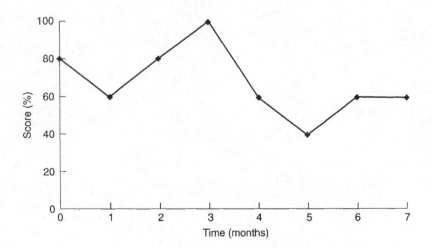

Fig. 14.6   Physical functioning score by time for an individual patient.

X_i is the design matrix of fixed covariates of patient i. It will generally include the times of measurement $(t_{i1}, \ldots, t_{iJ})$ as well as the treatment indicators and other explanatory variables such as age, sex, performance status, and so on.

M is a vector of indicators of the missing data pattern for patient i, where $M_{ij}=0$ if Y_{ij} is missing and $M_{ij}=1$ if Y_{ij} is observed.

β is a vector of parameter(s) which describe the distribution of the missing data mechanism.

For simplicity, in what follows we drop the subscript i and j from the notation. The joint distribution of M and Y is given by

$$f(Y, M \mid X, \theta, \beta) = f(Y \mid X, \theta) f(M \mid Y, X, \beta)$$

and the distribution characterizing the missing data mechanism or alternatively the probability distribution of the missing data pattern M is represented by

$$f(M \mid Y, X, \beta).$$

The distribution of the missing data mechanism reduces to

$$f(M \mid Y, X, \beta) = f(M \mid X, \beta) \text{ for data } \mathbf{MCAR} \text{ and}$$
$$f(M \mid Y, X, \beta) = f(M \mid Y^0, X, \beta) \text{ for data } \mathbf{MAR}.$$

15 *Using the Q-TWiST method for treatment comparisons in clinical trials*

Shari Gelber, Richard D. Gelber, Bernard F. Cole, and Aron Goldhirsch

Introduction

Quality of life (QoL) concepts have become increasingly important in clinical trials.[1-3] Investigators must utilize appropriate methods for incorporating QoL information when comparing treatment options. Such methods are especially useful when there is a trade-off between increased treatment toxicity and improved response. For example, a new therapeutic regimen may significantly delay disease recurrence or progression, but may also have undesirable side-effects compared with a standard treatment. It is important that the evaluation of QoL is made within the context of clinical outcomes related to the disease and its treatment.

The identification and grading of the side-effects of therapies were the first attempts at assessing the impact of treatments on QoL. Beginning with Priestman and Baum[4] subsequent efforts measured patients' perceptions of these side-effects and the symptoms of their disease. These efforts have resulted in the development of numerous QoL assessment instruments which have been reviewed for their psychometric properties and value for eliciting patient perceptions.[5-7] Further efforts focused on the integration of both quality and quantity of life into a single analysis to be used for treatment comparisons. This led to the development of the TWiST method[8] and its extension into Q-TWiST, 'Quality-adjusted time Without Symptoms of disease and Toxicity of treatment'.[9] The TWiST methodology made treatment comparisons in terms of survival time without symptoms of disease or toxicity of treatment (i.e. the survival time that remains after subtracting periods of time with symptoms or toxicity from the overall survival time). The Q-TWiST method permits a portion of the time spent with toxicity, relapse, or other clinical health states to be included in the comparison, as these health states frequently have some QoL value for patients.

Q-TWiST was originally designed to incorporate aspects of QoL into adjuvant chemotherapy and endocrine therapy comparisons for the treatment of operable breast cancer,[9-11] but the methodology has also been useful in other disease settings such as AIDS,[12,13] rectal cancer,[14] and malignant melanoma.[15] The objective is to include both survival and QoL in an analysis highlighting specific trade-offs using defined clinical events of interest. Thus Q-TWiST links aspects of QoL with the clinical outcomes (disease and treatment related) that are ordinarily used to evaluate separately the efficacy and toxicity of treatments. A Q-TWiST analysis can also be used to assist with treatment decision making when there is a trade-off between side-effects and a possible future benefit. It can demonstrate to a patient what the benefit might be depending on his or her tolerance for the treatment toxicities; this might improve patient compliance.

This chapter describes the Q-TWiST method and demonstrates how it can be used to compare treatments simultaneously in terms of survival and QoL outcomes. First we present the general methodology for conducting a standard Q-TWiST analysis and then provide an illustration using a clinical trial for melanoma. The next section describes additional applications in a variety of disease settings. Then several extensions of the standard methodology of Q-TWiST are presented. The chapter concludes with a discussion of guidelines for conducting a Q-TWiST analysis.

The Q-TWiST methodology

The Q-TWiST method makes treatment comparisons in terms of quality and quantity of life by penalizing treatments which have negative QoL effects and rewarding those which increase survival and have other positive QoL effects. As in an ordinary survival analysis, the focus of the method is on time, but rather than evaluating a single end-point such as overall survival or disease-free survival, multiple outcomes corresponding to changes in QoL are considered. The multiple outcomes partition the overall survival time into clinical health states which may differ in QoL. These clinical health states are selected to be relevant to the clinicians and patients. Each clinical health state is assigned a weight which corresponds to its value in terms of QoL relative to a state of best possible health. A weight of 0 indicates that the health state is as bad as death, and a weight of 1 indicates perfect health. Weights between 0 and 1 indicate degrees between these extremes. These weights are called utility scores. The Q-TWiST outcome is obtained by summing the weighted clinical health state durations and comparing the resulting amounts of Q-TWiST. Thus the method highlights trade-offs that result from different weightings of the clinically relevant health states.

The three steps of a Q-TWiST analysis

Defining clinical health states

The first step in the analysis is to *define* QoL-oriented health states that are appropriate for the disease setting under study. These should highlight specific differences between the treatments being compared. See Fig. 15.1 for an example from a melanoma study. The defined survival outcomes indicate transitions between the progressive states of health. The transition times may be unknown due to follow-up loss or patients surviving beyond the follow-up interval. Usually included among the clinical health states is TWiST (Time Without Symptoms of disease or Toxicity of treatment), a period of relatively uncompromised QoL,

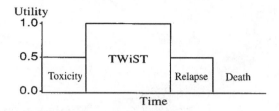

Fig. 15.1   Clinical health states for patients with high-risk, resectable malignant melanoma.

representing the best QoL available for the study patients. Each clinical health state is assigned a utility score, which may not be known. The utility score for TWiST is usually assumed to be unity because it characterizes a period of relatively perfect health. In some treatment comparisons TWiST might be assigned a value of less than unity, such as when one therapeutic regimen might return patients to a better state of TWiST (relatively good health) than another. The other clinical health states are generally associated with diminished QoL. Patients progress through the health states chronologically, possibly skipping one or more states, but never backtracking. This allows for a patient dying prematurely or not experiencing treatment toxicity. These states can be defined retrospectively at the time of data analysis or can be specified prospectively in the protocol document in anticipation of performing a Q-TWiST analysis.

Partitioning the overall survival

In the second step, Kaplan–Meier curves for the times to events that signal transitions between the clinical health states are used to *partition* the area under the overall survival curves separately for each treatment. See Fig. 15.2 for an example from a study of treatment for malignant melanoma. The areas between the curves are estimates of the mean health state durations.[16] For example, the area between the overall survival curve and the relapse-free survival curve is an estimate of the mean duration of time following relapse. In practice, censoring often precludes one from estimating the entire survival curve. In this case the average clinical health state durations (i.e. the areas between the Kaplan–Meier curves) are calculated within the follow-up interval of the study cohort. The resulting estimates are called restricted means[17] because they represent the mean health state durations restricted to the length of the follow-up interval. For example, if the median follow-up of patients in a breast cancer study were seven years, than it would be reasonable to calculate estimates of time spent in each clinical health state within seven years from randomization (i.e. average times restricted to seven years). As a useful visual display, the survival curves corresponding to the multiple outcomes that define transitions between health states for one treatment can be plotted on the same graph. Separate graphs can be produced for each treatment group. These are called *partitioned survival plots*.[16]

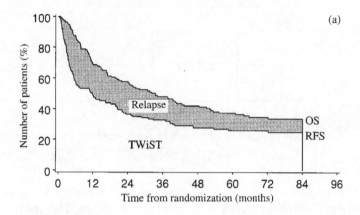

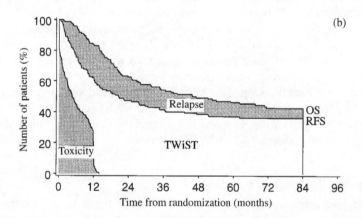

Fig. 15.2 Partitioned survival plots of (a) observation and (b) treatment with interferon-alpha-2b for ECOG 1684 study of patients with high-risk, resectable malignant melanoma. Survival curves are plotted for overall survival (OS), relapse-free survival (RFS), and treatment toxicity. Areas between the curves represent mean time spent with toxicity, with relapse, and without symptoms of relapse or toxicity (TWiST). From ref. 15, with permission.

Comparing treatments using Q-TWiST

The third step is to *compare* the treatment regimens using the weighted sum of the mean durations of each clinical health state as calculated in step 2. For example, in a disease setting involving TWiST and two other clinical health states,

$$Q\text{-}TWiST = u_1 \times \text{State } 1 + TWiST + u_2 \times \text{State } 2$$

where TWiST, State 1 and State 2 represent the average amounts of time spent in each state as estimated in step 2, and u_1 and u_2 represent the utility scores. Q-TWiST is calculated separately for each treatment group, and treatment effects are estimated by computing the differences in mean Q-TWiST. This quality-adjusted survival comparison offers the opportunity to include the utility weights to reflect the relative value to the patient of the different clinical health states. Treatment comparisons are made using a sensitivity analysis, called *threshold utility analysis*, which displays the treatment comparison for varying values of the utility scores.[16] When two treatments are being compared and there are two utility coefficients, the sensitivity analysis can be presented as a two-dimensional plot with a straight line, called a threshold line, indicating pairs of utility coefficients for which the two treatments have equal Q-TWiST. (See Fig. 15.5.) The threshold line is obtained by setting the treatment effect equal to zero and solving for the unknown utility coefficients, producing a linear equation. A confidence region for the threshold line can also be obtained by finding the pairs of utility coefficient values for which the confidence interval for the treatment effect captures zero. The plot shows which treatment is preferred in terms of Q-TWiST for each pair of coefficient values. Thus, a Q-TWiST analysis can provide information for treatment comparisons without requiring patient-derived preference measures.

A melanoma clinical trial example

Cole *et al.*[15] recently published a Q-TWiST analysis of an Eastern Cooperative Oncology Group (ECOG) melanoma trial evaluating the toxic effects (severe flu-like symptoms and fatigue) of high-dose interferon-alpha-2b (IFN-α) administered for one year against the improved disease-free survival and overall survival achieved with treatment compared with observation.

Recombinant IFN-α in high doses has been demonstrated to be an effective treatment for high-risk resected cutaneous melanoma. The ECOG trial (EST 1684) compared treatment (IFN-α administered for one year) with observation.[18] After a median follow-up of five years, the trial demonstrated a gain in median survival of 9.1 months and a gain in median relapse-free survival of 8.5 months for the IFN-α-treated group. This trial also demonstrated significant toxicity associated with IFN-α.

In step one of the Q-TWiST analysis the following three clinical health states were defined:

(1) *Toxicity* (TOX), the number of months during which patients experienced a grade 3 or worse toxicity;

(2) *Relapse* (REL), the number of months following relapse; and

(3) TWiST, the number of months spent without either grade 3 or worse toxicity or disease relapse. (See Fig. 15.1.)

These definitions enabled an evaluation of the trade-off between toxicity and clinical benefits of treatment with IFN-α.

The Q-TWiST model used the utility scores u_{TOX} and u_{REL} to reflect the diminished QoL of the clinical health states of Toxicity and Relapse, respectively. TWiST was assigned a weight of 1.0. Thus the QoL-adjusted survival rate was calculated as

$$Q\text{-}TWiST = u_{TOX} \times TOX + TWiST + u_{REL} \times REL$$

where TOX, TWiST, and REL denote the respective clinical health state durations. Fig. 15.1 shows an example of the different time periods with arbitrary utility coefficients of 0.75 for TOX and 0.5 for REL.

Step two used the clinical trial data to calculate separate Kaplan–Meier curves for the toxicity-free survival (TFS), relapse-free survival (RFS), and overall survival (OS) times. The first two curves partition the OS time into periods of time in TWiST, TOX, and REL. This is illustrated in the partitioned survival analysis for the observation group and for the IFN-α group shown in Fig. 15.2. The results were restricted to the first five years of follow-up corresponding to the median follow-up duration of the study cohort at the time of analysis. On average the patients treated with the IFN-α regimen spent less time in REL, but more time in TOX and in TWiST than the patients in the observation group. (See Table 15.1.) These differing amounts of time are illustrated by the areas between the curves representing the clinical health state durations in Fig. 15.2.

In the third step, the two groups were compared using a threshold utility analysis for all possible combinations of values of u_{TOX} and u_{REL} (ranging from 0.0 to 1.0). This is shown in Fig. 15.3. A threshold line can be obtained by finding the unknown utility values for which the treatments have equal Q-TWiST. In this analysis the IFN-α group experienced more Q-TWiST than the observation group regardless of the utility values. Therefore the threshold line does not appear on the figure. A confidence region for the threshold line can also be included. This is obtained by finding the pairs of utility score values for which the confidence interval for the Q-TWiST treatment effect captures zero. The 95 percent confidence interval for the threshold line is shown as a broken line in Fig. 15.3 and was calculated using the bootstrap method.[16] For values of the utility coefficients in the upper left of Fig. 15.3, the preference for IFN-α is statistically significant.

Table 15.1   Components of Q-TWiST for the ECOG 1684 study of patients with high-risk, resectable malignant melanoma

Outcome*	Treatment group		Difference	(95% CI)	P value
	Observation	IFN-α			
TOX	0.0	5.8	5.8	(5.0–6.7)	<0.001
TWiST	30.0	33.1	3.1	(−4.8–11.0)	0.4
REL	12.4	10.4	−2.0	(−6.2–2.3)	0.4
OS	42.4	49.3	7.0	(−0.6–14.5)	0.07
RFS	30.0	38.9	8.9	(0.8–17.0)	0.03

*The estimated period (months) within 84 months of randomization spent in each of the states TOX, TWiST, and REL are given according to treatment group. Average relapse-free survival (RFS) and overall survival (OS) are also provided.
Treatment differences appear with 95 percent confidence intervals.
From ref. 15, with permission.

Threshold Plot for Melanoma Study

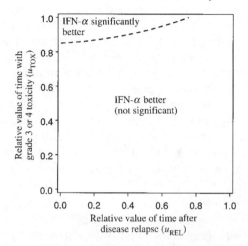

Fig. 15.3   Threshold utility analysis comparing IFN-α treatment versus observation for ECOG 1684 study of patients with high-risk, resectable malignant melanoma. The preferred treatment is shown for all possible values of u_{TOX} and u_{REL}. The area above the broken line indicates value pairs for which IFN-α treatment provided significantly more Q-TWiST compared with observation (two-sided $P < 0.05$). There are no utility coefficient pairs for which observation provided more Q-TWiST than IFN-α. From ref. 15, with permission.

Subjective patient judgements provide the weights for the components of Q-TWiST influencing treatment comparisons. A traditional efficacy analysis would consider the delay of disease progression or death as the main end-points. This is equivalent to assigning a value of 1.0 to the coefficient u_{TOX} and 0.0 to the coefficient u_{REL} to get a treatment comparison with respect to average RFS. For $u_{TOX} = u_{REL} = 1$, the comparison is of average OS. The threshold analysis indicates that regardless of the utility values placed on time with treatment toxicity and time following disease relapse, treatment with IFN-α provided more Q-TWiST than observation. For patients who place a high utility weight on toxicity (e.g. $u_{TOX} = 0.9$) and a low utility value on relapse (e.g. $u_{REL} = 0.4$), the benefit of IFN-α was statistically significant.

Extensions

Several extensions of the basic Q-TWiST methodology are described in this section. These extensions allow

(1) patient-derived preferences to be incorporated into the analysis;

(2) changes over time of the treatment comparison to be illustrated graphically;

(3) covariates to be included in the analysis by proportional hazards regression;

(4) parametric models to predict long-term treatment effects; and

(5) the Q-TWiST method to be used in meta-analyses.

Incorporating patient-derived preferences

A basic assumption of the Q-TWiST method is that the utility score for a clinical health state is independent of the duration of the health state.[16] This assumption can be checked by examining longitudinal utility scores. These scores can be obtained using specially designed questionnaires to collect these patient-derived assessments which can be mapped into utility score values using multi-attribute utility techniques.[19] An ongoing Intergroup study comparing surgical procedures for colon cancer is administering Spitzer's Quality of Life Index[20] which will be converted to utilities for a Q-TWiST analysis.[21] In addition, a childhood acute lymphoblastic leukaemia study is using the Health-Utility Indexes[22,23] to collect patient, parent, and clinician health status assessments of the child's QoL to generate utility scores for evaluation of treatment comparisons.

The Q-TWiST gain function

It is also possible to investigate how the Q-TWiST treatment effect unfolds over the course of follow-up. This is accomplished by performing the analysis at an evenly spaced sequence of times (restriction times) leading up to the follow-up limit. For example, if there are ten years of follow-up, then the analysis could be restricted to yearly intervals beginning at zero and ending at ten. The estimated treatment effect (i.e. Q-TWiST for treatment A minus Q-TWiST for treatment B) can be plotted on a time axis in order to display the results.[24] A single curve can be plotted for any specific utility score values, and a shaded region can be used to display the range of the treatment effect as the utility scores range between zero and unity. This is called the Q-TWiST *gain function* because it illustrates the amount of quality-adjusted survival time gained for one treatment compared to another. Figure 15.4 illustrates a Q-TWiST gain function comparing IFN-α

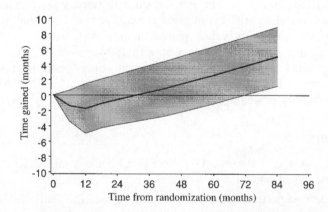

Fig. 15.4 Q-TWiST gain function comparing IFN-α treatment versus observation. The full line within the shaded region denotes the quality-adjusted months gained (for arbitrary utility values $u_{TOX} = u_{REL} = 0.5$) for the IFN-α treatment over the course of follow-up. The shaded region denotes the range of Q-TWiST gains as the utility coefficients vary between zero and one. From ref. 15, with permission.

treatment and observation in the previously described melanoma example. The unbroken line in this figure corresponds to utility coefficient values of 0.5 for both TOX and REL. The shaded region illustrates the range of results for the Q-TWiST gain function as the utility score values for TOX and REL range between 0 and 1. Early in the course of the follow-up, the toxic effects of the IFN-α treatment result in an initial loss in Q-TWiST compared with observation. This is because the advantages of the IFN-α treatment (i.e. increased disease-free survival and overall survival) do not appear until later in time. As the benefits are realized with additional follow-up, the Q-TWiST gain function begins to increase and will continue to increase provided the disease-free survival curves for the two treatments remain separated.

Incorporating prognostic factors

The Q-TWiST method has recently been extended to incorporate prognostic factors using proportional hazards regression models.[25] These models are used to predict the curves for the times to transitions between the clinical health states for various patient profiles, allowing one to look at how the prognostic situation affects the treatment evaluation in terms of Q-TWiST. In particular, separate threshold utility analyses are performed according to each patient profile.

As in the standard approach, the first step in the prognostic factor analysis involves defining the QoL-oriented clinical health states such as TOX and REL. It is also important at this time to define the patient profiles that are of interest. Typically, these will range from a good prognostic situation to a poor prognostic situation. As in the general method a threshold analysis illustrates how the gain in Q-TWiST might differ with respect to prognostic factors for each patient profile.

Forecasting treatment benefits

Treatment benefits are generally expressed as the amount of Q-TWiST gained within the follow-up period using restricted means. In some instances, however, it may be possible to forecast the future treatment benefit based on the available data. This has been done using parametric models to predict the tails of the Kaplan–Meier curves for times to transitions between the clinical health states.[26,27] The projected Kaplan–Meier curves can be used to increase the restriction time placed on the Q-TWiST analysis. This technique is designed to make the fullest possible use of long-term follow-up studies, and should not be used to make projections using premature data. For example, it might be useful to project the possible benefits of a treatment at 10 years using data with a median follow-up of five years, while it is not wise to make five-year predictions based on only one year of follow-up.

Meta-analysis

Meta-analysis, or overview, has become an increasingly important method for making treatment comparisons. This type of analysis combines the results of several randomized trials, each representing the same treatment comparison to increase the statistical power for the detection of treatment effects. The Q-TWiST method has been extended to incorporate aspects of QoL into meta-analysis.[28]

Two Q-TWiST meta-analyses of adjuvant chemotherapy for premenopausal and postmenopausal breast cancer have been performed[29,30] in collaboration with the Early Breast Cancer Trialists' Collaborative Group.[31] In the premenopausal study, data were analysed from 1229 node-positive breast cancer patients randomized in eight clinical trials comparing 'chemotherapy' versus 'no adjuvant systemic therapy'. The individual trial data were combined to produce an overall threshold utility plot at five years of follow-up and a Q-TWiST gain function for the 'chemotherapy' versus 'no chemotherapy' comparison. (See Figs 15.5(a) and (b), respectively.) This threshold plot of the meta-analysis indicates a difference between the two treatment groups favouring chemotherapy for most sets of patient preferences. The Q-TWiST advantage was statistically significant for some preference values. The delayed recurrence and improved survival balanced the early decline in QoL associated with increased toxicity, as illustrated by the gain function.

In the postmenopausal study data were analysed from 3920 node-positive breast cancer patients randomized in nine clinical trials comparing tamoxifen with and without chemotherapy. The threshold utility plot and gain function in Figs 15.6(a) and (b) indicate that adding chemotherapy provided more Q-TWiST for patients who value time spent with the toxic effects of adjuvant therapy more than the time after relapse. In contrast to the evaluation for the premenopausal patients,

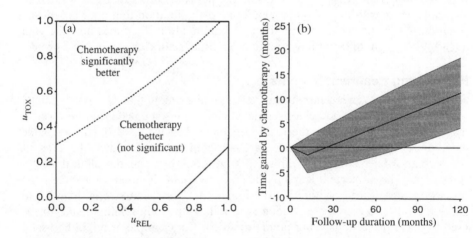

Fig. 15.5 (a) Threshold utility plot for 60 months comparing chemotherapy versus no adjuvant treatment for premenopausal breast cancer patients in a meta-analysis. The full line in the plot indicates pairs of utility coefficient values for which the two treatments have equal Q-TWiST. The dashed lines are the upper (95 percent) confidence limits for the threshold line. (b) Q-TWiST gain function for the meta-analysis of chemotherapy versus no adjuvant treatment for premenopausal breast cancer patients. The months of Q-TWiST gained for the chemotherapy group is plotted according to the follow-up duration. The shaded region indicates the range of months gained as the utility coefficients (u_{TOX} and u_{REL}) vary between zero and one. The full line within the shaded region corresponds to Q-TWiST with $u_{TOX} = u_{REL} = 0.5$. From ref. 29, all rights reserved.

(A) Threshold Plot for Postmenopausal Meta-analysis   (B) Gain Function for Postmenopausal Meta-analysis

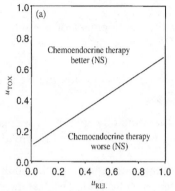
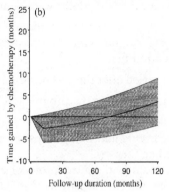

Fig 15.6   (a) Threshold utility plot for the meta-analysis of chemoendocrine therapy versus tamoxifen alone for postmenopausal breast cancer patients with a median of 84 months of follow-up. The full line in the plot indicates pairs of utility coefficient values for which the two treatment have equal Q-TWiST. (b) Q-TWiST gain function for the meta-analysis of chemoendocrine therapy versus tamoxifen alone for postmenopausal breast cancer patients. The months of Q-TWiST gained for the chemoendocrine therapy group are plotted according to the follow-up duration. The shaded region indicates the range of months gained as the utility coefficients (u_{TOX} and u_{REL}) vary between zero and one. The full line within the shaded region corresponds to Q-TWiST with $u_{TOX} = u_{REL} = 0.5$. From ref. 30, with permission.

the range of patient preferences for which adding chemotherapy to tamoxifen provided more Q-TWiST was narrower and the effect was not statistically significant for any utility pairs. Thus, patient preferences play a larger role in selecting chemotherapy plus tamoxifen for postmenopausal breast cancer patients than they do in selecting chemotherapy for premenopausal breast cancer patients.

Q-TWiST applications

The Q-TWiST method has been applied in a variety of disease settings. For each situation the definitions of the appropriate clinical health states have posed interesting challenges. When performing a Q-TWiST analysis, it is important to collaborate closely with clinicians treating the disease to ensure that the most relevant trade-offs are identified and appropriately accounted for in the analysis.

For instance, in Q-TWiST analyses in the setting of HIV infection[12,13] the trade-off examined was between the potential delay in disease progression and the toxicities (adverse events) associated with the use of zidovudine in patients experiencing little or no disease-related symptoms at the time of entry into the study. The original study was a double-blind, randomized, placebo-controlled clinical trial designed to assess the efficacy and safety of two different doses of zidovudine compared with placebo in asymptomatic, HIV-infected patients.[32] The QoL evaluation was especially important in this comparison because of the very similar survival experiences among the three arms in the study. The following three clinical health states were defined:

(1) TWiST, the number of months preceding the development of a grade 3 or worse symptomatic adverse event or HIV disease progression whichever occurred first;

(2) the period after the first occurrence of a severe symptomatic adverse event; and

(3) the period after the progression of HIV disease.

These definitions allowed for the evaluation of the trade-off between the increased adverse events and delayed disease progression, which are both characteristic of zidovudine therapy.

In a recently designed protocol evaluating treatment regimens for childhood acute lymphoblastic leukaemia (ALL), the major concern is the late adverse effects of the toxic treatments. Although prior to the 1960s ALL was almost uniformly fatal, currently it has a 70–75 percent cure rate.[33] Unfortunately, long-term survival has been associated with numerous late sequelae. These include late cardiac effects,[34] cognitive impairment,[35] growth abnormalities,[36] and second malignancies.[37] Thus the Q-TWiST analysis has to incorporate the reduced QoL for those children who were afflicted with one or more late toxicities. These late sequelae have been identified clinically, but the magnitude of their burden on the surviving population has not yet been determined. Thus the selection of which late events to include in a Q-TWiST evaluation has to be done prospectively.

For the treatment comparison of adjuvant radiation therapy alone versus combined radiation and chemotherapy for resectable rectal cancer it was necessary to include a clinical health state for late toxicities which occurred after the completion of adjuvant therapy.[38] In this case, the 'late sequelae' clinical health state could be followed by a resumption of TWiST. In this analysis the patients assigned to receive the combined therapy had more time with toxicity (3.1 months), shorter survival time after relapse (3.6 months), and more TWiST (6.1 months) than the patients who received adjuvant radiation therapy alone.[14] The Q-TWiST analysis indicated that the combined therapy provided more quality-adjusted survival time for a wide range of patient preferences for treatment toxicity and disease recurrence.

The treatment of non-small cell lung cancer presents different issues for a quality-adjusted survival analysis. The short survival time characteristic of this disease is the basis for extra concern on the acute treatment toxicities and associated decrease in QoL.[39] Since the treatments being evaluated may not return patients to relatively good health, this may be a situation where TWiST should be valued at less than one. One proposed Q-TWiST model includes six clinical health states as follows:

(1) time during treatment with chemotherapy, with or without radiation therapy, but without an objective (partial or complete) response;

(2) time during treatment with chemotherapy and with an objective (partial or complete) response;

(3) time off chemotherapy with an objective response (TWiST – assumed to be very infrequent);

(4) time with second-line chemotherapy;

(5) time off treatment following disease progression; and

(6) time with best supportive care prior to progression.

These states are progressive, but any state may be skipped; for example, non-responders will not enter the objective response or TWiST health states.

The Q-TWiST method has also been extended to other applications by Schwartz and colleagues. The extended Q-TWiST[40,41] is also a preference-based method that integrates the perspectives of the patient but in addition incorporates the perspective of the provider and social cost in the single analysis. The standard Q-TWiST method utilizes discrete and mutually exclusive health states while the extended Q-TWiST was developed for those situations where this model is not applicable because health state transitions are not easily defined. The extended Q-TWiST is a method of data analysis which incorporates information from measures of psychological, social, and functional status with preference values and the indirect or social costs of impaired health. It may, for example, highlight both the risks, benefits, and the costs of rehabilitation and palliative treatments for multiple sclerosis. Investigators are currently applying the extended Q-TWiST method to treatment evaluations for a range of chronic health problems, including diabetes; rheumatologic, sleep, and gastrointestinal disorders; and neurologic and infectious diseases.

Guidelines for performing a Q-TWiST analysis

A Q-TWiST analysis may be performed retrospectively after the completion of a clinical trial as illustrated by the melanoma example. The necessary data must be available for partitioning overall survival into the clinically relevant health states. These may be defined broadly, for example using the entire treatment period to represent toxicity.

If a Q-TWiST analysis is planned prospectively, more precise definitions of the clinical health states can be made and there is an opportunity to collect the specific end-points required to partition the overall survival time. As described above in the acute lymphoblastic leukaemia example, patient-derived utilities can also be obtained during the trial. We recommend that the threshold utility analysis be performed, even when estimates for utility scores are available within a trial, to allow the trial results to be interpreted for a range of individual patient preferences.

Toxicity is generally the most challenging component to define. Typically it is preferable to use criteria which focus on symptomatic rather than on laboratory events, as the former most directly influence patients' QoL. It may be difficult to accommodate intermittent toxicities precisely because the clinical health states are progressive. It is possible, however, to define toxicity as the time period from initial treatment until all toxicity has resolved. If there are long periods of time captured in this definition which are actually free of toxicity, this will be reflected by having a higher value for the average toxicity utility score.

Conclusions

The Q-TWiST method was specifically developed to provide treatment comparisons, within clinical trials, which incorporate both quantity and quality of survival. These comparisons are based on a utility approach to weighting different health states according to patient preferences. Q-TWiST integrates the subjective aspects of QoL assessment into a survival-time analysis to provide a range of outcomes useful for decision making in patient care. Incorporating patient-derived preferences into Q-TWiST sensitivity analyses is the next step in the development and generalization of the Q-TWiST method.

Acknowledgement

Partial support for this work was provided by grant PBR-53 from the American Cancer Society.

References

1. Schumacher, M., Olschewski, M., and Schulgen, G. Assessment of quality of life in clinical trials. *Stat. Med.*, 1991; **10**: 1915–30.
2. Cox, D.R., Fitzpatrick, R., Fletcher, A.E., Gore, S.M., Spiegelhalter, D.J., and Jones, D.J. Quality of life assessment: can we keep it simple? *J. Royal Stat. Soc. A*, 1992; **155**: 353–93.
3. Gelber, R.D., Goldhirsch, A., Hürny, C., Bernhard, J., and Simes, R.J. for the International Breast Cancer Study Group. Quality of life in clinical trials of adjuvant therapies. *J. Natl. Cancer Inst. Monographs*, 1992; **11**: 127–35.
4. Priestman, T.J. and Baum, M. Evaluation of quality of life in patients receiving treatments for advanced breast cancer. *Lancet*, 1976; **i**: 899–900.
5. Maguire, P. and Selby, P. on behalf of the Medical Research Council's Cancer Therapy Committee Working Party on Quality of Life. Assessing quality of life in cancer patients. *Br. J. Cancer*, 1989; **60**: 437–40.
6. Donovan, K., Sanson-Fisher, R.W., and Redman, S. Measuring quality of life in cancer patients. *J. Clin. Oncol.*, 1989; **7**: 959–68.
7. Moinpour, C.M., Feigl, P., Metch, B., Hayden, K.A., Meyskens Jr, F.L., and Crowley, J. Quality of life end points in cancer clinical trials: review and recommendations. *J. Natl. Cancer Inst.* 1989; **81**: 485–95.
8. Gelber, R.D. and Goldhirsch, A. A new endpoint for the assessment of adjuvant therapy in postmenopausal women with operable breast cancer. *J. Clin. Oncol.*, 1986; **4**: 1772–9.
9. Goldhirsch, A., Gelber, R.D., Simes, R.J., Glasziou, P., and Coates, A. for the Ludwig Breast Cancer Study Group. Costs and benefits of adjuvant therapy in breast cancer: a quality adjusted survival analysis. *J. Clin. Oncol.*, 1989; **7**: 36–44.
10. Gelber, R.D., Goldhirsch, A., and Cavalli, F. for the International Breast Cancer Study Group. Quality-of-life-adjusted evaluation of a randomized trial comparing adjuvant therapies for operable breast cancer. *Ann. Intern. Med.*, 1991; **114**: 621–8.

11. Gelber, R.D., Gelman, R.S., and Goldhirsch, A. A quality-of-life oriented endpoint for comparing therapies. *Biometrics*, 1989; **45**: 781–95.

12. Gelber, R.D., Lenderking, W.R., Cotton, D.J., *et al.* for the AIDS Clinical Trials Group. Quality-of-life evaluation in a clinical trial of zidovudine therapy in patients with mildly symptomatic HIV infection. *Ann. Intern. Med.*, 1992; **116**: 961–6.

13. Lenderking, W.R., Gelber, R.D., Cotton, D.J., *et al.* for the AIDS Clinical Trials Group. Evaluation of the quality of life associated with zidovudine treatment in asymptomatic human immunodeficiency virus infection. *New Engl. J. Med.*, 1994; **330**: 738–43.

14. Gelber, R.D., Goldhirsch, A., Cole, B.F., Wieand, H.S., Schroeder, G., and Krook, J.E. A quality-adjusted time without symptoms or toxicity (Q-TWiST) analysis of adjuvant radiation therapy and chemotherapy for resectable rectal cancer. *J. Natl. Cancer Inst.*, 1996; **88**: 1039–45.

15. Cole, B.F., Gelber, R.D., Kirkwood, J.M., Goldhirsch, A., Barylak, E., and Borden, E. A quality-of-life-adjusted survival analysis of interferon alpha-2b adjuvant treatment for high-risk resected cutaneous melanoma: an Eastern Cooperative Oncology Group Study (E1684). *J. Clin. Oncol.*, 1996; **14**: 2666–73.

16. Glasziou, P.P., Simes, R.J., and Gelber, R.D. Quality adjusted survival analysis. *Stat. Med.*, 1990; **9**: 1259–76.

17. Kaplan, E.L. and Meier, P. Nonparametric estimation from incomplete observations. *J. Amer. Stat. Ass.*, 1958; **54**: 457–81.

18. Kirkwood, J.M., Hunt Strawderman, M., Ernstoff, M.S., Smith, T.J., Border, E.C., and Blum, R.H. Interferon alpha-2b adjuvant therapy of high-risk resected cutaneous melanoma: the Eastern Cooperative Oncology Group Study Trial EST 1684. *J. Clin. Oncol.*, 1996; **14**: 7–17.

19. Torrance, G.W., Boyle, M.H., and Horwood, S.P. Application of multiattribute utility theory to measure social preferences for health states. *Operations Res.*, 1982; **30**: 1043–69.

20. Spitzer, W.O., Dobson, A.J., Hall, J., *et al.* Measuring the quality of life of cancer patients. *J. Chron. Dis.*, 1981; **34**: 585–97.

21. Weeks, J.C., O'Leary, J., Fairclough, D., Paltiel, D., and Weinstein, M. The 'Q-tility index': a new tool for assessing health-related quality of life and utilities in clinical trials and clinical practice. *Proceedings of American Society for Clinical Oncology (Am. Soc. Clin. Onc.)*, 1994; **13**: 436.

22. Feeny, D., Furlong, W., Barr, R.D., Torrance, G.W., Rosenbaum, P., and Weitzman, S. A comprehensive multi-attribute system for classifying the health status of childhood cancer. *J. Clin. Oncol.*, 1992; **10**: 923–8.

23. Feeny, D.H., Furlong, W.J., Boyle, M., and Torrance, G.W. Multi-attribute health status classification systems: health utilities index. *PharmacoEcon.*, 1995; **7**: 490–502.

24. Gelber, R.D., Cole, B.F., and Goldhirsch, A. for the International Breast Cancer Study Group. Evaluation of effectiveness: Q-TWiST. *Cancer Treat. Rev.*, 1993; **19**: 73–84.

25. Cole, B.F., Gelber, R.D., and Goldhirsch, A. for the International Breast Cancer Study Group. Cox regression models for quality adjusted survival analysis. *Stat. Med.*, 1993; **12**: 975–87.

26. Gelber, R.D., Goldhirsch, A., and Cole, B.F. Parametric extrapolation of survival estimates with applications to quality of life evaluation of treatments. *Cont. Clin. Trials*, 1993; **14**: 485–99.

27. Cole, B.F., Gelber, R.D., and Anderson, K.M. for the International Breast Cancer Study Group. Parametric approaches to quality-adjusted survival analysis. *Biometrics*, 1994; **50**: 621–31.

28. Cole, B.F., Gelber, R.D., and Goldhirsch, A. A quality-adjusted survival meta-analysis of adjuvant chemotherapy for premenopausal breast cancer. *Stat. Med.*, 1995; **12**: 975–87.

29. Gelber, R.D., Cole, B.F., Goldhirsch, A., *et al.* Adjuvant chemotherapy for premenopausal breast cancer: a meta-analysis using quality-adjusted survival. *Cancer J. Sci. Am.*, 1995; **1**: 114–21.

30. Gelber, R.D., Cole, B.F., Goldhirsch, A., *et al.* Adjuvant chemotherapy plus tamoxifen compared with tamoxifen alone for postmenopausal breast cancer: a meta-analysis using quality-adjusted survival. *Lancet*, 1996; **347**: 1066–71.

31. Early Breast Cancer Trialists' Collaborative Group. Systemic treatment of early breast cancer by hormonal, cytotoxic, or immunotherapy: 133 randomized trials involving 31000 recurrence and 24000 deaths among 75000 women. *Lancet*, 1992; **339**: 1–15, 71–85.

32. Volberding, P.A., Lagakos, S.W., Koch, M.A., *et al.* Zidovudine in asymptomatic human immunodeficiency virus infection: a controlled trial in persons with fewer than 500 CD4-positive cells per cubic millimeter. *New Engl. J. Med.*, 1990; **322**: 941–9.

33. Barr, R.D., DeVeber, L.L., Pai, K.M., *et al.* Management of children with ALL by the Dana-Farber Cancer Institute protocols – an update of the Ontario experience. *Am. J. Pediatr. Oncol.*, 1992; **14**: 136–9.

34. Lipschultz, S.E., Colan, S.D., Gelber, R.D., Perez-Atayde, A.R., Sallan, S.E., and Sanders, S.P. Late cardiac effects of doxorubicin therapy for acute lymphoblastic leukemia in childhood. *New Engl. J. Med.*, 1991; **324**: 808–15.

35. Waber, D.P., Bernstein, J.H., Kammerer, B.L., Tarbell, N.J., and Sallan, S.E. Neuropsychological diagnostic profiles of children who received CNS treatment for acute lymphoblastic leukemia: the systemic approach to assessment. *Develop. Neuropsych.*, 1992; **8**: 1–28.

36. Schriock, E.A., Schell, M.J., Carter, M., Hustu, O., and Ochs, J.J. Abnormal growth patterns and adult short stature in 115 long-term survivors of childhood leukemia. *J. Clin. Oncol.*, 1991; **9**: 400–5.

37. Kreissman, S.G., Gelber, R.D., Cohen, H.J., Clavel, L.A., Leavitt, P., and Sallan, S.E. Incidence of secondary acute myelogenous leukemia after treatment of childhood acute lymphoblastic leukemia. *Cancer*, 1992; **70**: 2208–13.

38. Krook, J.E., Moertel, C.G., Gunderson, L.L., *et al.* Effective surgical adjuvant therapy for high-risk rectal carcinoma. *New Engl. J. Med.* 1991; **324**: 709–15.

39. Grilli, R., Oxman, A.D., and Julian, J.A. Chemotherapy for advanced non-small-cell lung cancer: how much benefit is enough? *J. Clin. Oncol.*, 1993; **11**: 1866–72.

40. Schwartz, C.E., Cole, B.F., and Gelber, R.D. Measuring patient-centered outcomes in neurologic disease: extending the Q-TWiST methodology. *Arch. Neurol.*, 1995; **52**: 754–62.

41. Schwartz, C.E., Cole, Vickey, B., and Gelber, R.D. The Q-TWiST approach for assessing health-related quality-of-life in epilepsy. *Quality of Life Research*, 1995; **4**: 135–41.

VI

Interpreting and reporting results of QoL clinical trials

16 Clinical interpretation of health-related quality of life data

Eva Lydick and Barbara P. Yawn

There is measure in all things.
Horace

Not all therapies provide unequivocal benefit for all patients. With benefit often comes risk. Amelioration of some symptoms may result in different complaints. Preventive therapies provide enormous benefit to a few (unidentifiable) individuals at a price of slight risk, inconvenience, or cost to many. Health-related quality of life (HRQoL) is the term used to describe the integration of these various effects from the standpoint of the patient. Few question the importance of understanding the patient's health status and preferences; but confusion often arises in the form these HRQoL assessments take and in the interpretation of the results.

Quality of life has been defined as the gap between expectations and achievements.[1] The smaller the gap, the higher the quality of life. Only the individual is able to assess his or her own expectations and the consequent gap between them and his or her achievements. It is this subjective nature of quality of life that makes the uninitiated view quality of life measures sceptically. In addition, the measures themselves are unfamiliar to the average clinician; in fact, the available measures are proliferating at such a rate that even the most dedicated researcher in the field can not keep track of all of them. While subjective, HRQoL can be, and is, measured quantitatively with a precision that is equal to that of many familiar objective measures. Still, questions arise as to how well or accurately these measures reflect quality of life. One can only pity the poor clinician who must interpret HRQoL data when the construct of HRQoL itself is often poorly defined by the researcher and scores are reported in undefined units and in terms that are unfamiliar at best and unintelligible at worst.

Health-related quality of life, in its broadest terms, is not a new concept to clinicians. In this age of modern medicine, the majority of physicians' daily efforts are incapable of curing disease but are directed to modifying disease by reducing symptoms, preventing future complications, or increasing functional status, in other words, they seek to maintain or enhance a person's quality of life. It is not uncommon for the clinician to question the patient (or the patient's kin) regarding the impact of the disease or therapy on the individual's quality of life. 'How are you?' can be viewed as a 'global' quality of life question. While a start, this approach does not lead easily to quantitative assessment or comparisons. In addition, clinical assessments of HRQoL are often limited to a single area of interest or domain. A more inclusive evaluation of HRQoL may not be performed because of time limitations, lack of interest, lack of ease, or other reasons on the part of either the physician or the patient.[2]

Fortunately, collaboration between researchers in clinical medicine and psychometrics have developed numerous, perhaps too numerous, measures of HRQoL. While some generic tools, such as the SF-36, have been widely used across many disease states, it is unlikely that the average clinician will be familiar with the multitude of questionnaires, particularly those relevant only to a particular disease or condition, that they may encounter in the medical literature.

The purpose of this chapter is to aid the clinician who is relatively unfamiliar in the materials and methods of quality of life assessment in evaluating the meaning and usefulness of reports of HRQoL from clinical trials. By and large, HRQoL measures are easy to administer and score. Interpretation of those results may not be so easy. Clinical experience has taught that a blood pressure of 110/60 mmHg may be normal for a healthy adolescent but dangerously low for an accident victim. A 2 mmHg change in blood pressure probably has little clinical significance, but a 10 mmHg decrease can suggest impending shock or successful management of hypertension, depending on the situation. However, it is the rare physician who has developed any intuitive sense for any HRQoL score or clinically significant change in score. What is the clinical meaning of a HRQoL score of 48, or even 90, and what change in a score might be considered as clinically meaningful? That is, what score or change warrants consideration of modifying medical therapy either for an individual patient or to a standard of care?

As HRQoL units are undefined and vary from quality of life instrument to instrument, it is not surprising that it is difficult to assess the clinical significance of a score or a change in scores. However difficult, these problems must be addressed if quality of life measures are to become useful in every day practice or in the valuation of one therapy over another. In Table 16.1, we provide a summary checklist which we hope may be useful in determining the value to the clinician of HRQoL results in clinical trials reports. The checklist forms the framework for the information in this chapter.

Most trials are designed so that each patient serves as his or her own control and the comparison is between changes seen during or following treatment with two or more therapies. As such we will limit the discussion to assessment and application of *changes* in HRQoL scores reported from a *group* of patients. Absolute scores or change in an individual patient are discussed only as they relate to interpretation of group scores and changes in scores.

Table 16.1   Checklist for determining the value of HRQoL results

1. What is the value of the information?
   Does the quality of life information from this study add anything to your understanding of the preferences, desires, and needs of your patients?

2. How is quality of life measured?
   Are the measures used in the trial common measures, a new measure, a generic measure, a condition-specific measure, or a combination of measures such as a 'battery of scales'?

3. What information is available on the validity of the measures used?
   What scales are used? What domains are covered? What are the items in the various domains?
   Do the items and domains appear to cover most or all of the relevant dimensions?
   Does the instrument(s) have face validity?
   Were the measures used in a previously validated manner?

4. How generalizable are the results?
   Who are the patients included in the trial and how do they relate to the general population and to your population of patients? Do they have similar demographic and disease severity characteristics?

5. Are the analyses appropriate?
   Were all measurements, tests, and time periods reported?
   Were many of the patients at the floor or ceiling of the measures at the start of trial?
   Is there some indication of the distribution of change (difference between baseline and follow-up) in scores? Do only a few individuals account for all the change? Do some individuals show a marked change in the opposite direction from the majority?
   If means and standard deviations are reported (or medians), is there any evidence that the measure is linear?
   Do the authors indicate the number of drop-outs from the study and the reasons for discontinuation? Are the number of patients discontinuing or reasons for discontinuation likely to have affected the results?

6. What is the clinical significance (meaning) of the result?
   Has there been any effort to anchor the changes in scores reported to a more intuitive standard, such as disease severity, change over time, correlation with another measure, threshold for change, life events, or a global measure of health or health-related quality of life?

What is the value of the information?

> If you don't know where you are going, you will probably end somewhere else.
> *Laurence J. Peter*

HRQoL information should add to the clinician's understanding of the way in which the individual patient is likely to be affected by his or her disease, by the treatment provided, or by health care in general. The purpose of including HRQoL in clinical trials is to understand the patient's perspective on what they gain or lose from the treatment. This information should help in clinical decision making, that is, in deciding whether or not to modify specific elements of treatment such as medications, consultant care, patient education, or support services. The information should supplement information obtained during the medical history, physical examination, and laboratory testing.

Generic instruments that can be used in multiple populations and disease settings are particularly beneficial for developing physician familiarity with HRQoL measures. Developed from the RAND health insurance experiment and the medical outcomes study (MOS), the various MOS short and long forms (including the SF-36 and the new SF-12) have the advantage that scores are available for large numbers of healthy individuals as well as individuals with various chronic conditions.[3] With the recent and ongoing efforts to establish normative values for the SF-36[4-6] and other generic instruments,[7,8] the reviewer of clinical trial reports will benefit in being able to compare absolute scores to known disease states and levels of functional impairment. Repeated exposure to the measures will allow the physician to interpret HRQoL scores with the same ease as serum glucose measures.

Much effort has been expended in developing summary measures of HRQoL, but there are those who argue that HRQoL is inherently multidimensional and efforts to reduce it to a single score are misdirected.[9] Therefore, many clinical trials use multiple measures, each looking at a different aspect of HRQoL, rather than a single global score. Reporting scores for different domains aids in the understanding of the effect of the therapy on sleep, sexuality, or physical functioning and how different patients view decrements or improvements in these domains. Overall, HRQoL is the sum of a number of domains or dimensions weighted by the individual's own preferences. Patients differ not only in how they respond to particular diseases and therapies within these domains, but also how they value optimum health within specific domains. It is the difference in individual weighting and perception that argues against the use of a single summary score for HRQoL over multiple domains.

How is health-related quality of life measured?

You can observe a lot just by watching.
Yogi Berra

The methods section of any article should provide the name and description of the HRQoL instrument or, at a minimum, a reference that will provide the necessary information. While most clinicians may be unfamiliar with the specific measures, there should be clues within the publication itself regarding the origin of the HRQoL measure. For example, if the methods section talks about developing an instrument then it is likely the instrument was developed just for this study. New measures require extensive validation to ensure that the measure is testing what it is supposed to test and that the subjects understand the questions included in the measure. There will be no way to compare results in this trial with those reported in other trials or with other patient cohorts if a study-specific measure is used. When a previously used or validated measure is employed, representative scores and interpretation of changes can, and should, be provided.

Disease-specific measures are those tailored to query about items most affected by the disease in question and in terms that relate to the disease. As expected, these questionnaires are most sensitive to changes in the disease or condition under study. A statistically, or even clinically, significant change on these measures may not translate to significant change in overall HRQoL as measured by a generic instrument. In addition, disease-specific measures are unlikely to pick up distress unrelated to the disease that may be caused by the treatment. For example, if an effective treatment for arthritis causes gastrointestinal problems, the disease-specific questionnaire will probably show the significant benefit; however, the associated gastrointestinal problems will probably go undetected and unmeasured. Even generic measures may not include items on all the organ systems or functions of interest. Keep in mind the purpose of the trial. A measure that does not include any assessment of mood or fatigue may not be appropriate in assessing the impact on quality of life from a sedative hypnotic.

If the measure is referred to by name, references should be provided regarding the instrument and at least one validation study should be among those referenced. Measures should have been tested and validated in patients similar to those enrolled in this particular trial. For example, the Wisconsin brief pain index was developed for cancer patients.[10] Without additional testing and validation in a population of patients with herpes zoster,[11] this measure could not be used confidently to provide a comparative measure in a trial of therapies for herpes zoster. Similarly, the Katz adjustment scales developed for assessment of schizophrenic patients required validation and rescoring for use with epilepsy patients.[12] The term 'validated' requires a context. Scales and instruments are demonstrated to perform validly in certain settings; validation cannot be assumed when used in different cultures, patients, and with different modes of administration and for different purposes. There is extensive literature on what constitutes validation for different types of instruments.[9,13-15] The reader is also referred to Chapter 10 of this book.

What information is available on the validity of the measures used?

It certainly looked as if it were a rhinoceros.

Eugene Ionesco

Typically the methods section of any report describes the questionnaires used to assess quality of life and, for each instrument used, describes the domains or aspects covered by that measure. Less typically, the actual items within each domain are listed in the methods or in an appendix. While few clinicians will have time to become familiar with the psychometric properties of the questionnaires, they should expect that the instruments used and the results reported have some common sense, practical relationship to the disease and therapies tested. This is generally termed 'face validity'. Gill and Feinstein[16] describe face validity for a clinical instrument as 'the application of enlightened common sense, which is a mixture of ordinary common sense plus a reasonable knowledge of pathophysiology and clinical reality.' In their review of the quality of quality of life instruments, they relied on face validity rather than statistical or psychometric properties. There is no reason why, in most cases, the busy clinician should not follow suit.

Both individual items and domains included should have this face validity, that is they should appear to be measuring those areas of the disease and treatment that the clinician believes relevant. When it is possible to review the items or questions in the HRQoL instrument, common sense is a good standard against which to compare the items. Questions regarding the physical ability to rise from a chair might have little place in a study of depressed patients and the lack of any items on sleep or appetite would decrease the face validity of a HRQoL instrument in an antidepressant trial.

If portions or a description of the quality of life instrument are not included in the article, it may be difficult to assess face validity; in which case one wonders just how much the researchers wish the clinician to understand about the results and the applicability. Just as '*p* values' should not be enough to sway a clinician to adopt a new therapy where a new and poorly defined physiologic outcome measure is used, so statistical significance alone should not reassure a clinician that the therapy will provide a HRQoL benefit to the patient. Researchers can and should be required to describe their measures and results in such a way that they can be understood by their target audience.

> It may be that the race is not always to the swift, nor the battle to the strong—but that is the way to bet.
> *Damon Runyon*

Besides face validity, one should consider 'content validity'. To a large extent, the validity of the questionnaire depends on the extent to which items included are a comprehensive and representative sample of all possible items that could measure the effects of interest.[13,17] Responsiveness of the questionnaire may also depend on completeness of item identification. To the extent that the HRQoL measure does not capture all the problems of the disease or treatment side-effects likely to be experienced by the patient, it will not be possible to capture all the potential benefits of a new treatment.[18] Furthermore, completeness of item generation is also a hedge against having a disease-specific questionnaire that might be viewed as being biased towards a specific treatment.[18-20] Direct solicitation from patients of items that have an impact upon their quality of life has become the preferred method for identifying items for disease-specific quality of life questionnaires.[16,21]

Furthermore, the changes reported should seem reasonable in relation to other physiologic and objective measures. A treatment to reduce arthritic pain can be expected to have a positive impact on mobility, physical functioning, and perhaps sleep. It may have little or no impact on anxiety. In contrast, an antidepressant may show an impact on anxiety and not on physical functioning. As HRQoL is multidimensional, the lack of a positive change on every dimension should not be surprising or expected. Seemingly paradoxical findings may have very real and reasonable explanations. For example, patients newly diagnosed with catastrophic illnesses often report the greatest decrement on many emotional scales. Even as their physical condition deteriorates, their emotional response may improve as they learn to cope better with their disease.

Nevertheless, in most cases, the type, direction, and magnitude of change in HRQoL should appear reasonable in the context of the patients and therapy studied. It should be disconcerting to see substantial and significant changes in HRQoL in a trial showing no difference in any clinical or physiologic parameters.

How generalizable are the results?

Numbers ain't nothing, it's people that count.

Will Rogers

Regardless of the outcome measure used, the results from any clinical trial are often relevant only for a group of similar subjects. The study of an anti-seizure drug in the population of a university neurology clinic may yield little information of value to the family physician treating people with easily controlled epilepsy. The information is most likely to be generalizable if the patients in the study have age, gender, socio-economic, and disease severity characteristics that are similar to these of the patients considered for treatment.

In addition, HRQoL scores differ from many clinical test results in that they have an absolute top and an absolute bottom and the ranges do not necessarily incorporate the norms. If 85 per cent of the patients began at the bottom of the HRQoL scale, it is unlikely that the study can demonstrate an overall decline on this HRQoL measure regardless of what other outcomes may occur. It may be possible to state whether or not the treatment increases the subjects' quality of life, but no statement can be made regarding a decrement in the subjects' HRQoL. Conversely, little improvement can be expected in a group who are at the top or ceiling of the measure. The choice of an appropriate measure should permit demonstration of either a gain or loss in HRQoL.

In addition, HRQoL measures are rarely linear in their relationship to other outcome measures, making comparability between study population and target population(s) particularly important. For example, Ware[17] reports that for the range of 0 to 39 on the physical function domain of the SF-36, there is little difference in the percentage of individuals who report being unable to walk a block (8–16 per cent). And, over the 20 point range of 80–100, 98–100 per cent of individuals report being able to walk a block. However, as scores change from 40 to 79, the percentage of individuals who can walk a block rises from 32 per cent to 90 per cent. Thus a change of ten units in the steep part of the curve (40–79) could indicate a major change in physical mobility, while a change of ten units on either end of the scale (below 40 or above 80) may indicate little major change in physical functioning. The clinician (and others interested in interpreting the results) are cautioned that HRQoL results from any study are probably only valid for a very similar group of patients. Extrapolation of results to patients with worse or less disease or to a more diverse group of patients is probably not warranted.

Are the analyses appropriate?

Life is divided into the horrible and the miserable.
Woody Allen

As with any outcome measure, interpretation of the results requires attention to the study design and analysis. A previously validated instrument remains valid only as long as it is used in the same manner as it was in the validation study – that is, self-administered if validated self-administered, and with a full 36 items if it is a 36-item questionnaire. Whereas scores are reported for individual domains, it is questionable whether the domain taken out of context and used as a stand-alone instrument is valid.[4]

It is inadequate to report selective measures or domains from the battery of tests or domains and ignore other measures. All too often, trials involving HRQoL end-points include multiple questionnaires, each containing multiple scales and domains. Most or all questionnaires are administered at multiple time points. HRQoL is expected to fluctuate over time. There are statistical means to assess this fluctuation and obtain a summary score (Q-TWiST, repeated measures designs) whereby patients on different therapies can be compared. The reader is referred to Chapters 13 and 15 for a discussion of these techniques.

Results should be reported for all scales and domains tested and for each time period tested. It may indeed be that some scales are included for the same reason some laboratory measures are included – to assess whether there are unanticipated side-effects or harm from the therapy. If so, this needs to be stated and at least a brief mention made that no significant decrement was noted on those domains not expected to show any benefit with therapy. It may be that the researchers expected significant changes on only a few of the domains in the instrument. If that is the case, then it should be so stated. Beware the study report where numerous domains and scales were administered, but results are reported for only a few or at only selected time points. It needs to be questioned as to why the investigator felt it was necessary to include so many domains and scales.

Most clinical trials report summary results for the total population. There may also be a subtle change in the discussion to attempt to explain the relevance of the results to the individual patient. After all, a major objective of HRQoL is to individualize therapies and to account for different values. However, a significant change in mean HRQoL does not imply that all patients, or even most patients, can be expected to show a positive response to the therapy. Confusion between population and individual patient perspective is exacerbated by the emphasis of reporting clinical trial results in terms of mean difference of the change from baseline between treated and control groups. Often the mean change is within the test variance for an individual patient. The mean or median change reported for a group of patients may have little relevance to expected changes for a single patient.

I know who I was when I got up this morning, but I've changed several times since then.
Lewis Carroll

Changes in HRQoL are often evaluated by comparing the mean response with variance of a 'stable' population. This statistic is referred to as the effect size or responsiveness statistic. The stable population is variously defined as individuals in the run-in phase of the trial prior to assignment to the comparative treatments, placebo patients within the study, if the study has a placebo group, or an untreated population. As expected, the effect size will depend greatly on the variance. It is most important that the population be a truly stable one and that the variance be measured in such a way as to reflect the underlying day-to-day variation in self-reported HRQoL and the intrinsic measurement error under the conditions of the study.

As with objective measures, HRQoL scores can show regression to the mean; that is, on a subsequent assessment, patients originally selected because they had high levels tend to report lower levels (closer to the mean) and patients with low scores initially tend to report higher levels. For this reason, it is important that the trial include a run-in period that assesses HRQoL in addition to any clinical and physiologic measures more than once. As an example, in a study of patients with advanced stage cancer, Hadorn et al.[22] reported that the 146 patients who rated their initial quality of life as '8' or higher (relatively good HRQoL) experienced an average decrease in quality of life of 0.9 rating points. By contrast, the 168 patients who rated their initial quality of life at the very lowest levels of the scale (relatively poor HRQoL) experienced an average improvement in quality of life of 0.7 rating points. Such changes are compatible with regression to the mean and may not reflect any effect of therapy. Beware uncontrolled trials or trials where the control is an untreated population.

For both HRQoL and objective end-points, the greatest impact of an intervention is often in the tails of the distribution (the patients with the highest or lowest scores of the measure). Statistics that describe the tails or a cumulative distribution function would more clearly indicate how many patients are likely to have a significant benefit than simply reporting the mean or median. It would be easier to judge the likely value of the therapy to an individual patient and the number of patients likely to benefit. Besides the average change, it is also important to know the number of patients who benefited. Was the change such that almost all patients had a beneficial change in HRQoL or did only a small number of patients benefit substantially? For example, agent A may result in an overall statistically significant decline in quality of life, yet when each individual's data are reviewed it becomes clear that 10 per cent of the subjects account for 80 per cent of the decline in the quality of life score. The other 90 per cent either had no change or a clinically and statistically insignificant change. It may be unreasonable to withhold treatment from all people based on this decline in HRQoL in a small percentage of the subjects.

Alternatively, HRQoL studies may report no impact on the subjects' quality of life. However, examination of the distribution of the subjects' scores could reveal that some subjects had marked improvement. An equal number may show a decline and yet a third subset show no measurable impact. This could be just a normal variation around the mean or a marked difference in the impact of the treatment on different patients. If the latter, impact of the therapy on an individual patient would be difficult to predict unless further analysis can uncover some factors or patient characteristics highly associated with the low or high end results.

An increasingly popular way to quantify efficacy from a clinical trial is to report the 'numbers-needed-to-treat'.[23] This can be used for both beneficial and adverse events. Based on data from a clinical trial comparing auranofin versus placebo in arthritis patients,[24] we can estimate that a clinician will have to treat 10 patients with auranofin to obtain, on average, one patient who benefits from treatment (one who improves more than a quarter of their baseline level of activity and would not have improved without auranofin). Similar results could be reported for the 'number needed to treat' to move one person's HRQoL from a low to a moderate score.

Finally, it is probably unreasonable to expect that study discontinuation among patients in a trial is random with respect to HRQoL. A major reason individuals drop out of any trial are adverse reactions, deterioration of underlying condition, and lack of response to therapy. Caution must be used in interpreting any HRQoL results when there is an extensive amount of missing data and extreme caution is urged when there is differential missing data by therapy. When there are differential drop-out rates by treatment, the reader should be wary of *any* conclusions regarding comparative HRQoL.

What is the clinical significance (meaning) of the results?

> When I use a word, it means just what I choose it to mean—neither more nor less.
> *Lewis Carroll*

Clinicians may 'know' clinical significance for familiar tests when they see it and they may agree fairly well on what constitutes clinical significance, but they may not realize that their understanding of clinical significance of objective measures is based on their experience (or the experience of their teachers) with a large number of patients followed over time. Unfortunately, this experience is not available with HRQoL measures for most clinicians at this time. Faced with a completely new test and new units, interpretation of 'objective' measures are no easier than interpretation of HRQoL results, as witnessed by current controversy over the meaning of tests for prostate-specific antigen[25] and biological markers of bone turnover.[26]

What can be done to put results from HRQoL studies into context such that the relevance and impact of the changes seen can be understood by the clinician and the patient? One method is to 'anchor' the changes seen in HRQoL measures with other clinical changes or results.[27] The most commonly reported anchor is to relate changes seen on disease-specific questions to a global assessment of quality of life. A global question is one that asks about overall change, for example,

> Overall, has there been any change in your shortness of breath during your daily activities since the last time you saw us?[28]

The disease-specific measure might ask questions regarding changes in shortness of breath during multiple activities or query the patient regarding related symptoms such as wheezing and coughing. A minimal clinically significant change is then the summary score of the disease-specific questions which equates to a detectable change on a global (general) quality of life question. Thus, the changes seen in the longer disease-specific questionnaire are 'anchored' to reported changes in the overall disease state.

Why seek to anchor the disease-specific questionnaire? Why not use the single global? Longer questionnaires allow the definition of more levels, have greater reliability, and can represent individual domains of a health concept.[29] By anchoring to a more global response, the researcher shares the advantages of both – the interpretability of the single-item (global) question and the better psychometric properties of the longer questionnaire.

Changes seen with the same questionnaire in conjunction with a known therapeutic response can be used to assess the importance of changes with a new therapy. For example, patients with chronic heart failure who respond to digoxin report an improvement as measured by the chronic heart failure questionnaire of 1.6 to 2.1 points.[30] A change in the arthritis impact measurement scale (AIMS) with an experimental non-steroidal analgesic drug can be compared to changes on the same questionnaire reported by patients previously treated with injectable gold.[31] This anchor ties changes seen with other therapies to the clinician's understanding of the efficacy of digoxin.

These comparisons make clear the value of choosing validated questionnaires used previously in similar trials. In a summary of outcome measures for low back pain, Deyo et al.[32] conclude that

> Clinical research related to the treatment of back pain would be enormously facilitated if a small number of patient-oriented questionnaires become widely used. This would have the advantage of increasing the familiarity of clinicians with these measures, including the significance of a particular score or score change, and how they relate to other measures of clinical outcome.... We urge investigators not to 'reinvent the wheel' by developing new or *ad hoc* measures if more standard instruments can serve the same purpose.

Preference weighting by individuals can also calibrate and explain scores on selected questionnaires.[33] When preferences for various generic outcomes are reasonably consistent, interpretation of change from one health state to another is fairly straightforward. Hadorn and Uebersax[33] describe the calibration of a new brief questionnaire that divided patients into 16 disease state categories. States were consistently and appropriately ranked from 'no suffering' and 'no physical limitations' to 'severe suffering' and 'severe limitations'. Rankings were relatively unaffected by age, gender, ethnicity, or current quality of life or health status.

Responses of patients with a less well-studied or less well-understood condition can be put in context with responses of patients with more familiar diseases or conditions. From the analysis of the physical functioning scale administered to a large number of individuals, Brook *et al.*[34] concluded that a 10-point difference in the scale was equal to the effect of having chronic, mild osteoarthritis. The effect of an infectious disease, herpes zoster, at its peak is as devastating to the patient as such chronic diseases as congestive heart failure and clinical depression.[35] The rebound in HRQoL scores to values similar to those seen for the general population following resolution of zoster pain helps to interpret the meaning of these scores among zoster patients when used in a clinical trial setting.

Absolute scores on a questionnaire can also be related to health care utilization. Ware *et al.*[36] found that average predicted annual expenditures for mental health services were $10 and $34 for persons scoring in the highest and lowest third of the mental health index, respectively. This is more than a threefold difference between the two groups of individuals. While a change from a score in the lowest third to the highest third may not predict a decrease in annual expenditure for any particular person, the health utilization anchor is one that is easily understood by most clinicians.

Others have looked to calibrate changes or HRQoL results against reported life events.[34,37] This benchmarking or anchoring of changes in the less familiar HRQoL measures with more familiar life events could be valuable in the interpretation of HRQoL results. Unfortunately such comparisons are not easy. Whereas a change score may be available for every patient in the study, major life events are uncommon and their impact, like HRQoL, is not consistent between individuals. While intriguing, and having been suggested within several studies, full description of this calibration method is not available at this time.[37]

Prediction of future outcomes is another anchor that has been used. Marder *et al.*[38] describe levels at which changes on the brief psychiatric rating scale are predictive of a psychotic exacerbation within four weeks. Deyo and Inui[39] correlated changes in the sickness impact profile (SIP) with changes in more traditional measures of functional status in patients with arthritis. Changes can be related to disease progression. Spitz and Fries[40] benchmark the health assessment questionnaire (HAQ) with progression of disability with rheumatoid arthritis. For the first few years after diagnosis, disability, as measured by the HAQ, increases approximately 0.1 unit per year. Later, the rate slows to approximately 0.02 units per year. With a heterogeneous group of patients (with different starting values on the HAQ), it is less clear what a change of 0.1 may indicate. This latter example demonstrates not only the value of benchmarking with disease levels, but the non-linear relationship that often exists between scores and the anchor chosen to interpret them. Thus, the anchor may be valuable in interpreting changes in scores on the HAQ only when all patients in the study are newly diagnosed with rheumatoid arthritis.

The relevant anchor for the same questionnaire may need to be redefined for different populations. Just as one needs to validate the same questionnaire in different patient groups, one needs to find the appropriate anchor that will convey the significance of the observed change with therapy. Thus, alternative anchors may exist with the same questionnaire.

The common sense rule should also apply to any calibration. The resultant calibration and effects reported from the trial should make sense. While the HRQoL benefits of a new therapy should not go unheralded because of the unfamiliarity of the measure used, poorly documented claims of major effects do not further the field of quality of life research. For example, it is unlikely that the effects on HRQoL will be almost minimal for one antihypertensive agent, yet a second drug in the same class would have an impact similar to that of a mortgage foreclosure.[37]

> Let us not be too particular. It is better to have secondhand diamonds than none at all.
> *Mark Twain*

Exact correlation should never be expected for any calibration or benchmarking. If the benchmark or anchor were perfectly associated with the HRQoL measure, what would be the point of obtaining information on quality of life? Rather, these benchmarks are to provide general guidance in interpreting the value of the changes seen. Often benchmarks are available for only a proportion of the patients studied (life events, psychiatric exacerbations). An objective benchmark could never hope to capture the richness and variation of the construct of HRQoL. A benchmark is solely that – an aid in the interpretation of scores and changes. In the end, HRQoL measures are true outcomes in themselves and should never be viewed as measures of pathology or progression of underlying disease states. Who knows better whether a therapy has truly benefited a patient than the patients themselves?

> In a sense, patients' statements about how they feel about the quality of their own lives could be considered the gold standard itself. After all, can a patient think he has a good quality of life, and be wrong? Can he have a good quality of life without knowing it?[22]

Benchmarks should aid in the interpretation of results for health care providers, policy makers, researchers, and even patient groups themselves, but can not be expected to replace the HRQoL measure.

This is not to discourage the use of anchors in aiding the interpretation of HRQoL scores as these expressions often have more value than mere statistical significance. The ultimate goal of such anchors is to help the clinician gain familiarity with the more common measures. Over time and with increasing familiarity, the clinical significance of a particular level of change will become more obvious and less problematic to all.

> Everything's got a moral if only you can find it.
> *Lewis Carroll*

References

1. Calman, K.C. Quality of life in cancer patients—an hypothesis. *J. Med. Ethics*, 1984; **10**: 124–7.

2. Till, J.E. The Skeel article reviewed. *Oncology*, 1993; **7**: 66–7.
3. Stewart, A.L., Greenfield, S., Hays, R.D., Wells, K., Rogers, W.H., Berry, S.D., *et al.* Functional status and well-being of patients with chronic conditions: results from the Medical Outcomes Study. *J. Am. Med. Assoc.*, 1989; **262**: 907–13.
4. Ware, J.E. Jr, Snow, K.K., Kosinski, M., and Gandek, B. *SF-36 health survey: manual and interpretation guide*. Boston: The Health Institute, New England Medical Center, 1993.
5. Ware, J.E. Jr, Kosinski, M., and Keller, S.D. *SF-36 physical and mental health summary scales: a user's manual*. Boston: The Health Institute, New England Medical Center, 1994.
6. International Quality of Life Assessment Project. *Medical Outcomes Trust Bulletin*, 1995; **3**: 3.
7. The EuroQol Group. EuroQol—a new facility for the measurement of health-related quality of life. *Health Policy*, 1990; **16**: 199–208.
8. WHOQOL Group. Study protocol for the World Health Organization project to develop a quality of life assessment instrument (WHOQOL). *Qual. Life Res.*, 1993; **2**: 153–9.
9. Hyland, M.E. The validity of health assessments: resolving some recent differences. *J. Clin. Epidemiol.*, 1993; **9**: 1019–23.
10. Daut, R.L., Cleeland, C.S., and Flannery, R.S. Development of the Wisconsin brief pain questionnaire to assess pain in cancer and other diseases. *Pain*, 1983; **17**: 197–210.
11. Lydick, E., Epstein, R.S., Himmelberger, D., and White, C.J. Area under the curve: a metric for patient subjective responses in episodic diseases. *Qual. Life Res.*, 1995; **4**: 41–5.
12. Vickrey, B.G., Hays, R.D., Brook, R.H., and Rausch, R. Reliability and validity of the Katz adjustment scales in an epilepsy sample. *Qual. Life Res.*, 1992; **1**: 63–72.
13. Kirschner, B. and Guyatt, G. A methodological framework for assessing health indices. *J. Chron. Dis.*, 1985; **38**: 27–36.
14. Deyo, R.A., Diehr, P., and Patrick, D.L. Reproducibility and responsiveness of health status measures: Statistics and strategies for evaluation. *Control. Clin. Trial*, 1991; **12**: 142S–58S.
15. McHorney, C.A., Ware, J.E. Jr, and Raczek, A.E. The MOS 36-item short-form health survey (SF-36): II. Psychometric and clinical tests of validity in measuring physical and mental health constructs. *Med. Care*, 1993; **31**: 247–63.
16. Gill, T.M. and Feinstein, A.R. A critical appraisal of the quality of quality-of-life measurements. *J. Am. Med. Assoc.*, 1994; **272**: 619–25.
17. Ware, J.E. Jr. Content-based interpretation of health status scores. *Medical Outcomes Trust Bulletin*, 1994; **2**: 3.
18. Hyland, M.E. Selection of items and avoidance of bias in quality of life scales. *PharmacoEconomics*, 1992; **1**: 182–90.
19. Spilker, B. Standardisation of quality of life trials: an industry perspective. *PharmacoEconomics*, 1992; **1**: 73–5.
20. US Food and Drug Administration (Division of Drug Marketing, Advertising and Promotion). Draft principles for the review of pharmacoeconomic promotion. Workshop on comparing treatments: safety, effectiveness and cost-effectiveness, Washington, DC, March 23, 1995.

21. Yawn, B., Kurland, M., and Lydick, E. Item generation: the medium and the message. *Drug Inf. J.*, 1996; **30**: 961–963.
22. Hadorn, D.C., Sorensen, J., and Holte, J. Large-scale health outcomes evaluation: how should quality of life be measured? Part II—Questionnaire validation in a cohort of patients with advanced cancer. *J. Clin. Epidemiol.*, 1995; **48**: 619–29.
23. Wiffen, P.J. and Moore, R.A. Demonstrating effectiveness—the concept of numbers-needed-to-treat. *J. Clin. Pharm. Ther.*, 1996; **21**: 23–7.
24. Tugwell, P., Bombardier, C., Bell, M., Bennett, K., Bensen, W., Grace, E. *et al.* Current quality-of-life research challenges in arthritis relevant to the issue of clinical significance. *Control. Clin. Trial*, 1991; **12** (Suppl.): 217S–25S.
25. Walsh, P.C. Using prostate-specific antigen to diagnose prostate cancer: sailing in uncharted waters. *Ann. Intern. Med.*, 1993; **119**: 948–9.
26. Delmas, P.D. Biochemical markers of bone turnover. *J. Bone Miner. Res.*, 1993; **8** (Suppl. 2): S549–55.
27. Lydick, E. and Epstein, R.S. Interpretation of quality of life changes. *Qual. Life Res.*, 1993; **2**: 221–6.
28. Jaeschke, R., Singer, J., and Guyatt, G.H. Measurement of health status: ascertaining the minimal clinically important difference. *Control. Clin. Trial*, 1989; **10**: 407–15.
29. McHorney, C.A., Ware, J.E. Jr, Rogers, W., Raczek, A.E., and Lu, J.F.R. The validity and relative precision of MOS short- and long-form health status scores and Dartmouth COOP charts: results from the Medical Outcomes Study. *Med. Care*, 1992; **30**: MS253–65.
30. Guyatt, G.H., Sullivan, M.J.J., Fallen, E.L., Tihal, H., Rideout, E., Halcrow, S. *et al.* A controlled trial of digoxin in congestive heart failure. *Am. J. Cardiol.*,1988; **61**: 371–5.
31. Kazis, L.E., Anderson, J.J., and Meenan, R.F. Effect sizes for interpreting changes in health status. *Med. Care*, 1989; **27** (Suppl.): S178–89.
32. Deyo, R.A., Andersson, G., Bombardier, C., Cherkin, D.C., Keller, R.B., Lee. C.K. *et al.* Outcome measures for studying patients with low back pain. *Spine*, 1994; **18** (Suppl.): 2032S–6S.
33. Hadorn, D.C. and Uebersax, J. Large-scale health outcomes evaluation: how should quality of life be measured? Part I—Calibration of a brief questionnaire and a search for preference subgroups. *J. clin. Epidemiol.*, 1995; **48**: 607–18.
34. Brook, R.H., Ware, J.E. Jr, Rogers, W.H., Keeler, E.B., Davies, A.R., Donald, G.A. *et al.* Does free care improve adults' health? Results from a randomized controlled trial. *New Engl. J. Med.*, 1983; **309**: 1426–34.
35. Lydick, E., Epstein, R.S., Himmelberger, D., and White, C.J. Herpes zoster and quality of life: a self-limited disease with severe impact. *Neurology*, 1995; **45** (Suppl. 8): S52–3.
36. Ware, J.E. Jr, Manning, W.G. Jr, Duan, N., Wells, K.B., and Newhouse, J.P. Health status and the use of outpatient mental health services. *Am. Psychologist*, 1984; **39**: 1090–100.
37. Testa, M.A., Anderson, R.B., Nackley, J.F., Hollenberg, N.K., and the Quality-of-Life Hypertension Study Group. Quality of life and antihypertensive therapy in men: a comparison of captopril with enalapril. *New Engl. J. Med.*, 1993; **328**: 907–13.

38. Marder, S.R., Mintz, J., Van Putten, R., Lebell, M., Wirshing, W.C., Johnston-Cronk, K. Early prediction of relapse in schizophrenia: an application of receiver operating characteristics (ROC) methods. *Psychopharmacol. Bull.*, 1991; **27**: 79–82.

39. Deyo, R.A. and Inui, T.S. Toward clinical applications of health status measures: sensitivity of scales to clinically important changes. *Health Services Res.*, 1984; **19**: 275–89.

40. Spitz, P.W. and Fries, J.F. The present and future comprehensive outcome measures for rheumatic diseases. *Clin. Rheumatol.*, 1987; **6** (Suppl. 2): 105–11.

17 *Summarizing quality of life data using graphical methods*

Peter M. Fayers and David Machin

Introduction

A randomized clinical trial is the only form of scientific investigation that can be guaranteed to provide an unbiased comparison of the efficacy of different treatments, and QoL assessment is an essential component of this treatment evaluation. However, there are many problems regarding methods of analysis and interpretation of the results. Analysis of QoL data from clinical trials can be classified into two broad categories: confirmatory data analysis, and descriptive or exploratory data analysis. Confirmatory data analysis is used when a number of hypotheses are to be tested, and these should have been formulated before the study was commenced and should be specified in the clinical trial protocol. The testing of hypotheses can be based largely upon standard statistical significance testing, although there may be practical problems arising from the multidimensional nature of QoL assessments, the 'longitudinal' nature of the repeated measurements over time, and the occurrence of missing data for individual patients. Exploratory and descriptive data analyses, as their name suggests, are used to explore, clarify, describe, and interpret the QoL data. Frequently these analyses will reveal unexpected patterns in the data, for example suggesting differences in QoL with respect to treatment or other factors. However, exploratory analyses often consist of a large number of individual comparisons and significance tests, and some apparently strong effects may in fact arise out of chance fluctuations in the data – there is considerable variability and 'noise' when assessing QoL. Thus exploratory analyses may result in the generation of new hypotheses which should then be confirmed in subsequent studies; these exploratory analyses may lay the ground for future confirmatory analyses.

Because exploratory and descriptive analyses are less concerned with significance testing, graphical methods may be especially suitable. These largely visual methods have a number of advantages over purely numerical techniques. In particular, judicious use of graphics can succinctly summarize complex data which would otherwise require extensive tabulations, and can clarify and display the complex inter-relationships of QoL data. At the same time, graphics can be used to emphasize the high degree of variability in QoL data; this contrasts with numerical methods, which may often lead to results being presented in a format which causes readers to assume there is greater precision than the measurements warrant. Graphical techniques can highlight changes in QoL which are large and clinically significant, whilst making it clearer to readers which changes are unimportant (even though some clinically unimportant changes may represent statistically significant departures from zero).

Elements of good graphics

Before discussing the application of graphics to QoL data it is useful to review some principles of good graphical display. One consequence of the ready avail-ability of graphics from most analysis packages has been the proliferation of bad graphical display, since it is far too easy to produce inappropriate histograms, three-dimensional bar charts, and colourful pie charts. On the other hand, current computing facilities and modern publishing methods do offer unrivalled facilities for the production of extensive and high quality graphics.

What, then, are the basic principles of good graphics? One excellent source of background information is the now classic book by Tufte, *The visual display of quantitative information.*[1] Tufte provides a readable history of graphical practice, a wonderful display of good and poor plots and charts, and useful rules that should at all times be observed. In particular, five principles in the theory of data graphics are advocated as producing substantial improvements in graphical design; these principles apply to many graphics, and yield a series of design options through cycles of graphical revision and editing. These are

- above all else show data
- maximize the data–ink ratio
- erase non-data-ink
- erase redundant data-ink
- revise and edit.

Example data

Throughout this chapter we will illustrate the methods using data from the UK Medical Research Council (MRC) trial CH02, which compared conventional fractionation radiotherapy against continuous hyperfractionated accelerated radiotherapy (CHART) in patients with non-metastatic head and neck cancer. Since, at the time of writing, the final results of the study have not been published, the analyses presented here will focus upon one treatment arm, the patients receiving conventional radiotherapy. The QoL of these patients was assessed using the Rotterdam Symptom Checklist[2,3] (RSCL) and the Hospital Anxiety and Depression Scale (HADS).[4] Patients were scheduled to complete the question-naires pre-treatment (baseline), on days 21 and 28 during treatment, and then after treatment at six weeks post-randomization, six months and six-monthly until 30 months. The analyses included 237 patients, of which 168 (71 per cent) were male. Fifty-three per cent of patients had early (T2) stage disease, 39 per cent advanced (T3) disease, and 15 per cent more advanced (T4) disease.

The HADS scale[4] consists of 14 questions (items), which are first standardized so that 0 is the most favourable state and 3 is the least favourable. Seven of these items are then summated to produce the anxiety scale, and the other seven constitute the depression scale. Thus each scale ranges from 0 to 21.

The RSCL[2,3] consists of 30 questions on four-point scales ('not at all', 'a little', 'quite a bit', 'very much'), a question about activities of daily living, and a global question about 'your quality of life during the past week' with seven categories. It not only contains questions relating to general psychological distress but, as its name implies, it also places emphasis upon the symptoms and side-effects which are commonly experienced by patients. The RSCL has been widely used in European cancer clinical trials, and the MRC Cancer Working Parties have incorporated it in a number of their randomized trials.

Simple graphical summaries

Perhaps the simplest summaries of all are histogram and bar charts, which show the frequency distribution of the data. These are often used for the initial inspection of data, and to establish basic characteristics of the data. For example, prior to using a *t*-test one ought to check whether the data are distributed symmetrically and whether they appear to follow a normal distribution. Thus Fig. 17.1, which shows a histogram of the anxiety subscale, is a commonly seen method of displaying

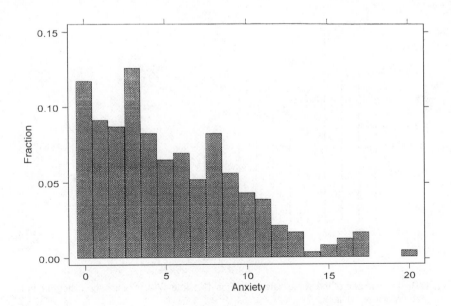

Fig. 17.1   Histogram of HADS anxiety levels (data from the CHART head and neck trial).

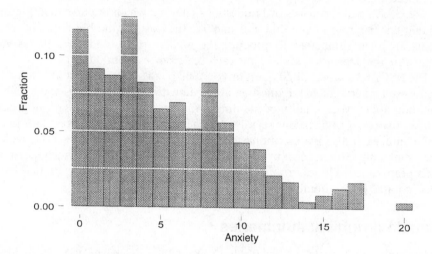

Fig. 17.2 A modified histogram, showing the same data as in Fig. 17.1. The shading is less dense, axis lines have been removed, and horizontal lines indicate 2.5, 5, 7.5, 10, and 12.5 per cent.

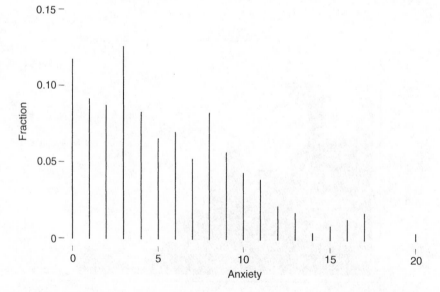

Fig. 17.3 A spike plot of the same data as in Figs 17.1 and 17.2, in which the histogram bars have been replaced by lines.

information. However, although this is a simple graphical display, there are a number of variations which may improve the presentation. Thus Fig. 17.2 shows the same information, but has added blank 'lines' making it visually easier to assess the height of the histogram bars. In addition, the unnecessary axis frame has been removed, and less dense shading used. These minor changes, which merely follow Tufte's precepts, greatly enhance the presentation.

However, many purists in graphical design argue that this can readily be improved by yet further minimizing non-data ink. Figure 17.3 contains the same level of information, and they argue that it is a preferable display because it is not only simpler but also avoids the arbitrary choice of bar widths. This form of display is sometimes called a spike plot. In addition to displaying data efficiently whilst minimizing non-informative ink, spike plots can be used when the equivalent histogram would have too many bars. For some forms of data, provided the sample size is adequately large, it might be useful to make spike plots of variables in which there are hundreds of categories instead of the 21 which are relevant for the HADS scale.

Comparison of two groups

Most clinical trials compare two or more treatments, and many other investigations and analyses are also of a comparative nature. Thus graphs comparing two groups are particularly common in publications. Using our data on anxiety, we shall consider such a comparison between males and females. This comparison is of interest since it has been suggested that there are differences in levels of anxiety experienced by patients according to both age and sex.

One common way of displaying the differences between two treatments or two groups of patients is a bar chart. A typical example is shown in Fig. 17.4, which displays the mean levels of anxiety for males and females, according to age group. Note that we again use blank lines to facilitate reading across the bars. This time these lines are especially helpful, since otherwise it is far more difficult to compare non-adjacent groups. Figure 17.5, however, in accordance with the above principles of good graphics, uses much less ink to show the same data. Here the lower unbroken line represents the males, and the upper line the females. The horizontal axis shows age. This display is not merely simpler than that of Fig. 17.4, but in addition it conveys its visual information far more vividly: it is easier to see the striking relationship between sex and anxiety. This figure could be further adapted to provide confidence intervals (CI) about each of the eight plotted points. When the groups are well spaced apart, as here, CIs can easily be distinguished and contribute useful information about the precision of the estimates; in general, however, the lines may be closer together or even overlapping, and CIs may become difficult to read. Since plots like Fig. 17.5 are so effective, it is curious that many publications continue to use the style of Fig. 17.4 instead of these simpler line plots.

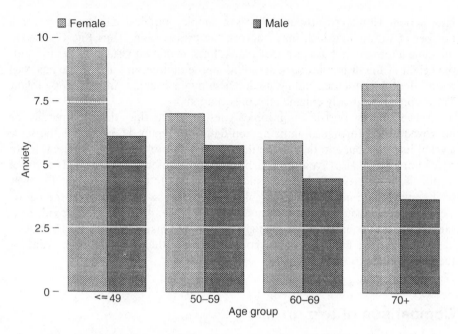

Fig. 17.4   Bar chart showing anxiety divided by age group and sex.

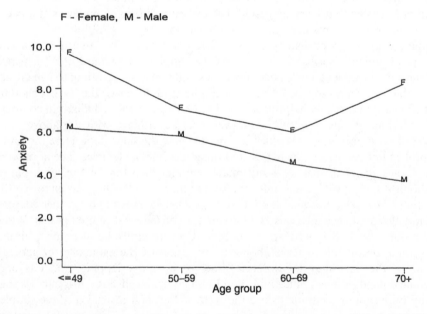

Fig. 17.5   Line plot of the same data as in Fig. 17.4 – a visually superior method of displaying anxiety by age group and sex.

Association of variables

When showing the association between two variables the simplest graphic is perhaps the scatter plot, as shown for age versus anxiety in Fig. 17.6. In this example we have superimposed a rangefinder box plot. The central cross marks the point of intersection of the two medians, and the lines all extend to cover the 25 per cent to 75 per cent quartile range. The outer lines show boundaries after excluding the extreme outliers.

Instead of a rangefinder box plot, an alternative addition to the scatter plot might be the regression line of anxiety for a given age. This could be more relevant whenever one is interested in the predictive aspect of a relationship: can we predict the expected mean anxiety level, for a given age?

However, it may be convenient to examine the relationship between one variable, such as anxiety, and another grouped variable, such as age group. This then leads to a variety of other potential graphics. Figure 17.7 shows a box plot (sometimes called a box-and-whisker plot) in which, for each age group, the median value is at the centre of the box, and the 25th and 75th percentiles are indicated by the edges of the box. In addition, there are 'whiskers' either side of the box, marking the range of the data after excluding extreme outliers. The dots underneath each box and whisker are a one-dimensional scatter plot, and are a convenient method of including information corresponding to histograms. Each dot represents one observation, and multiple observations with the same value are

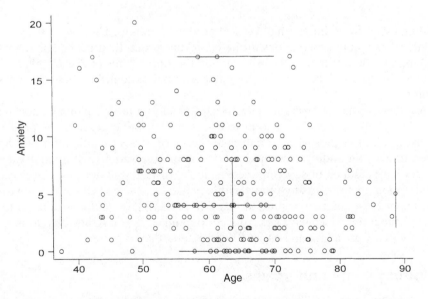

Fig. 17.6   A scatter plot with a rangefinder box plot. The central cross marks the intersection of the two medians, and the lines mark the interquartile range (25 and 75 per cent quartiles of each variable).

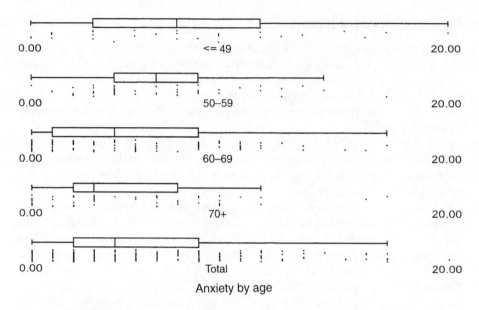

Anxiety by age

Fig. 17.7   Box plot with a one-dimensional scatter plot. The centre of each box indicates the median of the data, and the two edges mark the quartiles (25 and 75 per cent points). The 'whiskers' around the boxes extend to include all observations except extreme outliers. Below each plot is a one-dimensional scatter plot; in this, each observation is represented by a small dot.

distinguished by adding a small vertical random variation. Thus one can see that there are far more observations in the 60–69 age group than in the less than 49 group, and that although the whisker for the upper limit of the 60–69 group extends far to the right, there are very few data points contributing to this upper whisker.

Another, rather simpler yet effective graphic, is the dot plot as shown in Fig. 17.8. This is similar in concept to a scatter plot, but overcomes the problem of using a scatter plot when variables are grouped; if a straight scatter plot had been drawn, the multiple occurrences of many observations with equal values would have resulted in superimposed symbols. Instead, the dot plot places each observation adjacent to any others with equal value, thereby emphasizing where the majority of observations lie. In many respects the dot plot is analogous to a set of histograms which have been rotated to stand on side; it is, however, arguably more visually attractive and easier to understand than a histogram.

Plotting items and scales

One fundamental decision to be made when graphing aggregated data from QoL instruments is whether to plot the percentage of patients satisfying some characteristic, or whether to plot a summary statistic such as the mean or median.

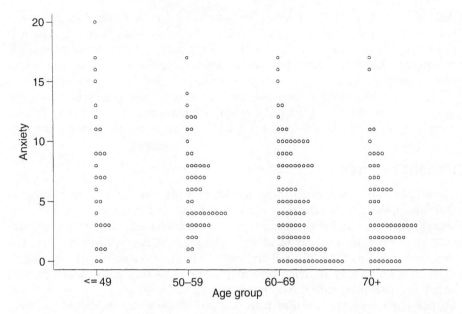

Fig. 17.8 Dot plot – a cross between a histogram and a scatter plot with grouped observations.

The three principal choices are to

(1) plot median scores of items and scales

(2) plot mean scores of items and scales

(3) plot the percentage of patients with values exceeding a certain level.

The RSCL and the HADS are typical QoL instruments. Many instruments use raw items with four-point categories[2–5], often with labels such as 'not at all', 'a little', 'quite a bit', 'very much' for the categories. Also, many items have strongly skewed distributions (asymmetrically distributed); for items representing rare symptoms and side-effects or infrequent problems, the majority of patients may report 'not at all' for; while for items concerning more common problems there may be a large proportion of patients reporting 'very much'. As a consequence, it is not uncommon for as many as half the patients to report the maximum for some items, and the minimum for others. Therefore the medians for these items would be the 'floor' or 'ceiling' values of either 1 or 4, which contains limited information for plotting. For such data it is better to plot mean values rather than medians, even though confidence intervals and significance tests should be based upon distribution-free methods and may make use of the median in preference to the mean.

An alternative is to classify patients into two (or possibly more) categories such as 'good status'/'poor status', or 'case requiring treatment'/'non-case', and use percentages. For example, considering an assessment of pain (on, say, a four-point scale of 1 = 'not at all', 2 = 'a little', 3 = 'quite a bit', 4 = 'very much'), one might either plot the mean pain score over time, or the percentage of patients reporting serious pain (e.g. pain categories 3 and 4). The concept of percentage plots could be extended to handle more than two categories, for example by superimposing plots corresponding to the percentage of patients in each of the four categories.

The figures that follow therefore use means and percentages in preference to medians. In addition, in accordance with common recommendations,[2,6] items have been standardized to scales of 0 to 100 for most of the plots in this chapter.

Patient profiles

The graphics described so far are applicable to many types of data, not merely to QoL measurements. One form of presentation that is particularly useful in QoL analyses is the profile plot. This attempts to display many dimensions simultaneously, divided by a grouping variable. An example is given in Fig. 17.9. The mean values of 16 of the RSCL items are shown, divided according to sex. These items cover a variety of symptoms and side-effects, such as lack of appetite, irritability, tiredness, nausea, vomiting, pain, difficulty sleeping, and so on. From Fig. 17.9 it is easy to see that there appears to be a sex difference for most items, with females scoring worse (higher) than males. A few items such as

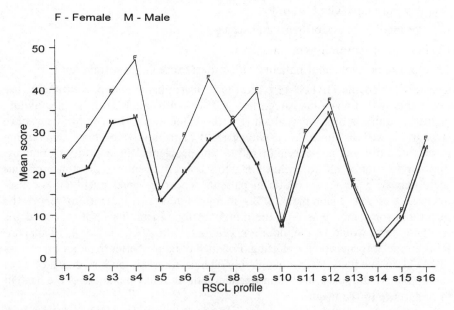

Fig. 17.9 A profile plot, with mean values of RSCL items s1–s16 transformed to a scale of 0 to 100. Most items show a difference between the two sexes, with females scoring higher (worse).

s5 (sore muscles), s10 (nausea), and s14 (vomiting) are equally low for both groups, since these symptoms were rarely experienced by this group of patients. Pain (s8) was more frequent, but experienced equally by males and females.

The profile plot could be extended further by adding confidence intervals about each point. This would make it easier to decide whether the observed differences are likely to be statistically significant rather than due to chance. However, it is important to remember that the sampling unit is the patient, and that most of the items are all inter-correlated; therefore any significance tests are not independent. One slight disadvantage to profile plots is that there may be a tendency for naïve readers of such plots to assume that the different dimensions may be compared (for example, in Fig. 17.9 to think that s1, lack of appetite, is less or 'better' than s3 and s4, tiredness and worrying). Readers might think this by analogy with the more familiar line plots in which lines join successive values of the same variable and where an upward shift in a line would indeed imply a change towards higher values. In general, however, items on QoL questionnaires will not have been scaled uniformly, and it is meaningless to describe whether one item or scale takes higher (or lower) values than other items and scales.

Profile plots are a convenient way to summarize changes in many dimensions, but can only handle a single, grouped explanatory variable. They may be particularly useful when a consistent and unambiguous pattern is seen across successive groups, such as successive age groups.

Incomplete longitudinal data

QoL measurements are frequently collected at repeated times before, during, and after treatment. Two of the most basic methods of graphical display of QoL over time are plots of percentages and plots of medians. However, this overlooks the problems of incompleteness of the data. When assessing QoL in clinical trials there may be large amounts of missing data, due to non-compliance, and also attrition of data caused by rapidly diminishing patient numbers with too few patients having a complete set of assessments, especially over the immediate period close to death. Analyses can be seriously distorted if the problems of incomplete data are ignored. Therefore in the remainder of this chapter we shall concentrate upon methods which can reveal patterns and consequences of missing data. Clearly the methods of Fig. 17.4 and Fig. 17.5 could be used if all one is interested in is displaying data over time; instead of age, one would use time. Also, clearly one can plot mean values, medians (if scales have more than a few categories), or percentages (such as 'percentage of patients with QoL score greater than 50', or some similar cut-off point). Such plots appear frequently in publications of QoL data – or, indeed, in publications of many types of longitudinal medical data. One example is in Fig. 17.10, taken from the MRC trial of palliative radiotherapy with two fractions (F2) or a single fraction (F1), in poor performance patients with inoperable non-small-cell lung cancer.[7,8] This shows the percentage of patients reporting, on a daily basis, dysphagia levels of 2 or worse (where 2 represents 'mild soreness when swallowing').

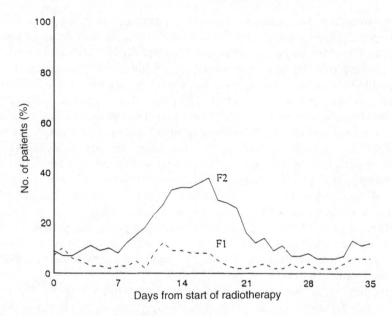

Fig. 17.10 A trial comparing two radiotherapy regimens for non-small-cell lung cancer, which used a daily diary card to assess QoL. There is a large difference in the percentage of patients reporting dysphagia (data from MRC Lung Cancer Working Party[7]).

Plotting all available data

One can regard each assessment separately, and plot all available data at each time point. Thus one might plot or tabulate the results across all patients at the baseline time point, using all completed baseline forms, and in the same analyses use all available forms for each of the other time points. This leads to different patients being used at each time point, according to whether or not they completed the questionnaire at that time. The main advantages of this method are its simplicity and the fact that it uses all available data. However, there are potentially serious problems: since different patients and different numbers of patients are used at each time point, the comparisons across assessments may be biased. Bias might arise if, for example, the more seriously ill patients tend to complete fewer forms. However, this not only affects graphical interpretation but also any general longitudinal analysis. One form of plot that is useful in examining attrition and departures from the assessment schedule simultaneously is to plot the QoL data for all patients and for all time points at which assessments are made. Thus Fig. 17.11 consists of scatter plots of the HADS depression scores for each patient of the CHART trial, plotted against the actual date of assessment. The critical values for clinical depression ('cases') and borderline depression scores have been indicated.

This information could also have been summarized on a single plot – Fig. 17.12. This plot indicates the attrition following the baseline QoL values as the density of the cloud of points reduces as time progresses. The increasing departures from

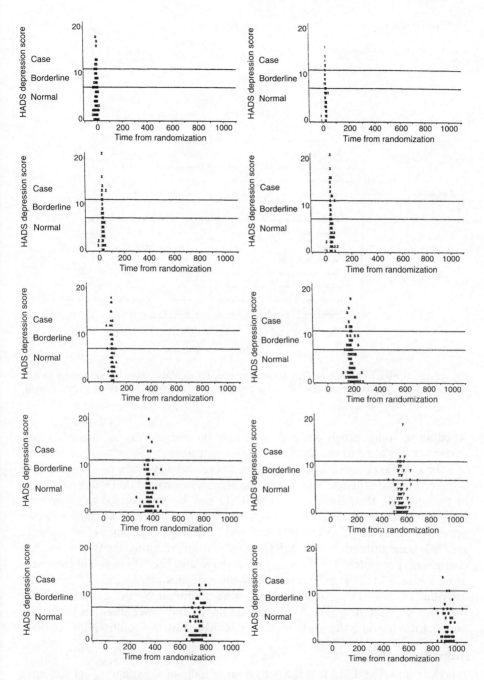

Fig. 17.11 Scatter plot of the HADS depression score for patients, against time of assessment, for patients receiving only conventional radiotherapy (data from the CHART head and neck trial).

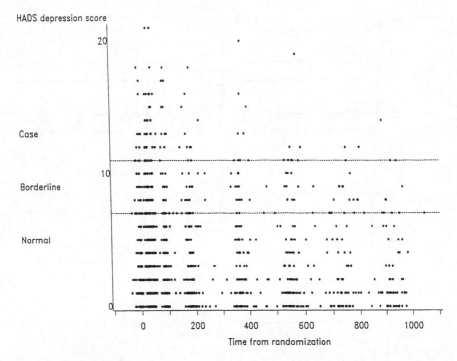

Fig. 17.12 Scatter plot of the HADS depression score for patients, against time of assessment, for patients receiving only conventional radiotherapy (data from the CHART head and neck trial).

schedule as time progresses are indicated by the increasing scatter of the assessments relative to the scheduled assessment times.

If the variation about the schedules is not regarded as serious, or if windows are imposed around schedule dates to define those assessments that can be included in the analysis, then the data of Fig. 17.12 can be summarized as a series of histograms for each scheduled assessment point. However, a more compact presentation can be given by using box and whisker plots in place of histograms; this has been utilized by the MRC Lung Cancer Working Party[9] to describe changes in time of RSCL values and which have also been divided into treatment groups (Fig. 17.13). The observed minimum and maximum values of the RSCL activities of daily living (ADL) score were indicated by the extremities (the 'whiskers') of the diagram. As usual, the upper and lower quartiles define the limits of the box and the median value is indicated by the point within the box.

Individual profiles

It is clear from Fig. 17.12 that the behaviour of individual patients is not indicated although if the numbers of patients was very small individual plotting symbols for each patient could be utilized and hence individual profiles identified and examined. To give some idea as to the variation in individual profiles, Fig. 17.14

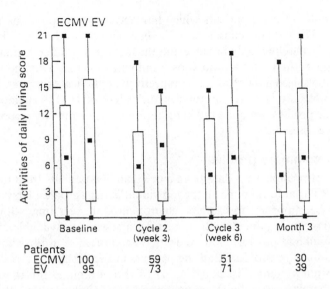

Fig. 17.13   Box plots of activities of daily living (ADL) of the RSCL at scheduled assessment times, by form of Chemotherapy allocated (ECMV or EV) (data from MRC Lung Cancer Working Party[9]).

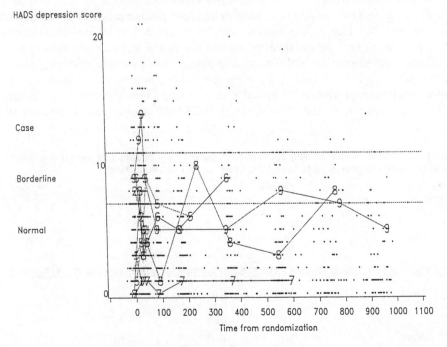

Fig. 17.14   Individual profiles of HADS depression score in selected patients, superimposed on the data of Fig. 17.12 (data from the CHART head and neck trial).

gives the profiles of eight patients which have been superimposed on the clouds of Fig. 17.12. The patients chosen were the first patients in the data file who had completed only baseline; only baseline and the first (post-randomization) HADS; only baseline, the first, and second (post-randomization) HADS; and so on. The plotting symbols used are 0, 1, 2, ..., 7 respectively, to indicate this fact. It is worth noting that not only is there variation in the values of HADS anxiety for these patients, their profiles are quite different, as are some of the completion times of the respective assessments.

Examining summary profiles

It is clearly not possible with data from more than 200 patients from the one arm of the CHART trial to examine all the individual patient profiles. However, it will nevertheless be important to examine changes in QoL over time, although it is recognized that those patients with the fewest assessments available may be the most severely ill and possibly close to death. A compromise in this situation is to present the summary profiles of all the patients in the groups represented by the individual profiles summarized in Fig. 17.14. For example, for those patients completing baseline plus four consecutive HADS (indicated by the plotting symbol 4 in Fig. 17.14), data may be summarized at each scheduled assessment. Table 17.1 shows the mean HADS anxiety score for patients from the MRC Lung Cancer Working Party trial comparing two forms of chemotherapy.[9] Patients are divided according to number of HADS questionnaires completed. The means of those 12 patients completing baseline plus first four assessments only is highlighted within the table. This profile suggests that the mean level of anxiety drops during the active treatment period then increases again at the last assessment.

These means, together with the corresponding values for the remaining profile groups, can then be plotted again superimposed on the clouds of Fig. 17.12. The plots (not shown) appear to be fairly consistent in that there is no systematic difference (relative to the total variation in HADS anxiety score) between the

Table 17.1   Mean HADS anxiety score at each assessment stratified by the number of assessments completed (data from MRC Lung Cancer Working Party[9])

HADS post-baseline	Number of patients	Baseline								
		0	1	2	3	4	5	6	7	8
0	72	7.99								
1	26	6.04	6.27							
2	34	6.62	5.29	4.65						
3	21	6.67	5.52	5.00	5.76					
4	12	6.17	3.75	3.33	3.25	5.42				
5	7	9.14	7.29	7.86	8.29	5.71	7.14			
6	10	6.80	4.90	5.80	5.50	5.70	5.10	4.50		
7	7	4.43	4.00	5.71	4.29	5.00	4.57	4.57	6.29	
8	13	7.00	6.15	6.69	7.23	4.77	5.77	6.77	7.46	6.92
All patients	n	260	185	164	119	88	65	55	40	27
	Mean	7.03	5.55	5.48	5.49	5.58	5.48	5.44	6.00	6.59

different profile groups. It seems reasonable therefore to take the next step and calculate an all-patient average for each time point (final row of Table 17.1). Figure 17.15 shows such a plot for the CHART trial, with the pattern of HADS depression scores as expressed by these pooled data. This suggests that therapy has been successful in reducing the mean HADS depression score, but this then gradually rises to baseline levels as time progresses.

The number of patients contributing to each point in this graph could also be shown beneath the time axis and 95 per cent confidence intervals for the mean at each schedule added. These would emphasize the increasing uncertainty attached to the values of each point with increasing patient attrition.

A final step in this graphical analysis will be to divide the data into treatment groups, calculate the means corresponding to those of the final row of Table 17.1 and plot these means for each treatment group separately (see Hopwood et al.,[10] Fig. 17.4).

As noted by Coates et al.[11] there are occasions when QoL measures may be indicative of prognosis. These profiles could differ between those patients who provide only early follow-up from those who provide detailed follow-up over a prolonged period since one is gradually left with the better prognosis patients over time. Indeed, Fig. 17.16 shows that if such profiles are summarized by shifting the

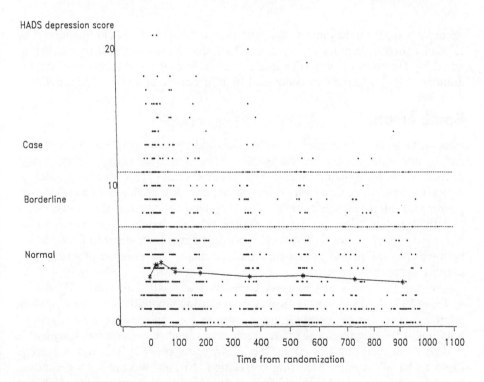

Fig. 17.15 Mean HADS depression score calculated for all patients completing each assessment, superimposed on the data of Fig. 17.12 (data from the CHART head and neck trial).

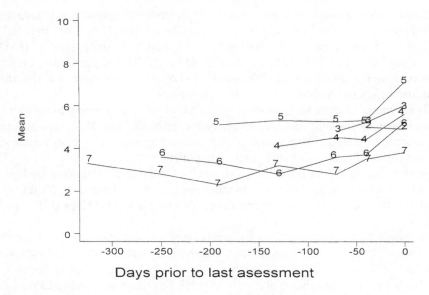

Days prior to last asessment

Fig. 17.16   Mean HADS depression score, reverse plotted from date of last QoL observation.

reference point from the date of randomization to the date of last information (close to death) then, at least for these patients, QoL deteriorates as death approaches, as noted by Herndon *et al.*[12] The integers used as plotting symbols indicate the number of QoL assessments completed by that particular group of patients.

Some errors

Finally, we finish with a naïve example of misleading use of graphics. A common – and, at first sight, apparently reasonable – form of analysis is to compare change in QoL scores for patients against their baseline values. Thus one might seek to determine whether patients who start with a poor QoL are likely to have an even poorer QoL after treatment, or whether they tend to improve. Hence one might plot the baseline score against the change between baseline and month three. A typical plot is shown in Fig. 17.17, showing a moderate degree of correlation between the change and the baseline measurement. One example of such a plot may be found in Rose *et al.*[13]

However, this plot is meaningless. Consider Fig. 17.18. This is broadly similar to Fig. 17.17. And yet Fig. 17.18 was drawn using computer generated random numbers! The reason becomes more apparent if one uses simple algebraic notation: if the first (baseline) measurement is x, and the second measurement is y, then we are plotting $(x-y)$ against x. Since x appears in both terms, there is likely to be a naturally occurring correlation. In fact, if x and y are random numbers, each completely independent of the other, then the expected correlation can be shown to be 0.4.

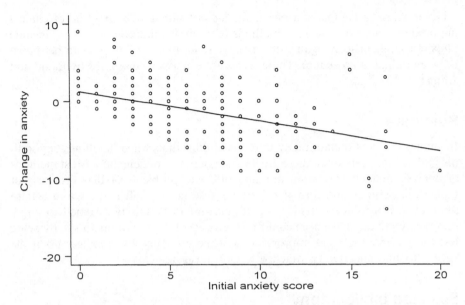

Fig. 17.17 Scatter plot of change in anxiety level against baseline measurement.

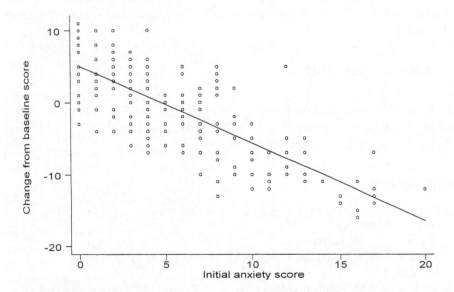

Fig. 17.18 Scatter plot of 'change in anxiety level' against baseline measurement – using randomly generated numbers in place of the second measurement.

Nevertheless, a comparison of change against initial value may be of clinical importance, and more rigorous methods of analysis are available. These include plots of change in score against the average score $(x+y)/2$, which can be shown to be an unbiased procedure. These issues are extensively discussed by Bland and Altman.[14,15]

Summary

In summary, there remain many unresolved difficulties when handling longitudinal QoL assessments when there are large amounts of missing data. Most methods of analysis and interpretation are susceptible to problems of bias. The use of numerical methods and formal hypothesis testing may lull readers into a false sense of security since statistical significance might be falsely assumed to imply that the hypotheses have been confirmed or rejected. Graphical methods, by being less formal, may be more appropriate and more readily lay emphasis upon the variability and uncertainty attached to QoL measurements.

Selected bibliography

Numerous papers have been published about graphical methods, and modern computer software is increasingly incorporating a variety of techniques. Excellent recent books include those by Edward Tufte,[1,16] William Cleveland,[17,18] and Anders Wallgren,[19] whilst the earlier books by Chambers[20] and Hoaglin[21] remain excellent.

Acknowledgements

The graphics in this chapter were produced using the packages SAS[22] and STATA.[23] The data used for illustrative purposes are from the Medical Research Council CH02 head and neck cancer CHART trial, and from trials of the Medical Research Council Lung Cancer Working Party.

References

1. Tufte, E.R. *The visual display of quantitative information.* Cheshire, Connecticut: Graphics Press, 1983.
2. de Haes, J.C.J.M., Olschewski, M., Fayers, P.M., *et al. The Rotterdam Symptom Checklist (RSCL): a manual.* Groningen: Northern Centre for Healthcare Research, 1996.
3. de Haes, J.C.J.M., van Knippenberg, F.C.E., and Neijt, J.P. Measuring psychological and physical distress in cancer patients: structure and application of the Rotterdam Symptom Checklist. *Br. J. Cancer,* 1990; **62**: 1034–8.
4. Zigmond, A.S. and Snaith, R.P. The Hospital Anxiety and Depression Scale. *Acta Psychiatr. Scand.,* 1983; **67**: 361–70.

5. Aaronson, N.K., Ahmedzai, S., Bergman, B., *et al*. The European Organization for Research and Treatment of Cancer QLQ-C30: a quality-of-life instrument for use in international clinical trials in oncology. *J. Natl. Cancer Inst.*, 1993; **85**: 365–76.
6. Fayers, P.M., Aaronson, N.K., Bjordal, K., and Sullivan, M. *EOTC QLQ-C30 scoring manual*. Brussels: EORTC, 1995.
7. Medical Research Council Lung Cancer Working Party. A Medical Research Council (MRC) randomized trial of palliative radiotherapy with 2 fractions or a single fraction in patients with inoperable non-small-cell lung-cancer (NSCLC) and poor performance status. *Br. J. Cancer*, 1992; **65**: 934–41.
8. Fayers, P.M. MRC Quality of life studies using a daily diary card – practical lessons learned from cancer trials. *Qual. Life Res.*, 1995; **4**: 343–52.
9. Medical Research Council Lung Cancer Working Party. Randomized trial of four-drug vs less intensive two-drug chemotherapy in the palliative treatment of patients with small-cell lung cancer (SCLC) and poor prognosis. *Br. J. Cancer*, 1996; **73**: 406–13.
10. Hopwood, P., Stephens, R.J., and Machin, D., for the Medical Research Council Lung Cancer Working Party. Approaches to the analysis of quality of life data: experiences gained from a Medical Research Council Lung Cancer Working Party palliative chemotherapy trial. *Qual. Life Res.*, 1994; **3**: 339–52.
11. Coates, A., Porzsolt, F., and Osoba, D. Quality of life in oncology practice: Prognostic value of EORTC QLQ-C30 scores in patients with advanced malignancy. *Eur. J. Cancer*, 1997; **33**: 1025–1030.
12. Herndon, II J.E., Fleisjman, S., Kosty, M.P., and Green, M.R. A longitudinal study of quality of life in advanced non-small cell lung cancer CALGB 8931. *Controlled Clin. Trials*, 1997; **18**: 286–300.
13. Rose, K.J., Derry, P.A., Wiebe, S., and McLaclan, R.S. Determinants of health-related quality of life after temporal lobe epilepsy surgery. *Qual. Life Res.*, 1996; **5**: 395–402.
14. Bland, J.M. and Altman, D.G. Statistical methods for assessing agreement between two methods of clinical measurement. *Lancet*, 1986; **i**: 307–10.
15. Bland, J.M. and Altman, D.G. Comparing methods of measurement: why plotting difference against standard method is misleading. *Lancet*, 1995; **346**: 1085–7.
16. Tufte, E.R. *Envisioning information*. Cheshire, Connecticut: Graphics Press, 1990.
17. Cleveland, W.S. *The elements of graphing data,* (Revised edn). Summit, New Jersey: Hobart Press, 1994.
18. Cleveland, W.S. *Visualizing data*. Summit, New Jersey: Hobart Press, 1993.
19. Wallgren, A., Persson, R., and Jorner, U. *Graphing statistics and data: creating better charts*. Newbury Park, CA: Sage, 1996.
20. Chambers, J.M., Cleveland, W.S., Kleiner, B., and Tukey, P.A. *Graphical methods for data analysis*. New York: Chapman and Hall, 1983.
21. Hoaglin, D.C., Mosteller, F., and Tukey, J.W. *Exploring data tables, trends and shapes*. New York: John Wiley, 1985.
22. SAS Inst Inc. *SAS/STAT user's guide, version 6*, (Vols 1 and 2). Cary, North Carolina: SAS Inst Inc, 1996.
23. StataCorp. *Stata reference manual: release 4.0*. College Station, TX, USA: Stata Corporation, 1995.

18 *Guidelines for reporting results of quality of life assessments in clinical trials*

Maurice J. Staquet, Richard A. Berzon, David Osoba, and David Machin

In recent years, the number of clinical trials incorporating measurement of health-related quality of life has substantially increased. However, due to the unfamiliarity of clinical researchers, editors of medical journals, and regulatory agencies with a field which has been until recently concentrated in the social sciences, several aspects of publications relating to quality of life assessment in clinical trials need to be improved. Important methodological issues related to the conduct and reporting of quality of life (QoL) studies have been published.[1-9] These papers show that weaknesses of the published reports of QoL clinical trials have been the lack of information on specific items such as the psychometric properties of the instruments and the handling of missing data, especially through patient attrition. Some of these deficiencies could have been corrected by more rigorous reporting.

The purpose of this chapter is to suggest general guidelines for the reporting of clinical trials which include a quality of life measurement. These proposals are intended for researchers reporting a new study as well as for those who are asked to critically evaluate the published reports. These guidelines are general in nature and, therefore, constitute a minimal set. More specific details may need to be added for particular diseases and types of treatments.

A QoL-specific checklist designed to assist authors is provided as an appendix. In addition, more general checklists[10-13] which are applicable to various types of clinical trials could be relevant.

Title and authors

The title must be concise and informative. Authors and their current primary affiliations should be referenced in conformity with the journal style. Appropriate keywords (such as the ones listed in the Index Medicus or in the Psychological Abstracts) should be given for indexing purposes.

The sponsor(s) of the research, if any, are to be disclosed as a footnote either here or at the end of the article.

Abstract

The abstract should present the purpose of the trial, the methods, the key results, and the essential conclusions.

Introduction

The objective of the trial needs to be stated in detail and its rationale must be supported with a comprehensive review of the literature relevant to the disease or the treatment of interest. Selective references supporting each statement should be provided.

The natural history of the disease and its treatment should be described succinctly so that it is clear why QoL is being assessed.

The pretrial hypotheses for QoL assessment must be stated briefly including which domains or scales were expected to show a difference between treatment arms. The author's definition of QoL should be presented. It must be disclosed here if the QoL trial reported is part of another research (e.g. a pilot study, a therapeutic trial, etc.).

Materials and methods

Population and sample

A description of the patient population, including the trial inclusion and exclusion criteria, is mandatory. The population sample must be described with appropriate demographic data, for example age, gender, and ethnicity depending on the context. Other variables, such as the clinical and mental status, if they are likely to alter the ability of the patient to answer a questionnaire, should also be included.

It is important to indicate how and from where the patients were recruited to the trial. For instance: indicate if the sample was random or one of convenience, the number of centres involved, and whether informed consent was obtained. If a subset of the total sample size is deemed to be sufficient for the QoL part of the trial, the method used to select the patients in the subset must be explained.

QoL instrument selection

The justification for the selection of a health profile (descriptive) and/or a patient-preference (utility) approach for the QoL assessment as well as of a particular questionnaire should be given. If the QoL instrument(s) is not well known or new, it must be described in detail and the psychometric properties (floor effects, ceiling effects, reliability, validity, and responsiveness to change) should be summarized with references. The rationale for creating a new instrument and the method by which the items were created is indispensable. For specific instruments, an indication as to whether or not the psychometric properties were established in the same type of population as the trial subjects is essential.

The time frame over which the subject has to assess their responses to the items of the questionnaire (e.g. yesterday, past week, or during the previous cycle of chemotherapy) needs to be indicated. If this varies from question to question, the details must be provided.

The method by which the instrument was administered (self-report, face-to-face interview, interviewer-supervised, telephone, proxy, other) must be supplied. It is important to give details of how the responses are scored, preferably by reference to a published scoring manual or other available source document. Any departure from such procedure should be detailed and justified. Information on how to interpret the scores is necessary, for example do higher scores indicate better or worse functioning or symptoms.

If appropriate, information on the process by which the measure was adapted for cross-cultural administration is to be given.

Sources relevant to the development and format of the QoL instrument(s) chosen should be included in the references. When an instrument (or item or scale) is being used in a new population or disease from that in which it was originally developed, the psychometric properties of the instrument in the new context must be reported.

Trial size

If a comparative trial is reported, the effect size planned to detect a difference between the arms of the trial is to be stated. An estimate of the required sample size for each arm calculated on the basis of the end-points of the trial should be provided. The alpha error (test size) and power are to be given. Specifically, the use of a one-sided test needs to be justified.

End-points

The dimension(s) or the item(s) of the instrument which were selected as end-point(s) before subject accrual need to be stated. End-points not chosen before the start of the trial are to be avoided. When QoL is not the primary end-point, the major end-points of the trial should be provided.

Timing of study assessment

The timing (schedule) of the QoL assessment in relation to trial onset, the treatments, including the scheduled times of instrument completion (e.g. every day, every month), must be given. The timing of the follow-up assessment should be specified: for instance at the completion of treatment or discontinuation of treatment, every three months, at the end of the trial, and so on.

Data

The means by which the data are collected and the procedure for evaluating their quality should be described. The criteria for what is to be considered adequate/inadequate must be specified *a priori*. A definition of the missing data should be given (see below).

Method of analysis

Ideally, only the QoL end-points defined before the trial commences should be used for the formal analysis. For these alone, confidence intervals and p values must be quoted. Other variables should be utilized for descriptive purposes only and can be used for generating hypotheses for testing in later studies.

The method(s) by which missing data were defined and analysed (including imputation methods) must be clearly stated. It is important to specify how data from patients who died before reaching the end-point were dealt with in the analysis.

The statistical methods of analysis must be described in sufficient detail so that other researchers could repeat the analysis if the full data were made available. When appropriate, the assumptions about the distribution of the data should be indicated. One must also indicate whether the analysis is by 'intention to treat' or otherwise. In case of multiple comparisons, attention must be paid to the total number of comparisons, to the adjustment, if any, of the significance level, and to the interpretation of the results. If applicable, the definition of a clinically important difference is to be given.

The authors should indicate if they are willing to make their data available to other researchers for the purpose of reanalysis or meta-analysis (give address, phone, fax, e-mail of the author responsible for providing the data).

Results

Presentation of data

The results of planned primary and secondary analyses should be presented along with the results of appropriate tests of clinical and statistical significance, such as p value, effect size, and other relevant parameters. The authors must report on all scales from all the instruments that were used in the study. In particular, authors should not pick and choose which scales to report from an instrument *post hoc* without indicating very clearly why this has been done. QoL data should include all time periods during which data were collected, as well as adequate information characterizing the distribution of data using typical statistics, such as means, medians, standard deviations, and ranges. When appropriate, a description of the distribution of enrolment time and the median follow-up time is helpful.

Patient data

All patients entered in the trial must be accounted for and their characteristics presented, for example, how many centres were involved, how many eligible patients were approached, how many were accrued, how many refused to participate, how many were unable to complete the questionnaires, and so on.

By and large, numbers of patients are needed separately in each arm of the trial for the patients in the following categories:

(1) eligible and entered

(2) excluded from the analysis

    (a) with inadequate data

    (b) with missing data

(3) adequately followed

(4) lost to follow-up

(5) died during the trial

(6) adequately treated according to protocol

(7) failed to complete the treatment according to protocol

(8) received treatments not specified in the protocol.

Scheduling of instrument administration

Descriptive information that contributes to an understanding of treatment schedules, patient compliance, time windows, median follow-up times, and other practical aspects of QoL data collection and follow-up are required. A table to provide the information by treatment group, such as Table 18.1, is desirable.

Missing data and compliance

It is imperative to document the causes of all missing data. Several types of missing data are possible and should be identified and documented separately in the publication:

(1) missing data due to non-completion of the questionnaire resulting from the death of the patient;

(2) missing data due to non-completion of the questionnaire for reasons other than death; and

(3) missing data due to non-response to items in the questionnaire.

It should be specified what missing data are due to informative (non-random) censoring (i.e. missing data due to the patient's health state or particular treatment) or to non-informative (random) censoring.

Table 18.1   Number of patients (pseudo data) in the trial and compliance in the completion of forms (two forms per patient) for treatment A* (after Hopwood _et al._, 1994[7])

Time schedule	Time window[†] (days)	Number			Number and percentage of expected[‡] forms received**
		Dead	Lost	Alive	
Day 0	−7 to 0	0	1	300	585 (97.5)
Day 21	14 to 28	5[∥]	10[∥]	295	501 (84.9)
Day 176	169 to 183	10[∥]	85[∥]	285	352 (61.8)
...	...	...	...	...	... ...
Total		...	...	...	... ...

* One form per treatment is needed.
[†] During which the questionnaires are filled and collected.
[∥] Number dead or lost between day 0 and day 21 or 176.
[‡] The number of expected forms is based on the number of people alive.
** 585/600 = 0.975; 501/590 = 0.849; 352/570 = 0.618.

Compliance with completion of the questionnaires can be defined as the percentage of completed forms received by the investigator from the number anticipated by the study design, taking due account of factors which would make completion impossible, such as the death of the patient.

A comparison between the percentages of missing data by item in the questionnaire (focusing on the major end-points as specified in the protocol) and by treatment group should be made and commented upon.

Statistical analysis

The main analysis should address the hypothesis identified in the introduction. Although it is recognized that there are often large numbers of items on a QoL questionnaire, the particular, and few, dimensions which were selected as design end-point(s) are to be the most relevant part of the report. Analysis of other variables as well as any subgroup analysis not prespecified must be reported only as 'exploratory' or tentative. If appropriate, the reasons for not adhering to the pretrial sample size must be discussed. In the case of a graphic presentation, it is important to specify the number at risk by treatment group beneath the time axis in the plot.

When 'survival' techniques are used for QoL data summary, the censoring mechanisms should be carefully documented. The number of interim analyses (planned or unplanned) and their results ought to be summarized briefly.

Discussion and conclusions

These topics can be separated under different headings or combined. The interpretation of the results, including any generalization, must be discussed in detail. The findings should be discussed in the context of results of previous studies and research. Some particular issues in the interpretation of QoL data should be addressed here:

(1) score improvement or deterioration irrespective of treatment;

(2) the relative importance of the observed changes;

(3) clinical meaning of the observed changes; and

(4) how the results increase knowledge in the field.

A summary of the therapeutic results should be reported alongside the QoL results so that a balanced interpretation of the trial results can be made.

References and bibliography

References should be given for all background material, the rationale, and the discussion. The format of the references should conform to the journal style to which the manuscript is submitted. If abbreviated, the title of journals must be abbreviated according to the 'List of journals indexed in Index Medicus', published annually, or according to the policy of the journal where the article is being submitted. 'Personal communications' and 'unpublished data' are to be avoided whenever possible.

Appendices

For instruments or battery of instruments or measure(s) selected for the trial which are not well known or which have been modified from the original version, it is appropriate to provide a copy here. For a copyright instrument, it is appropriate to give information about where the instrument can be obtained.

Acknowledgement

This chapter was adapted from Staquet *et al.*, *Qual. Life Res.*, 1995; **5**: 496–502; with permission of the publisher.

References

1. Sander, J.O. and Velduyzen Van Zanten. Quality of life as outcome measures in randomized trials. An overview of three general medical journals. *Controlled Clinical Trials*, 1991; **12**: 234S–42S.
2. Schumaker, M., Olschewski, M., and Schulgen, G. Assessment of quality of life in clinical trials. *Statistics in Medicine*, 1991; **10**: 1915–30.
3. Gotay, C.C. and Moore, T.D. Assessing quality of life in head and neck cancer. *Quality of Life Research*, 1992; **1**: 5.
4. Hunt, S. The credibility of quality of life claims in clinical trials. *Second Symposium on contributed papers in quality of life evaluation*, Charleston, USA, 1994.
5. Osoba, D. Lessons learned from measuring health-related quality of life in oncology. *Journal of Clinical Oncology*, 1994; **12**: 608–16.
6. Gill, T.M. and Feinstein, A.R. A critical appraisal of the quality of quality-of-life measurements. *Journal of the American Medical Association*, 1994; **272**: 619–26.
7. Hopwood, P., Stephens, R.J., and Machin, D. Approaches to the analysis of quality of life data: experiences gained from a Medical Research Council Lung Cancer Working Party palliative chemotherapy trial. *Quality of Life Research*, 1994; **3**: 339–52.
8. Coste, J., Fermanian, J., and Venot, A. Methodological and statistical problems in the construction of composite measurement scales: a survey of six medical and epidemiological journals. *Statistics in Medicine*, 1995; **14**: 331–45.
9. Fletcher, A. Quality-of-life measurements in the evaluation of treatments: proposed guidelines. *British Journal of Clinical Pharmacology*, 1995; **39**: 217–22.
10. Altman, D.G., Gore, S.M., Gardner, M.J., and Pocock, S. Statistical guidelines for contributors to medical journals. *British Medical Journal*, 1983; **286**: 1489–93.
11. International Committee of Medical Journal Editors. Uniform requirements for manuscripts submitted to biomedical journals. *Journal of the American Medical Association*, 1993; **269**: 2282–6.

12. The Standards of Reporting Trials Group. A proposal for structured reporting of randomized controlled trials. *Journal of the American Medical Association*, 1994; **272**: 1926–31.
13. The Asilomar Working Group. Checklist of information for inclusion in reports of clinical trials. *Annals of Internal Medicine*, 1996; **124**: 741–3.

Appendix: a checklist for authors reporting results of quality of life assessments in clinical trials

Title and authors

- Concise, informative and correct title.
- Nature of the study, i.e., randomized, controlled (phase III, phase II, a pilot or preliminary study, etc.).
- Authors and their institutional affiliations.
- Key words for indexing purposes.

Abstract

- Purpose.
- Patients and methods.
- Key results.
- Main conclusion(s).

Introduction

- Objective(s).
- Reason (rationale).
- Appropriately comprehensive literature review and selective references.
- Pretrial QoL hypotheses.
- Description of the disease(s) and treatment(s).

Patients and methods

Population and sample

- Description of the population sample.
- Inclusion and exclusion criteria.
- Source of patient sample.
- Requirement for consent form.
- Planned effect size and required sample size.
- Estimate of alpha error (test size) and power.

QoL instrument selection

- Type of assessment (health profile and/or utility) and its justification.
- Method and instrument(s) used.

- Psychometric properties, specially if not a well-known instrument.
- Time frame of questions.
- Scoring procedure.
- Cross-cultural adaptation, if applicable.

Trial size
- Anticipated effect size.
- Test size (alpha error) including one or two-sided power.
- Number of subjects in each arm.

End-points
- Dimensions or items used as end-points.
- Other end-points of study.

Timing of study assessments
- Schedule of assessments before, during, and after treatment (or other intervention), including frequency of follow-up assessments.

Data
- Method of collecting data.
- Procedures for quality control.
- Definition of adequate data.
- Definition of missing data.

Method of analysis
- Missing data defined and explained.
- Statistical methods.
- End-points analysed.
- Adjustments made (if any) for multiple comparisons.
- Definition of a clinically important difference.
- Planned effect size and required sample size.
- Estimate of alpha error (test size) and power.
- Adjustment for multiple comparisons.

Results
Presentation of data
- All important QoL data presented.
- Time required for accrual.
- Median follow-up time.

Patient data
Number of patients

- accrued and their demography
- eligible and entered
- excluded from the analysis with reasons
- with inadequate data
- with missing data with reasons
- adequately followed
- lost to follow-up
- who died during the trial
- adequately treated according to protocol
- failing to complete the treatment according to protocol
- who received treatments not specified in the protocol.

Scheduling of instrument administration

- Actual schedule followed.

Missing data and compliance

- Missing data must be documented fully with reasons, for example, missing due to death, missing for other reasons, missing due to incomplete response to items on questionnaires
- Compliance data, that is, number of questionnaires completed out of the number expected and number of items completed out of the number expected, should be given.

Statistical analysis

- Main hypotheses.
- Description of secondary (exploratory) analyses.
- Number of interim analyses, if any.
- Censoring mechanisms.

Discussion and conclusions

- Importance of any observed changes in QoL.
- Generalizability of the results.
- Clinical meaning of the results.
- Relationship of the results to those of other, similar studies.
- Summary of therapeutic results.
- How results advance knowledge in the field.

References

- Give all necessary references.
- Format to conform with journal style.
- Key words.

Appendices

- Copy of instruments used in the study, if appropriate/applicable, and their characteristics.

Index